THE ENCHANTMENT OF WESTERN HERBAL MEDICINE

THE ENCHANTMENT OF WESTERN HERBAL MEDICINE

Herbalists, Plants, and Nonhuman Agency

Guy Waddell

AEON

Aeon Books Ltd
12 New College Parade Finchley Road
London NW3 5EP

British Library Cataloguing in Publication Data

A C.I.P. for this book is available from the British Library

ISBN-13: 978-1-91159-756-8

Typeset by Medlar Publishing Solutions Pvt Ltd, India

www.aeonbooks.co.uk

CONTENTS

ACKNOWLEDGEMENTS

I would like to thank Dr Julie Whitehouse, Professor Volker Scheid, and Professor Tony Towell who supervised my PhD research at the University of Westminster, out of which this book grew. I could not have done it without them. Additionally, I would like to thank Nina Nissen, who has led the way in social science research into Western herbal medicine, and Luci Attala, who provided inspiration at just the right moment. I also offer thanks to my family. First, to Emma, whose narrative abilities are second to none and to whom I owe more than I can say. I thank our daughters, Minnie and Bea, who are finding their own strong voices and whose father spends too much time writing. I would also like to thank my parents, Peter and Yvonne, who have been extremely supportive throughout, and my brother, Mark, whose poems are already out there in the world. And thank you to Nick, whose wisdom is matched only by his kindness and his desire to get to the heart of the matter. While those thanked above have provided an environment for which I am grateful, I would now like to thank those who provided the primary material for the research, namely the herbalists involved in this research. Without their openness to having me spend time with them and their willingness to tell their stories the result would have been a thin soup indeed. I hope that some of the flavour of their narratives and lives is retained within these pages. I also offer my thanks to Oliver

Rathbone, Melinda McDougall, Cecily Blench, and James Darley at Aeon Books for their confidence in me and their guidance throughout.

This book is dedicated to Christopher Hedley, herbalist and teacher. I was lucky enough to know him for twenty-three years. I first met him when I went to an evening class in herbal medicine in the basement of Neal's Yard Remedies in Notting Hill, London. Each week, we did a tea tasting, then talked about the herb, its history, actions, phytochemistry, and different approaches to health care. He told wonderful stories and listened with his ears and heart wide open to all of ours. Christopher used to say, "Herbalism is about stories: people's stories they tell you and yours as you listen and think about how to treat them." Indeed, his stories were most likely responsible for many people deciding to study herbal medicine. Many of us owe our professions to Christopher. "How a plant is in the world is how it will be in you," Christopher would say. "Very generous things, plants. We don't deserve them, really." Along with his wife, Non, he developed a simple yet sophisticated tea-tasting methodology that he used with students and practitioners, arguing that differences of opinion about a herb could almost always be resolved by taking it as a tea.

On herb walks, he would point out a particular plant and say, "And here we have the most beautiful plant in the whole known universe," before moving on to the next plant, "And here we have the most beautiful plant in the whole known universe." He loved plants. His awe and love of green nature, combined with his willingness to truly listen and his knowledge about people and plants meant that his practice thrived. Despite never having a website or advertising, he developed a hugely successful practice. "When with patients, look closely and listen closely: they will tell you what's wrong with them; listen longer and they'll tell you what to do about it," he would say. "And then they pay you! It helps if you have white hair and look deeply into their eyes; they will think that you are wise!" While humour was a central part of his teaching, he was certainly wise, although he never claimed to have access to knowledge that anyone else couldn't cultivate. Christopher pointed out that the herbs we need are often under our noses, growing between the cracks in the pavement. He was an urban herbalist, and saw the city as offering up as many possibilities as meadows. He knew his patch like no one else.

People used to ask me how old Christopher was and I would reply that he was something between four and four hundred. He had the curiosity and twinkle of a four year old and the wisdom of the ancients. Non died in July 2017 and Christopher followed her on the autumn equinox. He always did have good timing.

PART I

INTRODUCTION, BACKGROUND, AND LITERATURE

CHAPTER ONE

Introduction

On the entrance door to a long-established complementary and alternative medicine clinic in the UK there is a sign that gives a menu of the therapies available. Amongst acupuncture, homeopathy, healing, and many others is "Herbal Medicine (Western)". This sign was put up in the late 1990s, with "(Western)" necessary to differentiate herbal medicine from Chinese herbal medicine that was making its presence felt on the high street in the UK. Eventually it became known as Western herbal medicine.

As a healing art that has persisted yet is barely acknowledged in the West, Western herbal medicine appears to be a mass of tensions. Being "Western" is partly a claim to modernity, yet it uses many plant species that would have been used hundreds of years ago. Stewart[1] suggests that while herbal medicine can be understood as a traditional medicine, putting "Western" before "herbal medicine" aligns it with a European philosophical basis. Most of its practitioners are not medical doctors, but their training includes much orthodox medicine. As a medical approach it transfuses much black-boxed knowledge from orthodox medical curricula, yet it prescribes "dirty pharmaceuticals" made from once living organisms, often including unknown and unquantified constituents.

Nissen and Evans[2] point out that there is no generally agreed-upon definition of Western herbal medicine. They argue that it is sometimes aligned with a scientific or "phytotherapeutic" approach to prescribing herbal medicines for patients, while others look to its American roots in the physiomedical and eclectic traditions which were taken up in the UK, or to the concepts of holism or vitalism, or to a practice that uses plants that are mostly native to Europe and North America.

Some of these plants can be found growing in the UK between cracks in the pavement as well as in parks and gardens and in the countryside, yet they may also be borrowed from other traditions such as Ayurveda and Chinese medicine. Jackson-Main[3] points out that Western herbal medicine can be a misleading term in that it breaches cultural and national borders and uses herbs and approaches from other traditions outside the West. He argues that it "almost defies definition".

As a Western healing art it is practised in the UK, America, and Canada, but also in the southern hemisphere countries of Australia and New Zealand. Western herbal medicine refers to a large geography yet practitioners often prefer to use medicines that they know as local plants. Its dominant language is English but some herbalists seek to understand what plants are telling them. Contradictions and tensions, of course, are not specific to Western herbal medicine. Referring to Chinese medicine and other medical traditions undergoing modernisation as well as to biomedicine, Scheid[4] states that "Wherever we look, syncretism and ambiguity abound." Despite the presence of plurality in diverse healthcare practices, Western herbal medicine has its herbal medicines—living plants that have somehow become medicinal. But what more can we say? This book seeks to unravel aspects of Western herbal medicine in the UK, arguing that a particular element of Western herbal medicine inherently produces differences within and between practices. However, a caveat is necessary here: despite Western herbal medicine being the subject matter, the reader is reminded that Western herbal medicine is a concept and does not exist as a bounded object. Rather, it is something to work with.

While much of the landscape and profession of Western herbal medicine is influenced by science, an intention of the current work is to investigate whether this involvement with science captures the experience of herbalists or whether something else is also going on. This necessitates bringing the herbalists themselves vocally into the presented material, something that has been largely missing from previous work. And if their voices are to be heard then their beginnings must be attended to. One aim is to identify why and how people come to be herbalists, to join a profession that is marginalised within healthcare practices, at the centre of modernity yet using age-old tools. Another aim is to consider what impact the once living-ness of herbal medicines has on herbalists, their practices and Western herbal medicine. A final aim is to contextualise this within wider conceptual and theoretical frameworks and to look for resonances in other knowledge practices.

From these aims the research question was eventually arrived at. How do people become drawn to learning and practising Western herbal medicine and what is the relationship between these entryways, the rest of their narratives, Western herbal medicine, and developments beyond Western herbal medicine? The objectives of the research thus became: to research the history of the development of the profession in the UK; to identify and critically evaluate the social science literature on Western herbal medicine; to identify herbalists with a wide variety of approaches to practice; to collect their biographic narratives using an interview methodology that seeks to cede control to the interviewee; to collect ethnographic data from the observation of consultations; to develop a theoretical and conceptual framework for the research that arises out of the primary data; to develop an approach to the analysis of the data collected that keeps the cases and voices intact but allows theoretical exploration; to compare the social science and historical data with the collected cases; and to identify spheres beyond Western herbal medicine that offer fruitful associations with the findings of the primary research.

Book outline

To state the obvious, Western herbal medicine is important to itself. In the UK, it is important to the 800 or so practitioners that make up its numbers as well as to their patients and the training institutions and professional associations. Beyond itself, Western herbal medicine is of interest to a powerful sceptic lobby in the UK that sees it lacking a solid evidence base and is opposed to its political recognition as a healthcare practice. However, looking beyond itself and its local politics, Western herbal medicine, in its engagement with living plants and with herbal medicines, will be shown to have relevance to those that seek to move the human from the epicentre of everything and look to new ways of working with the nonhuman.

This book will show that hidden experiences of meetings with plants, where the boundaries between herbalists and plants meet and are blurred, are important in some herbalists' routes to studying and practising and are also to be found in the later parts of these and other herbalists' narratives. This constitutes the "push" and "pull" of "enchantment", which will be seen to be a sensual affective energy that spreads throughout many, but not all, of the narratives and which embraces both more scientific and more traditional ways of doing herbal medicine. This enchantment sometimes starts before formal study begins, including at very young ages. It will be argued that herbalists' meetings with plants and herbal medicines allow herbalists to draw easily from a diverse range of influences that others may see as incommensurable, and challenges the view that Western herbal medicine is being "mainstreamed", "taken over" or "co-opted" by science. Despite the profession's engagement with science and politics, with modernity necessarily separating herbs from herbalists, it will be shown that herbalists meet with plants and herbal medicines in ways which challenge the assumption of human exceptionalism. Other traditions that use herbal medicines, such as Chinese medicine, Kampo, Ayurveda, and Unani Tibb, arguably have practices that have more solid and direct connections to, and articulations with, their histories, origins, and foundational philosophies. This book suggests that at least a part of Western herbal medicine is formed gravitationally by the herbs themselves as living plants in relationship with the herbalists who prescribe them. Meadowsweet, horsetail, yarrow, lady's mantle, hawthorn, betony, black cohosh, sage as well as species not indigenous to the West such as the various ginsengs, as living plants and as medicines made from them, are in relationships with their herbalists. And this has arguably been the case for a long while, meaning that the tradition of Western herbal medicine is made up of, at least partly, herbalists' relationships with plants.

The centrality of herbs and their sensual ability to enchant herbalists raises questions about the agency of living plants and of herbal medicines. It also raises questions about how the relationship between herbalists and plants may be reconceived. There are developments in plant sciences as well as in the social sciences and humanities that resonate with the cases and with the current exploration of Western herbal medicine, and these will be considered in the later sections of this book. Recent work in the plant sciences relates plant physiology to spheres of interest that had previously been restricted to the animal and human sciences, including the study of behaviour and communication, raising questions as to how plant intelligence and agency should be considered. There are also signs of change in the social sciences and humanities, where the journey to nonhumanism, aspects of posthumanism and various ontological turns have permitted the decentring of the human to include plant-specific concepts such as "plant thinking" and "plants as persons". These new ways of looking at the world resonate, to varying degrees, with the cases of individual herbalists discussed, and with Western herbal medicine.

In order to explore Western herbal medicine a route has been chosen that starts with what has been largely absent from the limited research that has been carried out to date: the voices of herbalists themselves, presented as words in "thick" cases. The backbone of the research is a narrative approach to gathering interview data, namely that found in the biographic narrative interpretative method that allows the subjects to tell their stories without interruption. This minimalist-passive approach to interviewing reduces the likelihood of the researcher missing elements and themes that are important to the subjects. Without this method, it is unlikely that the research question would have been arrived at. Ethnographic methods were also used to provide both background information and substantive descriptions, particularly of consultations. The research is then presented as selected cases of individual herbalists.

Part I of the book starts with a look at the fragmented history of Western herbal medicine in the UK. It is fragmented because it has not had a clarified position within the academic field of the history of medicine, rather than because it has not been persistent, if marginal, as a medical practice. The book will then address the political history of herbal practice in the UK, which looks at the profession's fight for survival and recognition, before exploring the profession's engagement with science. The social science research on Western herbal medicine is then reviewed, where Nina Nissen's work resonates with directions that will become important for the development of arguments in this book. Part II begins with an account of the methodology used. The reasons for herbalists being drawn towards studying and practising herbal medicine are then described, with some herbalists having "visible entryways" that are arguably unsurprising. This is contrasted with the "hidden entryway" herbalists, who had various "meetings" with plants, often at a young age, including being "called" by plants. These accounts are presented here because they form the foundation for this book and for the selection of its conceptual orientations, which are then described. The starting point for this is Max Weber and his arguments about the disenchantment of the modern world. David Abram, Bronislaw Szerszynski, and Jane Bennett are then drawn on to suggest that enchantment is alive and well in the modern world, including in Western herbal medicine. Josephson-Storm is turned to, in order to suggest that, just as the social sciences have historically promoted both humanism and looked beyond it, so Western herbal medicine is a patient-centred practice that radically embraces nonhumans.

The cases are then presented in part III, first the visible entryway herbalists and then the hidden entryway herbalists. Each case is first made up predominantly of the herbalist's own words, followed by a reflective section that looks at how the entryways relate to the rest of the narrative. The book then looks beyond the cases, arguing that it is the enchanted meetings with plants, that is, with creatures from another kingdom, and with medicines made from them, that allows difference to be easily brought into practices and into Western herbal medicine. The argument is also made that enchantment is a sensual affective energy and is found in both scientific and traditional approaches to practice, with both often easily existing within the same practitioner. The cases are also compared to social science research as well as the history of Western herbal medicine and the profession's engagement with science.

In part IV the enchantment of plants is explored through recent developments in plant science and in vegetal philosophy which point, respectively, to the enchanting power of similarities and of differences between humans and plants. This turn to plants is then situated within the growing field of critical plant studies and established academic disciplines before locating this, more broadly, within growing attention to the nonhuman in academia. Finally, the implications of increased plant agency are considered for understanding Western herbal medicine, resulting in the proposal, following Michael Marder, that the concept of "grafting" can help us understand something about the agency of herbalist-plant-herbal medicine assemblages in Western herbal medicine.

CHAPTER TWO

A fragmented history of Western herbal medicine

At the very least, herbal medicine as orthodox and unorthodox medicine in the West has a long history. Tobyn, Denham, and Whitelegg[5] have traced its historical textual sources. This journey starts with the classical medicine of Celsus, Dioscorides, Pliny, and Galen in the first two centuries AD and its fertilisation of Arabic medicine and then moves to Anglo-Saxon and late Middle Ages texts including those of Hildegard von Bingen and the Physicians of Myddfai. The Renaissance and early modern period brought the "herbals" (texts that describe herbs and their medicinal properties) of Leonhart Fuchs, William Turner, John Gerard, John Parkinson, and Nicholas Culpeper before the Anglo-American connection was cemented in the works of Cook, Ellingwood, and Coffin in the nineteenth century. Notable twentieth- and twenty-first-century texts include those by Maud Grieve, A. W. Priest and L. R. Priest, and Thomas Bartram, that then drew more and more heavily on scientific sources and approaches in the work of Rudolf Weiss, Elizabeth Williamson, David Hoffman, Simon Mills, and Kerry Bone as well as organisations such as the German Commission E, European Scientific Cooperation on Phytotherapy (ESCOP), and the British Herbal Medicine Association (BHMA).

Historians mostly treat herbs like any other object in the hands of the physician. Even those historians who are also herbal practitioners, such as Tobyn, Denham and Whitelegg,[5] and Barker,[6] are keen to place those who prescribe herbs as medicines within the history of physicians and medicine in general. What makes this history distinctively "herbal" is rarely considered. Just as the herbs are often unseen and silent in the fragmented histories, so are the herbalists, unless they are physicians that have authored herbals. This book will argue that herbalists, as well as their plants that become herbal medicines, have more agency in shaping Western herbal medicine than has been previously considered.

Stobart and Francia[7] suggest that the history of herbal medicine lacks a coherent identity with much relevant scholarly research being hidden from view. With the exception of the broad overview of Griggs,[8,9] Stobart and Francia point out that the development of Western herbal medicine in the context of the rise of modern medicine after 1800 has not been considered. The history of herbs as orthodox medicines both before drug medicines and after them has not developed sufficient momentum to become a sub-discipline within the history of medicine. Recently there have been attempts to remedy this, particularly by the establishment of the UK-based Herbal History Research Network.

Of course, herbs as medicine are to be found within diverse written histories of medicine, but they are scattered, not given prominence, and have not generally gathered those around them who identify as scholars of the history of Western herbal medicine. And most of those scholars that may self-identify as such, for example, MacLennan and Pendry,[10] Pitman,[11,12] Tobyn, Denham, and Whitelegg,[5] Barker,[6] and Stobart[7] are also herbal practitioners, mostly outside academic history of medicine departments, seeking to understand the history of Western herbal medicine partly to inform their and other herbalists' practices.

Stobart and Francia[7] point out that the historiography of herbal medicine suggests that in medieval and early modern times writers emphasised the status and lineage of medical knowledge, while with the success of modern medicine in the nineteenth century, descriptions shifted towards locations within antiquarian and folklore studies and that by the twentieth century herbal medicine had come to be regarded as part of alternative or folk medicine or "quackery". Hence there was a movement of writings on herbal medicine, from one being concerned with medical lineages, practice, and status to one being concerned with herbs as tools, often negatively conceived, of cultural activities outside the perimeter of true medical knowledge.

Orthodox and herbal medicine: a long goodbye

Identifying when orthodox and herbal practice separated is a tricky business. MacLennan and Pendry[10] argue that despite herbs being prescribed by orthodox medics well into the 1900s, the separation of herbs from orthodoxy had already begun by the time that the staunch supporter of herbal medicine, Henry VIII, came to the throne in 1509. This was largely due to the influence of Arabic practices on medical thinking, with the later development of an educated medical elite as well as regulatory legislation cementing this separation. On the other hand, Griggs[9] notes that the influence of Paracelsus resulted in chemically prepared medicines entering the apothecary shops by the end of the sixteenth century and the editor of *A Modern Herbal*,[13] writing in 1931, suggests that "botany and medicine came down the ages hand in hand and then parted company in the seventeenth century". Taking another leap through time, Williamson[14] argues that the history of herbal medicine is, up until the eighteenth century at least, largely the history of medicine itself. William Withering's[15] identification, in 1785, of foxglove as the "active" ingredient in a formula for dropsy may also be the beginning of a point of separation between herbal medicine and orthodox medical practice. And Douglas Guthrie, a surgeon, medical historian, and member of the Botanical Society of Edinburgh, locates the date of this separation as coinciding with his penning an article, that was published in 1961, in which he reflects on his own education in botany by his professor. He writes:

> The age-old alliance between Botany and Medicine has come to an end this year. No longer will the first-year medical student rush sleepily to the Botanic Gardens Lecture Hall in order to be in his seat by 8 a.m. when Professor Bayley Balfour will arrive and lock the door behind him. How clearly one can recall these days, although the details of the lectures have long since faded from one's memory.
>
> Anatomy still remains the basic foundation of Surgery, but Botany is not now the basis of medicine, as it was for many centuries.[16]

Indeed, botany was last taught to University of Edinburgh medical students in 1957.

The wide variations of these dates, from Henry VIII in the early sixteenth century, to 1957, suggest two things: that the separation of orthodox practice from herbal practice was indeed a process, rather than a moment, and that medicine has to varying extents always been about pluralism. However, beyond rare instances of both NHS and private "integrated" healthcare practices, such as the Royal London Hospital for Integrated Medicine, or medical doctors prescribing herbal medicines in private practice, contemporary orthodox practice and the practice of Western herbal medicine are today separate entities.

Herbalists defined by their medicines

Although there is little historical research into British herbalists, in a rare paper, Brown[17] looked at the period from the last quarter of the nineteenth century to the early years after WWII, and argues that herbalists in Britain were defined by two factors. First, they rejected inorganic medicines, only using "vegetable substances" in the belief that it was remedies from the plant kingdom that operated in harmony with the simple laws of nature. "Poisonous" medicines were avoided. W. H. Webb,[18] writing in the 1916 foreword to his *Standard Guide to Non-Poisonous Herbal Medicine*, argues that "As the true Herbalist rejects the inorganic substance from his store of remedial agents, so does he, and with equal persistence, reject the poisonous, life-destroying drug ..." The remedies were either whole plant materials or simple extracts, likely emphasised in direct opposition to the "regular" practitioners who were increasingly isolating "active principles" through chemical methods. For example, Harry Orbell wrote in 1939, that "when some active principles of herbs are used separately their therapeutic action is totally different to that obtained when the whole of the properties of the plant in question are employed".[17] Taking the example of lobelia, writing in 1915, Scott explains that "Lobelia inflata, so freely used by botanic doctors, contains an alkali which is poison, lobeline, but it also contains an acid which destroys its poisonous property; and the two properties, as combined in the plant, form a medicine which is harmless, and yet powerful in rooting out disease."[17]

British herbal medicine in harmony with nature and with America

As well as these herbalists being defined by the safe, whole plant medicines that they used, they also believed that it was the driving force of nature that kept people healthy as long as the laws of nature

were obeyed. As such, therapeutic endeavours must aid the processes
of nature and the "vital force". This emphasis on the "vital force" was
partly due to the American influence of Samuel Thomson on British
herbalists, who argued that his medicines "harmonized with the law
of life".[17] Barker[6] describes how Thomson (1769–1843) based his system
of therapeutics on the idea that all illness came from cold; heat was
synonymous with the "vital force": "Heat is life, cold is death." Healing
required using vapour baths and hot water plus the removal of toxins
via sweat, purging, and emesis. While "heroic" by today's standards his
methods were reportedly successful in treating commonly fatal infectious diseases such as typhoid fever, influenza, yellow fever, diphtheria,
measles, whooping cough, and malaria. The best known of Thomson's
formulae, "Composition Powder (formula number 2)", increased "vital
heat" and was used widely for influenza, dysentery, and gastrointestinal pain and included barberry bark, hemlock inner bark, ginger,
cayenne, and cloves.[19] These treatments were gentler than the bleeding and toxic heavy metal medicines of the orthodox medicine of the
time. Thomson sold "patents" of his system to those who then practised
it, and became a very wealthy man. Caldecott[20] shows how Thomson
attracted young intellectuals like Alva Curtis to his approach. However,
while Curtis was drawn to the simplicity of Thomson's system he was
additionally interested in the latest medical discoveries of the day. This
was too much for Thomson who had anti-intellectualism at heart and
eventually a "New Light" Thomsonianism, later to be called "physiomedicalism" was born, with Alva Curtis and William Cook establishing
training institutions. The scientific discoveries that were particularly
taken on board were the autonomic nervous system and understandings of the blood circulation.

Physiomedicalism developed a complex theoretical knowledge
to underpin their practice, part of which included an energetic diagnostic system similar to the yin and yang of Chinese medicine.[19]
Patients were seen as either "asthenic"—deficient and underactive,
or "sthenic"—excessive and hyperactive, with herbs prescribed based
on physical examination that included pulse and tongue diagnosis.
Caldecott[20] notes that Alva Curtis translated Thomson's understanding
of hot and cold into more scientific terms, such that interference with the
vital force was causing either "over-contraction" or "over-relaxation".
William Cook[21], writing in 1869, applied knowledge of the autonomic
nervous system, with "irritation" being a sympathetic response leading

to "contraction", and "depression" being a parasympathetic response leading to "relaxation". J. M. Thurston,[22] writing in 1900, developed Cook's ideas in his *The Philosophy of Physiomedicalism*. Wood[23] describes Thurston's understanding of various "tissue states" of the body along with their treatment. Thus "irritation" requires plants to reduce heat, "constriction" requires antispasmodics, "atrophy" requires "trophores-toration", "relaxation" requires astringents, "stagnation" requires blood purification and "depression" requires warming stimulants. Central to physiomedicalism was the key concept of the "vital force", the belief that every living system is maintained by this force, with disease being due to its disruption.[20,24] According to British physiomedicalists Priest and Priest,[25] "the vital force is always resistive, eliminative and recon-structive in intent"—referring to what may now be seen as the immune, elimination and repair functions of the body. Particularly key was the promotion of the function of the bowels, lungs, kidneys, and skin, and the encouragement of "alterative" activity via elimination and diges-tive function. Further emphasis was on "equalizing the circulation"—ensuring arteries, veins, and capillaries are working well in relationship, as well as promoting "trophorestoration"—that is, restoring function to organs and tissues with herbs that have particular affinities for them.[20,24]

American herbal medicine came to Britain with Dr. Albert Coffin in 1838.[26] He had been successfully treated by an Indian woman in America for a serious lung condition, which set him on his journey to becoming a doctor. He settled in England, and brought his herbal medi-cines and journals of self-help to the industrial North, particularly to Yorkshire, Lancashire, and the Potteries and was reportedly success-ful, especially in treating infectious diseases like cholera.[27] He travelled widely in England, teaching "medical botany" and appointing "agents" to sell his remedies, books, and journals. He set up various "medico-botanical" societies, particularly in the North, where he had a following among the temperance and non-conformist movements. He was said to have successfully treated a cholera epidemic in 1849 using Samuel Thomson's approach that included oak bark, cayenne, raspberry leaves, and lobelia.[26] The success of "medical botany" can partly be attributed to its uptake by those who were witheringly opposed to orthodox medi-cine, as well as to the growth of self-help approaches to healthcare.[28] Brown[29] shows how Englishmen, including John Stevens, John Skelton, Joseph Nadin, and William Fox also brought American Thomsonian practices to England, which retained an "intense antagonism towards the medical establishment".

British herbalists also identified with American counterparts due to the professional status that the derivatives of Thomsonian medicine enjoyed in the States, namely the physiomedical and eclectic medical traditions.[17] British herbalists travelled to America to exchange information, contributing to the use of indigenous North American plants in the British *materia medica*.[30]

CHAPTER THREE

A political history of the profession

As noted above, until modern times the history of herbal medicine was in many ways the history of medicine itself.[5,7,31] McIntyre[31] points out that the herbals of Dioscorides and Galen were the major European medical sources for over twelve centuries, which were then taken up by Arabic culture and eventually fed back into Western Christian medicine. Medicinal herbs were often grown in walled gardens of medieval monasteries and given the species name of "*officinalis*", meaning the official medicinal species.

However, by the end of the medieval period, English herbalists, who had no officially sanctioned position in the various institutions of medicine, were given protection by Henry VIII in the Herbalists Act of 1542. Footler[32] reveals the words of what became known as the "Herbalists Charter":

> … it shall be lawful to every Person being the King's subject, having Knowledge and Experience of the Nature of Herbs, Roots and Waters, or of the Operation of the same, by Speculation or Practice, within any part of the Realm of England, or within any other of the King's Dominiuns, to practice, use and minister in and to any outward Sore, Uncome Wound, Apostermations, outward Swelling

or Disease, any Herb or Herbs, Ointments, Baths, Pultess, and Emplaisters, according to their Cunning Experience and Knowledge in any of the Diseases, Sores and Maladies beforesaid, and all other like to the same, or Drinks for the Stone, Strangury or Agues, without suit, vexation, trouble, penalty or loss of their goods.

Despite this support, the Act provided no legal definition of who someone "having knowledge and Experience of the Nature of Herbs" might be. This lack of definition continues to this day. The resulting uncertainty for herbalists can be seen in the political history of the profession. While herbalists' individual voices, other than of those who have authored texts, have rarely been heard in either the history of medicine or in other academic disciplines, the profession of herbal medicine is more visible and has responded to its predicament. This will be considered below.

Herbalists in search of a (consulting) room of one's own

With this background we now turn to look at developments, from the mid nineteenth century to the present day, of the profession of Western herbal medicine in the UK, as a marginalised alternative medical practice.

Saks[33] locates the formal creation of alternative medicine with the passing of the 1858 Medical Act, which gave medical doctors protection of title and the ability to self-govern via the General Medical Council that was established in the same year. Prior to this date, from the sixteenth century, while there were limited monopolies such as those established with the Royal College of Physicians, the Society of Apothecaries, and the Royal College of Surgeons, there was a relatively open entrepreneurial contest between the different purveyors of health that included herbalists, bonesetters, healers, and those seeking to sell their proprietary medicines. Thus, Saks sees the 1858 Act as pushing non-orthodox practitioners, including herbalists, to the margins of legitimacy.

One swift response to this was a meeting, also in 1858, of nationwide medico-botanic practitioners in Manchester that formed the British Medico Botanic Society.[26] This was to be the foundation for the National Association of Medical Herbalists (NAMH), initially known as the British Medical Reform Association, which was established in 1864 in

Shirley's Temperance Hotel in London and later became the National Institute of Medical Herbalists (NIMH) in 1945.[26]

In 1885 there was an attempt to include lobelia, a much-favoured Thomsonian remedy, on the Poisons Schedule. However, this was successfully resisted by the NAMH. In 1886, an amendment to the Medical Act of 1858 was proposed that would make it illegal to practise medicine unless a medically qualified doctor. However, herbalists successfully campaigned against this Bill.[31] The recognition of the need for formal training led to a series of short-lived training institutions in the North, including in Leeds, Rochdale, and Southport. The Metropolitan Medico-Botanic College was opened in London in 1891 although it is unclear how long it existed, and in 1931 the NAMH opened its College of Botanic Medicine in London, which closed in 1940.[26]

In 1894 the Medical Herbalists Defence Union was established to defend herbalists from attacks by the allopathic establishment. In 1895 the NAMH was registered as a limited company, with all its subscribers being from the north of England. The NAMH amalgamated with the United Society of Herbalists and Midland Botanic Society and formed alliances with other organisations to have a more powerful voice in the representation of medical herbalists.[26] Its memorandum of association was codified and sought to demarcate qualified from unqualified practitioners and to "repress malpractice" through a General Council on Safe Medicines.[17]

In 1901, the NAMH formed sub-committees: a publishing sub-committee; an examinations sub-committee that oversaw the exams that all prospective members had to pass; a school sub-committee to oversee training curricula; and a parliamentary sub-committee to lobby for state recognition of medical herbalists.

Fred Fletcher-Hyde, a past president of NIMH, who held two degrees, one in chemistry and another in botany, and who completed the NAMH tutorial course in 1941, reports that between 1901 and 1922 herbalists tried for registration three times—a Private Members' Bill, a Charter of Royal Incorporation in 1907, and a 1922 Medical Herbalists (Registration) Bill, but none of these attempts was successful.[34] In 1902 William Henry Webb and his wife Dr Sarah Webb, who had qualified as a physiomedical doctor in America, started the School of Herbal Medicine in Southport, drawing American lecturers to teach on its four-year course. It was referred to by the NAMH as The Botanic Sanatorium and Training School of the NAMH of GB Ltd.[26]

In 1911, the National Health Insurance Bill was passed into law, which required insured persons to register with one of a panel of medical practitioners. Initially, the selection of medical practitioners was left in the hands of the local insurance committees. However, Insurance Act regulations subsequently made it clear that these practitioners could not include herbalists.[17] In the NAMH's 1911 secretary's report it was stated that "The most serious thing which has happened to affect Herbalists is the National Insurance Bill. The handing over to the absolute mercy of the allopaths of about fifteen millions of people, without any appeal against their decision, is a most serious matter."[26]

In lobbying for a Medical Herbalists Bill in the early twentieth century the NAMH argued that "It is our desire to compel a standard of Education and Regulation so that the public can differentiate between Bone Fide herbalists and those who trade on the name."[9] More than 130 MPs signed up to this 1923 Private Members' Bill, which enjoyed an unopposed first reading. However, the government refused to make time for the Bill to progress, which McIntyre[31] notes is unsurprising given the comment of the chief medical officer, Sir George Newman, that "It is doubtful whether a trained herbalist is any less dangerous than an untrained one."

In 1941, a new Pharmacy and Medicines Act withdrew the rights of herbalists to supply herbal remedies to patients on the grounds of public safety. While herbalists could still diagnose, give advice, and prescribe they could no longer dispense, effectively making it illegal to practise. However, many herbalists did continue to dispense herbal medicines to their patients.[9] Fred Fletcher-Hyde reports, in an interview, that while some prosecutions were brought against herbalists "no jury would convict so the matter was dropped. Like other herbalists I felt I was not breaking the law but merely using the herbs God provided to heal the ills of mankind. We were practising under a form of Divine Principle."[34]

When the NHS was launched by Aneurin Bevan in 1945, herbalists initially sought inclusion. However, Bevan said that herbalists could be incorporated only if subordinate to the medical profession. Herbalists chose to stay outside the NHS rather than lose their independence.[35] In 1948, the NIMH and the Hospital for Natural Healing in East London founded the School of Herbal Medicine, offering clinical training similar to orthodox hospital outpatient departments.[26]

Saks[33,36] notes that the countercultural movements of the 1960s and 1970s contributed to the popular critical engagement with orthodox medicine, motivated partly by drug safety scares as well as a desire for increased patient choice. This was reflected in the political popularity of such authors as Ivan Illich,[37] who argued that the medicalisation of life often added to burdens of ill health, rather than relieved them. During this time, there was a related increase in demand for alternatives to conventional medicine. However, the medical establishment continued to defend its territory, arguing that only medical doctors should be able to practise alternative medicine, particularly homeopathy and acupuncture. Even so, there was growing political support for complementary and alternative medicine within Parliament, and royal support from Prince Charles, who eventually established the Prince's Foundation for Integrated Health in 1993.

The drug tragedy that impacted most on herbalists was the introduction of thalidomide in the early 1960s. The resulting iatrogenic deformities led to a public and political outcry over the lack of appropriate drug safety measures. The government rushed in legislation that addressed drug testing and licensing. McIntyre[31] notes that herbal medicines were caught in the middle of this and would be licensed in the same way as drugs. Furthermore, Fred Fletcher-Hyde noted that the legislation would have meant that consultations with herbalists could only take place at the same location as herbal medicines were manufactured and that there were no provisions for tinctures, creams, and ointments, saying that "This would have closed us down."[34]

This led to a huge response by the public and herbalists alike, with thousands of letters written to MPs by patients, and hundreds by herbalists, arguing for the public right to choose herbal medicines and to consult herbalists. Amongst others it was the energetic political work of Fred Fletcher-Hyde that helped secure the exemptions to the Act. He remembers that "In the Lords, I was so familiar a sight that often when visiting the chamber I would be greeted by the various staff as, 'M'lud'."[34]

This work paid off and Fred Fletcher-Hyde notes that many of the MPs "had not received so many letters on any issue since Mr Enoch Powell's racist statements".[34] The result was that when the 1968 Medicines Act was passed into law it carried special provisions. These exemptions were Section 12.1 and 12.2. Section 12.1 specified an exemption for herbal medicines from licensing provided that they are supplied following a one-to-one consultation. Section 12.2 exempted herbal medicines as long as they are produced according to standard traditional, non-industrial methods and for which no written claims are made. Barker[6] notes that the law implicitly separated the consulting herbalist from the retailing herbalist.

However, critically and similarly to Henry VIII's "Herbalists Charter", it did not set out any professional definitions of what or who a herbal practitioner is. McIntyre[31] reveals that Fred Fletcher-Hyde later recalled that, when he requested that the term "herbalist" should be defined, he was told that the definition would be provided after consultation with the pharmacists and doctors. Realising that this was likely to lead to damaging restrictions, he avoided mentioning the subject again and the term "herbalist" remains undefined to this day.

After 1968, formal herbal education grew in line with what came to be seen as an increasing crisis in modern medicine, including its paternalism, lack of humanism, and reductionism. This arguably arose out of modernisation that included urbanisation and globalisation,[38] with the "revival" of herbal medicine tapping into environmental concerns.[39] Indeed, herbal medicine is often seen as the "greenest" of medicines, with a supply chain that starts in the soil, and is reflected in the disposition of many herbalists.

In 1991, the NIMH introduced a binding code of ethics and disciplinary procedures. In 1994, the NIMH established an accreditation board to assess training standards and in the same year the University of Middlesex took its first intake of students for a BSc degree in herbal medicine. By the beginning of the new millennium, herbal medicine was considered one of the "big five" complementary alternative medicine (CAM) practices and was to become a candidate for regulation.[39] The House of Lords Select Committee on Science and Technology was ordered to report to Parliament on CAM in the UK, and published its report in November 2000. Saks[33] notes that the authors used a tripartite system to categorise alternative medicines into a hierarchy. The first group had their own diagnostic approaches, organised practitioners, and a credible evidence base. Herbal medicine was in this group, along with osteopathy, chiropractic, homeopathy, and acupuncture. The second group was said to complement orthodox medicine and as such did not have therapy specific diagnostic skills. This group included aromatherapy, hypnotherapy, massage, and reflexology. The third group was identified as having very different philosophical principles when compared with conventional medicine and included radionics, iridology, and, incongruously, given acupuncture's placement in the first group, traditional Chinese medicine (TCM). The report identified herbal medicine and acupuncture as being suitable for state regulation—the state licensing of practitioners to practise on the basis of their training and compliance with continuing professional development—due to the existence of a credible evidence base, consensus among practitioners to move forward to statutory regulation, well organised professional associations and a risk to the public if practitioners were unqualified.

Subsequently, two Department of Health working groups have made proposals for the statutory regulation of the herbal medicine profession as a whole, which is made up of Western herbal medicine, Chinese herbal medicine, Ayurveda, and Tibetan herbal medicine. About 800 of these 1500 herbalists practise Western herbal medicine. These reports have looked at how a self-regulating council could be given the legal right to establish minimum levels of competence, ethical practice, and disciplinary regulations.[39] The regulating authority that was suggested is the independent regulator the Health and Care Professions Council (HCPC). In 2011 the health secretary, Andrew Lansley, backed the statutory regulation of herbalists. However, since then, progress became slow for a number of reasons, including a perception by the European Commission that the UK government, by granting statutory regulation, was seeking to avoid European medicines legislation in order to allow access of herbalists to unlicensed herbal medicines that had been removed from the market by European herbal medicines legislation, namely the Traditional Herbal Medicinal Products Directive.[40] Herbalists' representatives were given governmental reassurance that registration remains a government objective. However, a third working party report[41] has argued, in contradiction to previous reports, notably the House of Lords report of 2000, that there is insufficient evidence of efficacy. This assessment, along with a reduced risk profile of herbal medicine products, largely due to tighter EU legislation via THMPD, meant that voluntary self-regulation was recommended over statutory registration. Since this report no further political statements have been forthcoming from the government over the future of the herbal medicine profession and this is unlikely to be addressed in the near future.

While the historical desire for (unfulfilled) political recognition continues to this day, there was a linked but more immediate recent impingement on herbal practice in the UK that came in the shape of EU legislation. During the time frame of research for this book the UK, as a member of the EU, was subject to EU objectives of harmonisation, including in health care. The EU's legal basis is in Napoleonic Law, requiring specific legislation to allow CAM practitioners to practise medicine. This can be at variance with UK Common Law, where historically practices have been legal unless prohibited by law. Anticipating such conflicts and how they may affect herbal medicine in the UK, in 1993 the EHPA (European Herbal Practitioners Association), later to become the EHTPA (European Herbal and Traditional Medicine Practitioners Association), was established as an umbrella organisation of professional associations to address these issues and how they affect herbal practice. In October 2005, the EU Traditional Herbal Medicinal Products Directive 2001/83/EC (THMPD) came into effect, albeit with a seven year transitional period, requiring Section 12.2 products from the 1968 Medicines Act to be registered herbal medicines that have to meet specific standards of safety and quality and be accompanied by indications and patient information. In the UK, responsibility for these assurances rests with the Medicines and Healthcare Products Regulatory Agency (MHRA). The EU THMPD replaced section 12.2 of the 1968 Medicines Act, which had permitted "finished herbal products" to be supplied to patients by a third party. With the loss of Section 12.2, herbalists may only supply herbal medicines that have not been "industrially produced", in other words, that have been prepared by herbalists on their own premises, as laid out in 12.1 of the 1968 Medicines Act. However, this legislation affects Western herbal medicine practitioners less than other traditions because it is mostly "non-industrially produced" medicines that are used anyway, namely dried herbs and tinctures, that are made up by the practitioner for the individual patient. This is compared with Chinese herbal medicine where proprietary formulae are often also used. However, it has affected practitioners who use a third party "prescription service" for their patients, although these practitioners are likely to have been relatively few in number.

From the above it can be seen that herbalists, since the inception of what would become the NIMH, the largest of the current professional bodies of practitioners, have had to organise politically in order to maintain their abilities to practise. While herbalists are by no means unanimous in their desire for statutory regulation—as Michael McIntyre points out, "Herbalists of all persuasions are generally sceptical of 'Big Brother' and jealously guard their professional independence"[35]—professional organisations have been vocal and active in their desire to see the distinction between bona fide practitioners and unqualified practitioners enshrined in law in order to give their members legal recognition in a rapidly changing world.

Western herbal medicine hidden by CAM, and herbs hidden by politics

The political organisation of the profession has made Western herbal medicine more visible, extending public awareness beyond herbalists and their patients. However, this politicisation has arguably made herbalists' tools, namely plants used as medicines, less visible. The reasons for this are now discussed. Western herbal medicine in the UK, where it is mentioned, is often found in both academic and popular debates on complementary and alternative medicine (CAM), with "CAM" used as an umbrella term to define all therapies that are outside orthodox medicine. One of the consequences of using this umbrella term is that the specificities of individual therapies become less visible. CAM becomes a unifying category and an object of enquiry in its own right. In the political sphere the component parts of CAM and their meanings can remain hidden. Although plenty of discussions as to what separates orthodox medicine from CAM are to be found elsewhere, the focus here is on how governmental attention to what Wahlberg[42] calls the "field of CAM" means that once a CAM practice is seen to have the prerequisites for regulation, the specificities of it as a medical system are positioned outside the concern of regulators. Such is the case for Western herbal medicine. Wahlberg contrasts the rapid development of CAM in the UK since the 1980s with early twentieth-century implementation of "strategies of marginalization, subordination and exclusion" by orthodox medicine against non-orthodox practices. Thus, Wahlberg suggests that CAM may be analysed as a Foucauldian "field of problemitization" where, instead of restricting access to non-orthodox practices, as was done in the past, it is "responsible" practice that is encouraged through the "normalization" of practice. Wahlberg describes how, over the last three centuries the battleground of who is a recognised practitioner has shifted from the commercial field of miracle cures (in the eighteenth and nineteenth centuries), to competing theories of health (in the late nineteenth and early twentieth centuries), to the situation today, where it is practitioner qualifications, competency, responsibility, conduct, and development that constitute an "ethical field of battle".

From this perspective practitioners become competent partly by their organisation into associations of practitioners as well as the unification of these associations. This is certainly true for herbal medicine in general and Western herbal medicine in particular. Of the 1500 or so listed herbalists, about 800 are practitioners of Western herbal medicine, with the remaining being mostly Chinese herbal medicine practitioners, along with Ayurvedic and a small number of Tibetan practitioners. Of the eleven professional bodies representing these 1500 herbalists, four of them represent 800 Western herbalists, with the NIMH representing about 500 herbalists. The professional bodies of Western herbal medicine are generally well organised, with established codes of conduct and disciplinary procedures. The four Western herbal medicine professional bodies, along with their Chinese medicine, Ayurvedic, and Tibetan colleagues, initially came together under the umbrella of the EHPA (European Herbal Practitioners Association, later the EHTPA) partly to negotiate with the government over statutory regulation, although only two smaller professional bodies of Western herbalists are now left within the EHTPA, due to political differences.

Wahlberg[42] argues that, beyond organising and unifying themselves, competency can be further advanced by defining qualifications and skills. Thus, the Herbal Medicine Regulatory Working Group (2003), set up by the EHTPA, the Prince's Foundation for Integrated Health (FIH), and the Department of Health in 2001, has suggested procedures to protect patients and public from unfit practitioners.

Professional bodies have engaged with these concerns. The NIMH requires that new members must have graduated from specific training courses, comply with its memorandum and articles of association, codes of ethics, practice, and disciplinary procedures, including health and fitness to practise, and must be of "good character".

Interestingly the NIMH code of ethics and practice[43] could very nearly be taken up as it is and applied to other therapies. Apart from saying that members must keep up with developments in herbal medicine, there is barely any mention of herbal medicine in the entire document that covers the member's obligation to her or his patients, ethical/professional boundaries, legal obligations, and good practice, commercial obligations, obligations in practice, relationships with professional colleagues and obligations as a teacher.

Furthermore, the continuing professional development (CPD) requirements of the NIMH[44] describe how herbalists must comply with

CPD each year, keeping a record of what they did, what was learnt from it and what impact it had on their practice. The CPD scheme is based on reflective learning, with members identifying their own learning needs and how these are met. The CPD scheme could equally be taken up by any professional body of any discipline.

Even the long-established oath (affirmation of herbal practice) that new members of NIMH take, barely mentions herbs, suggesting that it is the skills rather than the tools that define the profession:

> I solemnly promise that I will keep this affirmation and this stipulation—to follow the profession of herbal medicine according to my ability and judgment, for the benefit of my patients and to abstain from all that is deleterious and mischievous. I will give no deadly medicine to anyone if asked, nor suggest such counsel.
>
> With purity and holiness will I pass my life and practise my art.
>
> Into whatever houses I enter I will go into them for the benefit of the sick and will abstain from any voluntary act of mischief or corruption.
>
> Whatever in connection with my professional practice or not in connection with it, I see or hear in the life of any person, which ought not to be spoken of abroad, I will not divulge as reckoning all such should be kept secret.
>
> While I continue to keep this affirmation inviolate may it be granted to me to enjoy life and the practice of herbal medicine, respected by all persons and all times.

Although it is looking unlikely, should Western herbal medicine eventually be granted statutory regulation, it is likely that the Health and Care Professions Council (HCPC) would be the legal regulating agency. If we look at the HCPC's "standards for prescribing", which sets out the knowledge and skills a practitioner should be able to demonstrate, and which Western herbal medicine would also be covered by, it is clear that what is prescribed is not the focus. Thus, knowledge of pharmacodynamics, pharmacokinetics, pharmacology, and "therapeutics relevant to prescribing practice" is required, along with making a "prescribing decision based on relevant physical examination, assessment and history".[45] Herbs would be treated like any other therapeutic substance. If Western herbal medicine is not to be regulated by statute, then it is likely to be recommended that the Professional Standards

Authority (PSA) set the standards for a voluntary register of herbalists.[41] Similarly to the HCPC, the PSA's Standards for Accredited Registers[46] do not reveal a concern with the specific tools of any particular therapy.

Thus, as Wahlberg[42] suggests, the "problem of quackery is increasingly located in an ethical field of practitioner competency, qualifications, conduct, responsibility, and personal professional development, almost (but not quite) regardless of the form of therapy in question". In the case of Western herbal medicine, the generic nature of the standards taken on by governing bodies and potential regulators means that the herbs themselves are invisible in the political regulation of unified and competent herbalists. Instead, herbalists are visible as a cultural phenomenon in need of some form of political regulation.

Bruno Latour can help us to understand the invisibility of herbs and herbal medicines in the political landscape just described. Latour,[47] using Shapin and Schaffer's[48] *Leviathan and the Air-Pump* as his main resource, locates the beginning of modernity—the "Modern Constitution"—very specifically at the time of Thomas Hobbes and Robert Boyle in the mid-seventeenth century. Latour argues that "the Moderns" were born when a particular "purification" was instigated—when knowledge was split between knowledge of people and knowledge of things, with Boyle and science and objects and nature on one side of the man-made fence, and Hobbes and politics and subjects and society on the other. This purification may be summarised as the nature/culture divide, with nature addressed by science and culture addressed by politics. Pickering[49] argues that Latour's *We Have Never Been Modern* is an attempt to explain the grip of the human/nonhuman dualism on our imagination, originating with Boyle's separation of nature from the speaker, and with Hobbes's theorising of social order independent of material circumstances. Thus, with nature separated from culture, modernity was born. However, Latour's second point is that "hybrids" are produced out of this purification: modernity's demand for sharp demarcations between nature and culture means that more things necessarily become hybrids. Latour gives the ozone layer as an example of a hybrid, with it being understood through diverse actors including gases, the sky, upper-atmosphere chemists, meteorologists, measurements, heads of state, the rights of future generations, desperate patients, and industrialists. Thus the ozone layer, like any "thing" is the product of relationships and associations rather than existing a priori. Even though the Modern Constitution attempts to produce only subject or object, culture or nature, which can be dealt with either by politics or science, it is hybrids that proliferate. As Latour says: "Everything happens in the middle, everything passes between the two, everything happens by way of mediation, translation and networks, but this space does not exist, it has no place. It is unthinkable." While modernity is defined as this process of purification and hybrid creation, the former process is valued and claimed, while hybrids are discounted and denied. Therefore, as Bennett[50] observes, modernity, a paradoxical combination of claims, presents itself as a shiny, consistent, and enlightened alternative to a messy world, with the superior moderns not making the primitive mistake of muddling up the human with the nonhuman, the natural with the cultural. Hybridisation must be swept under the carpet to avoid accusations of an archaic animism. Thus, as we will see, the hidden entryways of herbalists, where nature and culture meet, are, well ... hidden. Latour's concept of "purification" can help us understand how herbalists, as part of culture, have been assigned to the political sphere of near-regulation, where the herbs themselves are barely visible, while herbal medicines, as part of nature, have been "normalized" to become "a distinct object of expert bodies of knowledge".[51]

Latour's observation that while modernity proudly purifies, it is hybrids that proliferate, can help explain another observation: that consternation occurs in Western herbal medicine when hybrids come into the open. Hybrids made up of shorter networks are likely to be less visible than those in longer networks. The herb-herbalist network which will be described in the cases is a short network and less visible than the longer network that makes up traditional herbal registrations (THRs): non-enchanting herbal hybrids that mix both nature and culture. We will take the case of St John's wort as a THR. A brief review of THRs is necessary. As mentioned previously, since 2011 the EU's Traditional Herbal Medicinal Products Directive (THMPD) has been in operation requiring "medicinal herbs" to be sold as THRs. However, herbs are also sold as "food supplements" with it being the responsibility in the UK of the MHRA to authorise the THRs and to distinguish between products that should be THRs and those that are food supplements, with this being done on a case-by-case basis. THRs are required to have been in safe use for thirty years, including at least fifteen years in the EU. Clinical evidence is not assessed by the MHRA in the approval process. THRs are to be used for minor self-limiting conditions without the supervision of a doctor. The EU motivation was to improve quality, provide consumers with accurate information and to harmonise practices across the EU. THRs have a less costly registration process than drug medicines and it is proof of safety, including in the manufacturing process, along with proof of traditional use, that are required of each product, rather than efficacy. Instead, efficacy is plausible on the basis of traditional use. Schwabe is one of the leading suppliers of THRs in the UK. They have a St John's wort product called "KarmaMood". This product is sold in a blister pack with a THR registered trademark logo as well as braille lettering and an information leaflet inside, which add to the apparent authority of the KarmaMood, although the packaging design does include a picture of a herb.

So, what makes KarmaMood a Latourian hybrid? In the terms of Latour, the purification of nature from culture has not happened in KarmaMood. It is a "medicinal product" (nature), regulated by the MHRA, the government agency that also regulates drug medicines, but its use is based purely on the safety of "traditional use" (culture). Its production is governed by technical standards (science) that arose out of EU legislation to harmonise trade, improve quality, and protect consumers (politics). Furthermore, there is a much larger evidence base for St John's wort's use in "mild to moderate depression" rather than "low mood and mild anxiety". However, because depression is not a "mild, self-limiting condition", it cannot be recommended for the use for which there is most evidence. So KarmaMood, with its network of herb farms, blister packs, braille, official MHRA approved THR logos, "traditional use" claims, EU legislation, German phytomedicines companies, distributors, and retail outlets can be regarded as a hybrid, created out of this network. The lengthened network has brought it greater attention and has antagonised some, particularly those who want herbal medicines to be approved by the same standards as drug medicines and insist that traditional use is no indication of efficacy. Thus, David Colquhoun, professor of pharmacology at UCL, in a TV interview, asks, "Why should there be different rules for herbals, which after all are just pharmacological agents of a particular subgroup, and for other ones? It's crazy to have two systems."[52]

He also says, "There is no need to supply any information whatsoever about whether they work or not. That itself is very odd, given that the MHRA's strapline says: 'We enhance and safeguard the health of the public by ensuring that medicines and medical devices work and are acceptably safe.' In the case of herbals, the bit about ensuring that medicines work has been brushed under the carpet."[53] Mixing culture and nature, or tradition and science just doesn't make sense to moderns.

CHAPTER FOUR

The profession and science

We have seen how the profession of herbal medicine has acted politically to protect itself, and how the regulatory impulse separates the herbal profession from its herbs, replacing them with skills and competencies. We will now look at how the profession has become increasingly allied with science, with herbs becoming an object of scientific investigation. Brown[17] notes that, as far back as the end of the nineteenth century, herbalists aspiring to professional status "needed to dispel some elements of their traditional image. First it had become necessary to purge herbalism of association with astrology," with the term "Culpeperism" being used to belittle and distance authors from the astrological aspect of Nicholas Culpeper's seventeenth-century work that was still influential two centuries on. Brown also highlights the embarrassment caused in the 1920s and 1930s by the image of the herbalist as a disreputable stallholder or someone who works in a dark, dusty shop decorated with the trappings of apothecaries. Herbalists saw attending to the sick to be a superior calling when compared to the retail supply of herbal medicines. This view remains prevalent in more recent times. For a decade from the late 1980s, in a continuing attempt to separate the professional consulting medical herbalist from the health shop supply of herbs, the NIMH had a requirement that its members should have a separate entrance for their patients that was not via a shop. Just at the time when Chinese medicine, which included the use of herbs, was opening its shop doors to passers-by on the high street, Western herbalists were shutting some of theirs. Although the number of herbalists who had shops was probably small, the requirement of separate doorways is reflective of the continuing concern of professional bodies to be aligned with the professionalism of orthodox medicine.

Journals

The possession of specialised knowledge is key for any group's claim to be a profession. Brown[17] points out that at the start of the twentieth century, texts on *materia medica* were not written by contemporary herbalists but relied on "out of date" sources. In response, the NAMH issued an updated *National Botanic Pharmacopoeia* in 1905, the second edition of which, produced in 1921, had all "poisonous remedies" removed.[5] Students and practitioners had other difficulties: in the 1880s the only British works recommended to students were by Skelton and even Webb's 1916 *Standard Guide to Non-Poisonous Herbal Medicines*[18] was reliant on American material. While the NAMH purchased the rights to Skelton's *Science and Practice of Herbal Medicine* in 1904 the text was thirty-four years old by the time students read it as course material. Brown reports one herbalist who said in 1929 that "We are sadly deficient in published works. We have none written by men of authority possessing British medical and scientific qualifications ..."[17] One way of generating specialised knowledge is through research. Brown shows that herbalists at the beginning of the twentieth century were aware of the importance of research to practice. Hence the NAMH awarded a medal for the best paper reporting original research at the annual conference. Shelley[26] points out that in 1909 the NAMH council agreed to award a number of prizes for an essay on "herbalism", giving "a) its scientific (or best) definition, b) the best means of making it scientifically effectual in the prevention and cure of disease", with the purpose of giving these prizes being that herbalism may be seen as worthy of state recognition. However, there were few opportunities for clinical research without holding medical qualifications. One way, however, to improve the scientific and professional status was through the publication of official journals. Thus, the NAMH initially published *The Botanic Practitioner*, which was replaced by *The Herbalist* in 1902 and by *The Medical Herbalist* in 1925.

Later, in 1938 *The Medical Herbalist* was combined with *Health from Herbs* before *The Herbal Practitioner* became the professional journal in 1940.[17]

The first issue of the *British Journal of Phytotherapy* was published in 1990 by the College of Phytotherapy. Hein Zeylstra was both the principal of the college and editor-in-chief of its journal. It was published quarterly or six-monthly until 2001. The first issue included a statement that the book *Herbal Medicine* by Rudolf Weiss,[54] published in 1988, "provides a good example of what phytotherapy stands for or should stand for ... The text speaks for itself."[55] This issue then presents reproductions of the prefaces to both the first and sixth editions of Weiss's text. In the first edition, the preface states that "A deliberate break has been made from the traditional approach still widely used today, which has its roots in history and folk medicine."[54] The *British Journal of Phytotherapy*, in its eleven-year life, published pharmacological and phytochemical studies, literature reviews, monographs, clinical notes and case reports, herbal approaches to particular biomedical conditions, and contemporary debates on phytotherapy. While traditional knowledge is referenced, it is rarely referenced alone when presenting information on particular herbs. Rather it is the evidence of science that is considered to be authoritative, with the traditional sources providing background. Whether it is barley, liquorice or sage that is the focus, it is the pull of science that allows these articles to be published in this journal rather than the push of tradition.

The *European Journal of Herbal Medicine* was published by the NIMH from 1994 to 2004, producing three issues per year. Its aim was to create "a forum for sharing information and opinion about developments in the field, including scientific, professional and political issues of importance to us as medical herbalists".[56] Compared with the *British Journal of Phytotherapy* it included more papers on historical aspects of herbal medicines, with a section designated "Traditions" that included considerations, for example, of the history of Scottish herbal medicine, Culpeper, Gerard, humoural medicine, Hildegard von Bingen, vitalism, folk medicine, and Chelsea Physic Gardens. It also included more clinical notes than the *British Journal of Phytotherapy* and the monographs presented generally contained more references to traditional sources, although there were regular updates on "research news". In the first edition David St George argues that herbal and other CAM modalities should not seek to force themselves into the biomedical model but should "be looking to the complementary therapies to help us gain insight into why and how orthodox medical science is limited."[57]

In 2011, the NIMH launched its new journal, the *Journal of Herbal Medicine*, this time a peer-reviewed Elsevier journal. The editorial of the first edition states:

> To consolidate our future position as registered healthcare profession-als and advance our profession it is vital to recognize that research is no longer an optional extra ... research is an essential activity and we must underpin our practice with sound scientific evidence. As a profession, in addition to the generation of data on the individual actions of herbs, we need to focus on the creation of sound evidence that takes account of the individualized nature of herbal practice.[58]

No longer is it possible for the profession to survive simply by looking back to the wisdom of the past, but a scientific evidence base must be created in order to facilitate herbalists' anticipated future recognition by the state. While there are a handful of papers in this journal that look at practitioner prescribing and experiences, thus investigating the "individualized nature of herbal practice", the vast majority of papers are concerned with other aspects of Western herbal medicine, including preclinical laboratory studies, the occasional clinical trial, reviews, monographs, and historical and opinion pieces. For the *Journal of Herbal Medicine* it is the indications from scientific studies that are emphasised, although traditional knowledge sources may be used to "support" such evidence. Even though scientific evidence and traditional knowledge are often presented as mutually reinforcing, it is only science that can stand on its own: this is the nature of peer-reviewed scientific journals. In this sense, the more recent *Journal of Herbal Medicine* is more like the *British Journal of Phytotherapy* and less like the *European Journal of Herbal Medicine*, with clinical experience and tradition being less emphasised in the search for an objective knowledge that will satisfy science and regulators. These differences between older and newer journals are also broadly reflected by Evans[59] who, in reviewing herbal therapeutic articles in a contemporary Australian herbal medicine journal, suggests that there is a similar move away from traditional knowledge to scientific knowledge in clinical discussions.

Pharmacopoeias

Treasure,[60] a herbalist and author, describes Kuhn's argument that science progresses non-linearly with crises or revolutions interrupting "normal science". Observations and data lead to a "paradigm" of "normal science". Eventually, however, anomalous findings accumulate which are "incommensurable" with the existing paradigm, leading to a crisis and the emergence of a new paradigm that can explain the anomalous findings. This is followed by another period of normal science. Applying such a framework to Western herbal medicine, Treasure additionally brings in a modern web-based analogy. He argues there has been a move from "Herbalism 1.0" to "Herbalism 2.0". Herbalism 1.0 is characterised by "the Herbal". In fact, notes Treasure, "The Herbal is the Paradigm." "The Herbal", authored by the expert practitioner, is an authoritative knowledge base of botanical remedies, pharmacy, and therapeutics. Treasure sees Dioscorides's *De Materia Medica* as being the first authoritative herbal. Other herbals central to the tradition include those described by Tobyn et al.[5],—Greco-Roman and Arabic herbals such as those written by Galen and Avicenna; in the Middle Ages those written by Hildegard von Bingen and the Physicians of Myddfai; in the Renaissance and Early Modern period those written by Paracelsus and Culpeper; and in the nineteenth century, those authored by Cook, Thurston, Ellingwood, and Felter. Treasure argues that these "expert practitioners express a specific conception of the nature of a herbal remedy", often in terms of "virtues", where the herb is not defined by what it does so much as what it has "the power to do".

Herbalism 2.0, on the other hand, was presaged by the period of crisis in the last decades of the nineteenth century and the first few decades of the twentieth, when there was an urgent need to legitimise herbal medicine in the face of a pharmaceutical industry that was closely aligned with a confident orthodox medical profession. Treasure argues that the expert author and the herbal have been replaced by the monograph, often presented in pharmacopoeias: "Eminence based medicine was replaced by evidence based medicine," with monographs designed to oppose "legal-regulatory initiatives intended to minimize the credibility and availability of herbal medicines". The monograph became based on objective scientific data, even if there were variations in the monograph's focus on either more analytical or more therapeutic orientations. While herbals considered the virtues of herbs, monographs revealed the actions of herbs based on reductionist science.

The British Herbal Medicine Association (BHMA), an interest group of retailers, manufacturers, and herbalists, was established in 1964 to address regulatory controls on herbal medicines. Part of its response was to create a pharmacopoeia-based record of plant monographs in use by medical herbalists. The publishing of the *British Herbal Pharmacopoeia* began in the 1970s, and was motivated partly by the recognition that the 1968 Act was only a stopgap, with the absence of a legal definition of a herbalist and continuing medical opposition leaving herbalists open to attacks that may partly be addressed by putting herbal practice on a sounder scientific footing.[6] In fact, Griggs[9] tells how the BHMA had been told by the government, in the drafting of the 1968 Medicines Act, that non-poisonous herbs that were included in standard reference books might be exempted from expensive requirements of safety and efficacy that were applied to drug medications. The BHMA then established its Scientific Committee, resulting in various editions of the *British Herbal Pharmacopoeia*. The 1983 edition[61] provides quality criteria and therapeutic information for 232 plants or "botanical drugs". It represents a collation of material from the 1976, '79, and '81 editions. It includes sections on identification and macroscopical and microscopical descriptions before outlining the actions, indications, combinations, preparations, and dosages of the herbs, with these therapeutic aspects being based on the clinical experience of key herbal practitioners of the day, although the authors included those with specialist knowledge of pharmacy, pharmacognosy, science, and medicine as well as herbal practice. Tassell[62] reports that ten key members were closely reported in the survey, with up to sixty consulted on specific areas.

The dosages sections of the entries reveal what can be seen from a non-clinical perspective as demonstrating inconsistencies or contradictions. For example, if we take the herb *Cimicifuga racemosa* (black cohosh), the dosages recommended include 0.3 to 2g of the dried material or the same by decoction, representing more than a six-fold variation. If taken as a liquid extract of a 1:1 strength, meaning 1g was used to make 1ml, then the dose is 0.3 to 2g, which is consistent with the dose of the dried material. However, a tincture dose made using a tincture of one part dried plant to ten parts of 60% alcohol is recommended to be taken in a dose of 2 to 4ml, which is equivalent to 0.2 to 0.4g of the dried plant material. This is less than the decoction or liquid extract dose. These differences in dosage are duplicated within the various monographs, and are hardly surprising as these dosages were based on the clinical experience of an unspecified number of practitioners. This dosage range obviously leaves open to question what is the "right" dosage for a particular individual. This uncertainty was removed by the time that the 1996 edition of the *British Herbal Pharmacopoeia*[63] was published, with no dosages being recommended at all. This was not the only difference between the earlier and later editions. While the '83 edition contains therapeutic information as discussed above, the '96 edition contains only information on actions, which for most of the herbs is limited to simply one word. *Cimicifuga racemosa* has the following actions in the '83 edition: antirheumatic; antitussive; sedative; emmenagogue. It is also has the following "indications": rheumatism, rheumatoid arthritis, intercostal myalgia, sciatica, whooping cough, chorea, tinnitus aurium, dysmennorrhoea, uterine colic, and has "specific indications" of muscular rheumatism and rheumatoid arthritis. In the '96 edition however, the therapeutic section describes its action solely as "anti-inflammatory" and provides no indications. While both editions have information on botanical identification and macroscopical and microscopical descriptions, the latter edition ignores the less biomedically acceptable terms of "antitussive", "sedative", and "emmenagogue", and substitutes "anti-inflammatory" for "antirheumatic".

The desire for the scientific status of herbs can also be seen in the publication of the *British Herbal Compendium* in 1992[64] with its comprehensively referenced summaries of constituents, phytochemical structures, therapeutic uses, and regulatory status. Like the *British Herbal Pharmacopoeia* the therapeutic indications of the *British Herbal Compendium* are based on senior NIMH members' clinical experience. However, they are supported by pharmacological research. As Swale[65] notes, the monographs contain less information on therapeutic indications than was presented in the 1983 edition of the *British Herbal Pharmacopoeia*, with information on herb combinations being omitted. She argues that "Presumably this is because of the BHMA Scientific Committee's wish to give as far as possible only information which can be substantiated by solid research evidence."

The 1992 edition of the *British Herbal Compendium* does give a fuller and referenced description of the actions of black cohosh than the 1996 edition of the *British Herbal Pharmacopoeia*—"endocrine (pituitary, oestrogen-mimetic) activity [6, 9]: emmenagogue; antirheumatic". It also gives the indications as "menopausal disorders [8, 10–17], premenstrual complaints, dysmenorrhoea, uterine spasm [18]".[64] What can be noted from this is that when the *British Herbal Compendium* gives references to actions or indications they are all related to its hormonal activity, which had been increasingly researched since 1983. The actions and indications in the *British Herbal Compendium* do not include the traditional "antitussive" and "sedative" actions of the 1983 edition of the *British Herbal Pharmacopoeia* that are less evidenced by science. Similarly, rheumatic complaints that were once the staple area of application of *Cimicifuga racemosa* are not given as primary indications, but as "other uses".

Training

Graham-Little[66] reports that the NAMH, in 1935, gave instruction via its four "principal" tutors, located at 46 Bloomsbury Street, London, in "anatomy and physiology, materia medica and therapeutics, pathology and physical diagnosis, diseases of women and children, chemistry", and that there was an additional postal course in these subjects. There was an oral examination based on a curriculum divided into three periods of three months. This curriculum included thirty-two subjects, with twelve lectures in each subject. In addition to the subjects mentioned above the course covered "bacteriology, general medicine, general surgery, gynaecology and obstetrics, paediatrics, orthopaedics, urology, dermatology, oto-rhino-laryngology, ophthalmology, radiology and electricity, venereal diseases, and infectious diseases ..." The fee for the whole course was 25 guineas. After successful completion of the examinations and oral test, the student was awarded the "conjoint" degree, made up of "degree of LCBM" and "degree of MNAMH", which qualified the recipient for practice. After a year, if the practitioner presented a thesis of at least 5000 words, he would be awarded a higher degree of doctor of botanic medicine. While the exact content of these courses is unknown, the NAMH had embraced what appears to be a fairly conventional approach to the development of its curriculum.

W. Burns Lingard helped develop the NAMH postal course. His 1958 book *Herbal Prescriptions from a Consultant's Case Book*[67] was an attempt, "at any rate as far as I am concerned", to refute a statement made at the Scarborough conference of 1955 that "All the old Herbalists who have died have taken their knowledge with them." He alphabetically lists his formulations by conditions. Throughout the book there is no mention of any theoretical or philosophical considerations. It is a purely empirical work, addressing bio-medically defined illnesses. Thus, for example, for "Blood pressure—hypertension" he writes: "Abnormal tension of the walls of the arteries" and recommends, per dose:

Fl. Ex. Cactus ……....………m.15
Fl. Ex. Crataegus…...………m.5
Fl. Ex. Salix Nig……………m.30
Fl. Ex. Passiflora…...………m.20
Fl. Ex. Menyanthes …………m.30

The addition of Fl. Ex. Valerian is suitable in many cases but the remedy is not well tolerated by many patients. Diet should be mainly fruitarian and vegetarian. Avoid salt, red meats, pork and all rich food. Avoid alcohol.

While the formula, like many others in the book, reflects a *materia medica* drawing on both European and North American herbs, the American concern with concepts drawn from Thomsonianism and physiomedicalism was absent, being replaced by the empiricism of formulae applicable to diseases. On the other hand, at the same time, A. W. Priest[68-70] was producing teaching material for the NIMH that continued to emphasise physiomedical approaches to diagnosis, medication, and *materia medica*. Concepts of vitality, relaxation and contraction, stimulation and inhibition, and trophorestoration, remained central, as did a focus on the circulatory and autonomic nervous systems. Priest and Priest[25] eventually produced a condensed book in 1983 that drew together some of these teachings.

It is likely that the move away from physiomedical influences was a gradual one. Barker[6] notes that in Britain training to be a medical herbalist had been conducted from Hyde's Herbal Clinic in Leicester with training via correspondence and seminars. This training was established in 1969 and ran until 1978 when Hein Zeylstra was appointed as the new principal of the School of Herbal Medicine in Tunbridge Wells on behalf of the NIMH education fund.[30] The course was entitled "The Full Time Course" and was undertaken over four years. It drew heavily from European scientific approaches to herbal practice and marked the end of NIMH training in what had been influenced by the physiomedical tradition.

Phytochemistry replaced the vital force. Traditional use of herbs became less of a justification for their clinical use in training as more evidence was sought from scientific research. The School of Herbal Medicine became an independent college, the College of Herbal Medicine, in 1982, and finally the College of Phytotherapy in 1991. By 1990 the NIMH had approved training clinics in Brighton, Bristol, Coventry, Exeter, London, Manchester, and Winchester.[30]

The 1980s and 90s saw a rise in the number of herbal organisations: the College of Practitioners of Phytotherapy was established in 1991, with Hein Zeylstra as its first president, as a body of professional herbalists that sought to represent those herbalists who practised on a scientific, phytotherapeutic basis, and for whom herbal medicine was seen as being a complete approach to health, not requiring other modalities. Indeed, those who today apply for membership and who practise additional therapies to herbal medicine are likely to be turned down. Other practitioner organisations emerged in the 1980s seeking to represent those herbalists who had trained outside NIMH or CPP courses. These herbalists had diploma qualifications from courses that emphasised influences such as iridology, naturopathy, and energetic systems of medicine such as Chinese medicine and Ayurveda. They included the Unified Register of Herbal Practitioners, the Association of Master Herbalists, and the International Register of Consulting Herbalists. The umbrella organisation of the European Herbal Practitioners Association (EHPA), introduced above, was established in 1993 (later to become the European Herbal and Traditional Medicine Practitioners Association in 2006), when it became clear that the legislative framework for herbal practice in the UK was likely to be challenged by the EU.

Eventually there were to be seven degrees in herbal medicine available in the UK as training to degree level was taken outside the auspices of the NIMH and the College of Phytotherapy. The seven courses were at Middlesex University, the University of Westminster, the College of Phytotherapy (externally validated and subsequently moved to the University of East London), Napiers University, the Scottish School of Herbal Medicine, the University of Central Lancashire, and the University of Lincoln. Today, only two degrees remain—at Westminster and Lincoln. This reduction is likely due to a number of factors, including the burden of student fees (up to £9000 per year), a saturated higher education market providing herbal medicine degrees, and the influence of a powerful sceptic lobby that sees CAM and BSc degrees as being mutually incompatible.[71-74]

Since the 1980s, just as evidence-based medicine has sought to influence orthodox medical practice, there has been an increasing emphasis on grounding the practice of herbalists in a scientific evidence base, thus facilitating the awarding of BSc degrees in herbal medicine. This apparent scientisation of herbal medicine training, where scientific discourses are emphasised and given more validity than traditional ones, may be seen in the requirement of the European Herbal and Traditional Medicine Practitioners Association[75] that recognised training courses teach a core curriculum based on nine modules in order that the graduates of these courses are eligible for membership of the professional bodies that make up this association.

Most of these modules (e.g., human sciences, clinical sciences, plant chemistry and pharmacology, pharmacognosy) are based around the conservatism of orthodox medical training with its basis firmly in the reductionist cause-effect model that assumes human physiological uniformity. Less conservative biomedical content, such as psychoneuroimmunology, has at times been variously taught but has eventually been reduced or squeezed out of courses.

However, one of these nine modules is a module specific for each tradition of herbal medicine. For Western herbal medicine this module suggests "using appropriate conventional and complementary diagnostic skills to select herbs". In fact, all the degree courses teach orthodox medical diagnostics via physical examination and case history taking and include 500 hours of clinical practice. At the level of diagnosis of biomedical disease there appears to be little non-orthodox conception of diagnosis in training although student herbalists often use the information gained from long consultations to treat a broader understanding of "what is the matter" with any particular patient.

Beyond the question of diagnosis, in both its 2007 and 2014 versions the module specific for Western herbal medicine recognises that "designations that may describe a particular approach may include but not be limited to, physiomedical, vitalistic, holistic, energetic, phytotherapeutic and biomedical",[75,76] and that it is up to each teaching institution to make its approach clear.

The reading list supplied with the "module specific to Western herbal medicine" does contain texts that broadly fit into these different designations but, as with all categories, they tend to oversimplification. An examination of many of these and related texts reveals that they often contain elements of other "designations". Thus "phytotherapy" texts[54,77-79] which comfortably turn to science, are not alone in their attention to cutting edge physiology, as this was a hallmark of nineteenth-century-originated physiomedicalism[25] and its application of the then-recent discovery of the autonomic nervous system. In its modern variant physiomedicalism also turns to more contemporary science, for example immunology and pharmacokinetics.[24] "Vitalistic" approaches that explain health in terms of activation of the vital force and trophorestoration of tissues and organs are found explicitly within physiomedicalism but also, more implicitly, within holistic approaches where herbs are described as being tissue and organ-specific.[80,81] The consideration of physical, mental, emotional, and spiritual dimensions in such holistic approaches are often addressed in "energetic" approaches[82] where these different levels are connected via the movement of energy. And such energetic approaches that use various understandings of "constitutions" and of the qualities of heat, cold, damp, and dry are not averse to taking into account the phytochemical constituents that are the bread and butter (or gluten and butyric acid, if you will excuse the pun) of biomedical evidence-based approaches.[83,84] It is notable that the biomedical texts are the only texts that remain closed to other designations. Most texts that students come into contact with will be hybrids of different designations.

The textbook most frequently emphasised in training courses, Mills and Bone's *Principles and Practice of Phytotherapy*,[77] was reworked into a second edition.[78] It amasses the weight of scientific evidence within it and can be identified by the number of scientific references and bibliographic sources. As Owen[85] notes, the first edition of this text, published in 2000, was a landmark event with its blending of traditional Western herbal medicine and evidence-based scientific research, clinical approaches, and awareness of regulatory concerns over safety and dosage. The second edition, published thirteen years later, is expanded and revised to take account of the increased research on medicinal plants, pharmacology, and pathophysiology and is twice the size of the first edition. Barker[86] describes the first edition as representing the culmination of the hope that herbal medicine will come to be accepted as an authoritative academic and clinical discipline—"the whole thrust of this enterprise is to match reputation with scientific evidence", and that "The writers are afflicted with a condition that besets all of us in this field: the voice of unrecognition—a complaint for the world to turn to an appreciation of the qualities we husband for the greater good." This is equally true for the second edition, in its resourceful marshalling of even more science for the phytotherapeutic endeavour.

While tradition, on its own, is less likely to be seen as sufficient to justify a herb's use in the context of a profession that is seeking recognition, a sense of how easily both science and tradition are resourced is best demonstrated with quotes from a talk by Kerry Bone given after the publication of the second edition. Kerry Bone[87] talks about saffron, describing how research is validating traditional use documented by Avicenna in the eleventh century.

Now saffron is the world's most expensive spice, and when you think about it, you have this small little crocus growing in a field and people have to go and hand pick just the 3 stigmas from every flower, you can understand what sort of yield you get from each acre, it is not going to be high, and that is why it is so expensive. But the good news is, because it is so concentrated, you don't necessarily need a very high dose. And in the saffron, in particular, we have the carotenoids in a form as glycosides, and what that means is it's not just a concentrated extract, it's a concentrated enhanced bio-available extract for carotenoids, because when you get the crocins via the saffron tincture, the bacteria in your large bowel take the sugar part off the glycoside. That leaves the carotenoid there to be absorbed. Now the thing that sparked my interest in saffron was the clinical trials that started coming through in its use in depression. … we have a number of trials with saffron, … trials where it has been compared with SSRIs and so on, but it doesn't just stop there, and it shows that saffron has a sphere of influence on the nervous system, because there are some promising early trials on Alzheimer's disease and there is a trial in PMS. And, fairly recently, a very interesting trial, and it is probably neurological, showing that saffron can regulate appetite.… it reduces snacking behavior in people who are overweight … Also we know of course that the eye is the extension of the nervous system, and we are now seeing some promising early trials in age-related macular degeneration. In fact in one open label trial, patients over a 3, 6, 12 month period were able to improve their visual acuity by up to 2 lines on the Snellen chart … I am certainly giving saffron, about 4 or 5ml a day to my patients with AMD … Also recently we have had some clinical trials of saffron where it was used in patients already on SSRIs … It was found in two separate trials, one in men and one in women, that it reduced sexual dysfunction in patients taking SSRIs … it demonstrates that saffron is quite safe to take with SSRIs …

I'd like to close by looking at what Avicenna wrote about it in the Cannon of Medicine, and he wrote this more than a thousand years ago. He said oral use of saffron improves the complexion. Well we know that carotenoids do this and there is a carotenoid supplement being developed overseas … called Astaxanthin the pink colour in krill, and it has been shown in clinical trials to improve the complexion and it's a property of carotenoids. He also said it strengthens the eyesight and is useful in day blindness and he could well have been referring to some sort of variant on AMD that may have occurred many years ago. "It is a stimulant of sexual desire" and we had those studies of SSRI-induced sexual dysfunction. And he also further said that it reduces the appetite. Isn't it extraordinary that the uses documented by Avicenna over a thousand years ago for saffron are being validated by modern research.

While herbalists can talk about a herb in ways that draw from both science and tradition, it is scientific sources, as seen in the journals, pharmacopoeias, texts, and training of herbalists that have been emphasised. It is this, along with a powerful desire for political survival, as seen in the precarious and tenacious history of Western herbal medicine, that has enabled the profession to progress as far as it has today in its venture to gain political recognition, independence, and credibility. Let us now turn to the social sciences to see how scholars from these disciplines understand contemporary Western herbal medicine.

CHAPTER FIVE

Practice, concepts, and knowledge: views on Western herbal medicine from the social sciences

While much of the history of herbal medicine, particularly since the nineteenth century, remains hidden, there is a small but growing social science literature investigating contemporary Western herbal medicine. In a 2012 review article, Nissen and Evans[2] identify twenty-five academic papers from the social sciences addressing Western herbal medicine in Europe, North America, and Australasia. Since this review, there have been at least eleven further additions.[88-98] Of these thirty-six publications, twenty are authored by fourteen scholars who are qualified in herbal medicine, with thirteen of these being trained in the UK. This raises several points: that thirty-six publications is a low, but rising, absolute number of social science inquiries into Western herbal medicine; that such academic inquiry, similarly to the history of Western herbal medicine, is fuelled to a considerable part by herbalists themselves; and that without this curiosity from within herbal medicine, it would be more difficult to discern its presence within the social science literature at all. Some of these papers, that provide background and are relevant to the arguments of this book, will now be discussed.

Nissen and Evans[2] identify two themes in the literature. The first theme is the "mapping" of practice that investigates the professional titles that are used, the clinical practice, the demographics of herbalists and their patients, and the therapeutic relationship. The second theme is a concern to engage with theoretical issues regarding the development of herbal knowledge. Both themes shall be considered here, including consideration of the work done since their review, with an additional emphasis on the development of theoretical concepts relating to herbal practice.

"Mapping of practice" and conceptual understandings

Looking to the first theme, Nissen and Evans[2] draw on Nissen[99] to suggest that UK herbalists prefer the term "medical herbalist"; about 80% of herbalists are female; a typical UK herbalist is between forty-one and fifty years of age, Caucasian, works part time, and gains her patients by word of mouth. They suggest that a typical patient is a woman with a wide range of women's health concerns. Additional practice-related information may be seen from a "snapshot survey" by the NIMH of its members' practices over a week in March 2012.[100] The NIMH is the largest body of herbalists in the UK. All 630 members of the NIMH were sent a survey document and asked to record information about patients that consulted them between 5 and 12 March 2012. With a response rate of 31%, 195 herbalists participated. The largest group of responders fell into the 45 to 55 years old age range, followed by 55 to 65 years, then 35 to 45 years, and finally the 25 to 35 years. Of those who responded, 41% had been in practice for between three and ten years. Most of those surveyed (55%) practise from one location, although 28% practise from two locations. Most herbalists work either from multidisciplinary practices or from home, with 34% of herbalists having a retail outlet attached to their clinic. Looking at the regions where herbalists practise, the North-West, South-West, Scotland, and South-East have the highest prevalence of herbalists, ranging from 12% to 16%. The fees for a first consultation predominantly range from £25 to £45, with only 25% charging over £45. A similar picture is seen in the follow-up fees, with 66% of herbalists surveyed charging under £30. The herbalists surveyed had an average of seven consultations during the week, with 72% of the patients being female. The presenting symptoms of patients showed a dominance of nervous system complaints (especially anxiety, insomnia, depression and low mood, and high stress levels), and gastrointestinal complaints (especially bloating, abdominal pain, and constipation).

This was followed by "general" complaints (especially fatigue and low energy), and by gynaecological symptoms (especially hot sweats/ flushes and premenstrual symptoms). Referrals to herbalists were nearly equal in number by other healthcare professionals and by patient self-referral. If self-referred, other patients and family played an important role in this process.

Looking to clinical practice and the therapeutic relationship Nissen and Evans[2] argue that most herbalists characterise their practices as "traditional Western herbal medicine", "Western European", or "Western herbal medicine". Furthermore, the consultation is largely made up of taking the case history, as well as diagnosis and development of a management plan and dispensing. Beyond the prescription of herbs, the joint construction of patients' stories is highlighted as being an important part of the therapeutic process.

The medicines that are prescribed and dispensed are mostly minimally processed herbal preparations such as tinctures, or dried herbs to be prepared as water extracts.[90] This will be seen to make sense in the context of the importance to herbalists of knowing the living plants from which their medicines are made, where minimal processing keeps the herbalists closer to their medicines' living origins. Denham[27] notes, drawing on her thirty years of clinical experience as well as on Conway,[79] that herbalists take a broad clinical history. They may examine the patient, and discuss a wide range of factors including diet and lifestyle, as well as emotional and spiritual meanings. At the same time, they develop a diagnostic rationale for the treatment plan that includes an individualised prescription. Whitehouse[101] adds that herbalists work within the context of "shared care" as most patients arrive at a herbalist's door having already visited an orthodox doctor and received a medical diagnosis.

It is interesting, and relevant for this book, that it is commonly noted that approaches to practice are diverse,[97] plural,[96,99,102,103] and that treatment is individualised.[104,105] This is something that will be confirmed by the cases in this book, although a novel reason for such variety will be suggested.

Looking beyond the demographics and mechanics of practice, to more theoretical concerns, Stewart,[1] in an interpretative phenomenological case study approach to understanding herbal practice and Asperger's syndrome, suggests that herbalists' "ways of being" are made up of ethical and reflexive "ways of knowing"; that herbal medicines, diet, and lifestyle make up their "ways of doing"; and that "ways of being practical" are seen by the rapid decisions that are made. In Yates's[97] study of the treatment of distress by herbalists the therapeutic process was composed of "being heard" which was enabled through accessibility, time, and talk; "being held", facilitated by rapport, support, and reframing; and "being treated", arising out of patient empowerment and holism. West and Denham[94] investigated the clinical reasoning of UK herbalists and concluded that they use complex thought processes when formulating prescriptions for patients. They identified both analytical and non-analytical thinking by herbalists. Hypothetico-deductive reasoning, pattern recognition, and intuition were all employed. The ease with which herbalists utilise these diverse resources in their internal clinical reasoning may also have a parallel in the way that herbal practice may be seen to be an assemblage of diverse elements beyond the bounded practitioner. Snow,[88] for example, suggests that the characteristics of herbal preparations, the patient-practitioner relationship as well as the physical environment, combine to produce important context effects that affect patient health. The non-hierarchical relationship between herbalists and patients that Snow refers to, and is confirmed by Nissen[102,103] and Little,[106] will be seen to resemble herbalist-plant relationships that will be discussed later in this book. Snow argues that the herbal medicines themselves act as symbols of tradition and natural healing and that their sensory qualities may affect biology. Of course, the sensory qualities of herbal medicines originate in the sensory qualities of the living plant, something that will also come to be seen to be important to the herbalists found later in this book. Snow[107] suggests a framework for studying physiology that is relevant to Western herbal medicine. This includes a perspective that emphasises body-wide coordination of physiology; a psycho-biological perspective that resources developments such as psychoneuroimmunology, stress physiology, and context effects; a socio-biological perspective that looks to concepts such as empathy and compassion; an evolutionary and ecological perspective that draws from, for example, consideration of co-evolution, epigenomics, and broad exposure to phytochemicals; and a perspective that seeks connections across scales, for example from the gene to the organism, or from moments to years, and utilises concepts such as emergence and levels of causation. Each of these perspectives seeks to make connections across boundaries, bringing areas together that had previously been separate, something that also resonates with the narratives of herbalists that we will encounter later.

Nissen,[102,108,109] in feminist ethnographic fieldwork of women herbalists in the UK, suggests that the bodies and selves of female patients in these practices exist at the place where self-care and self-fulfilment meet the tensions of women's lives, necessarily making Western herbal medicine a politicised form of health care. Herbal practice affords an opportunity for renegotiating and revaluing women's identities and selves. The patient-practitioner relationship is a "storied relationship" through which both Western herbal medicine and patients' narratives are constructed out of the patient-practitioner negotiated partnership. However, such partnerships may not be limited to human-human relationships but can be extended to herbalist-plant relations, as we will see.

To summarise, the accessing of different ways of making clinical decisions,[94] the entanglement of the medicine and the context,[88] the connection-making of a specifically Western herbal medicine approach to physiology,[107] and the importance of relationship[102,103,108,109] will be seen to be in keeping with herbalists who know plants differently.

Continuing with the theme of relationship, Niemeyer[90] conducted a grounded theory exploration of how American herbalists arrive at their herbal formulations. She identified a five-step process of "personalization" of the medicine to the patient that occurs as "weaving a tapestry of right relationships" to explain how "concordance", or the fit between the person and the medicine, results in the "restoration of dynamic equilibrium". Niemeyer argues that right relationship "describes the parts in reference to the whole" and that this is sought in the client, in prescribing for the client, and in the process of practising personalised Western herbal medicine "as an integrated and interconnected whole". She suggests that this includes the whole person, the social, the environmental, and the universal. "Right relationship" is said to create an emergent order and increases the coherence of the whole. Herbalists do this with their clients when they gather and interpret information, formulate the medicine for the client and assess outcomes.

While Niemeyer avoids direct engagement with "holism" in Western herbal medicine, Nissen[102,103] identifies and describes three distinct holistic perspectives within women's practice of Western herbal medicine in the UK—the homeostatic, the bio-psycho-social, and the spiritual that, in the movement from the material through the social to the immaterial, are nevertheless contained within each other, rather like Russian dolls. Importantly, Nissen suggests the existence of "multiple and co-existing practices", and describes how individual practitioners can variously draw on more than one perspective, although the homeostatic perspective allows less fluidity with other perspectives than the other two. This is similar to the findings of this book, as will be seen in the cases below, with herbalists drawing on diverse influences that sit easily together, with the reason for this being explored in herbalists' relationships with plants and herbal medicines. Nissen suggests that the accommodating nature of the term "holism" allows the diversity of approaches to practice to hang their cloaks on the same peg and argues that this is more attractive to herbalists than the use of the controversial concept of vitalism. Hiller[92] examines the concept of vitalism and argues, albeit with little empirical evidence, that Western herbal medicine continues to adhere to this "discredited" concept, suggesting that this "actively impedes" the development of an evidence base. It will later be argued that Western herbal medicine easily, and maybe even necessarily, retains diversities of approaches within itself and within individual practitioners.

However, this book will not pursue holism within Western herbal medicine. This is partly because it is a slippery term. Scheid[110] argues that holism can be opposed to reductionism or can be complementary to it, it can have a specific meaning tied to gestalt psychology or be the trope of "the whole is greater than the sum of its parts", it can be conservative or progressive. Scheid reveals the lineage of the term as arising out of eighteenth-century Germany, as inflected differentially through both Kant and Engels, with the term "holism" eventually being coined by Jan Smuts in 1926 in South Africa and used to justify apartheid, and later taken up by Nazism, yet also was associated with vitalist thinking in France and neo-Hippocratic medical thought. The tendency of holism to reduce life to systems, with their explicit or implicit boundaries, is felt to too easily contain Western herbal medicine, simplifying some of its complexities. Additionally, and perhaps most importantly, the term holism was not significantly brought up by the herbalists themselves in the current research, which prefers to follow threads within narratives rather than focus on categories. However, the diversity of approaches to practice is something that this book also demonstrates. Having said this, where a flicker of holism may be detected in this book is in the enchantment of herbalists by plants, with such meetings pointing towards a greater sense of completeness for humans, if not for plants, as well as in the identification of threads that connect different parts of a narrative into a whole case.

Nina Nissen has been central to the development of social science perspectives on Western herbal medicine. There are two areas of her work, beyond the recognition of the diversities of practice within Western herbal medicine, which resonate with the focus of this book. They are her concern with narrative and elements of "biographical holism", and her excavation of the meaning of "naturalness" in Western herbal medicine. For Nissen,[2,102,109] the stories of women herbalists are valid objects of inquiry, with the narrative co-construction of patients' stories being important in the practice of Western herbal medicine. Similarly, narrative is important in this book, where the relationship between how people become herbalists and the rest of their stories of involvement with herbal medicine leads to a previously unconsidered formulation of what Western herbal medicine may be. Related to narrative, Nissen introduces the term "biographical holism", to refer to the "merging of practitioners' life stories, personal experiences, values and beliefs with their adopted framework of holism".[102] While the current book does not adopt holism as an analytical tool, the biographies are certainly important for how practice and Western herbal medicine may come to be seen. Looking to "naturalness", Nissen[96] explores this concept as the nonhuman element that is bound to herbalists and patients. She finds that Raymond Williams's three definitions of nature—as essence, material world, and force—are all present in Western herbal medicine and argues that this is positioned to help displace humans from the epicentre of everything. Nissen's position resonates with this book's consideration of herbalists in relation to the nonhuman but here the focus is more specifically on plants and their agency as well as, as we shall see, in recent developments in the plant sciences and social sciences, rather than broader concepts of nature or naturalness.

Herbal knowledge: paradigms and beyond

We now turn to the second theme identified by Nissen and Evans[2]: a concern to engage with theoretical issues to do with the development of herbal knowledge. Much of this social science research suggests that the tradition of Western herbal medicine is being taken over by science—moving from one paradigm to another, from herbalism to phytotherapy or from expert practitioner to evidence-based herbal medicine. This research, which has been conducted mostly in the UK, Australia and Canada, often includes a sense of loss about this process.

Jagtenberg and Evans[111] suggest that: "In short, the so-called globalization of society and culture has influenced contemporary Western herbal medicine in a number of ways that challenge the rationale of traditional herbalism. As herbal medicine becomes an international industry—*global herbalism*—it is pushed toward a positivist and reductionist philosophical appreciation of the use of medicinal plants." Looking at the Australian context from the mid 1980s they argue that while traditional Western concepts of toxicity, enervation, and suboptimum organ function are of use to herbalists alongside knowledge of pathology and physiology, it is globalisation "in the guise of science, technology and progress that is more likely to destabilize the traditions of Western herbal medicine. This is the direction from which an industry led profession will come." Hence, they see good manufacturing practice (GMP), new industrial techniques, and governmental regulation of herbal products as likely to have detrimental effects on the traditional practice of Western herbal medicine in Australia.

The UK situation has similarly seen the interconnected influences of legislation (most notably the EU's Traditional Herbal Medicine Products Directive), GMP, and industrial techniques on the retail supply of herbal medicines. However, businesses that supply herbalists with tinctures and dried herbs, because these are not classified as "finished products", face less stringent requirements in that GMP is not a legal necessity. Despite this there is concern among smaller producers that more and more will be demanded of them by governmental agencies in the future. Casey,[104] in a survey and interview study of Australian herbalists, argues for the concept of "mainstreaming" in order to understand Western herbal medicine in Australia. Mainstreaming is a social process where the boundaries between Western herbal medicine and orthodox health care are seen to be shifting, but with the latter becoming dominant. The movement is one way, with Western herbal medicine taking on orthodox concepts and practices. Just as Jagtenberg and Evans argue for the deterministic effect of global herbal medicine on herbal practice, Casey similarly argues that Western herbal medicine is being mainstreamed and, in the process, losing its identity. Similar to Casey,[104] and to Jagtenberg and Evans,[111] Evans[112] argues that

Australian herbalists' traditional philosophical basis is being replaced with a science knowledge base, which weakens the ability of herbalists to maintain their professional identity. Evans uses Gross's model of "cultural location" to suggest that Western herbal medicine, in placing itself close to the power of science, has trouble maintaining its own identity. Evans,[59] after comparing a herbal text from 1931 with one from 2007, and journal articles from 1989–2008, suggests that Australian herbalists are moving towards the use of evidence-based medicine rather than traditional knowledge in their clinical discussions, with phytochemistry and clinical trials being favoured over traditional use. Evans argues that evidence-based medicine "encourages the development of herbal knowledge based on products made from plants rather than on the plants themselves". Later it will be seen that plants may have more say in herbal knowledge than this statement suggests.

VanMarie[105] argues that Western herbal medicine in the UK assumes the features of orthodox science, particularly in the favouring of a science base, in the search for acceptance. VanMarie suggests that this biomedical emphasis was a tactic consciously adopted by leaders of the profession, while also arguing that there is an anomaly between the "phytotherapeutic" education of herbalists and the actual "traditional" practice of Western herbal medicine. Although formal knowledge is not necessarily discarded, practice draws on clinical experience and the various traditions of herbal medicine.

Like Casey,[104] Singer and Fisher[113] turn to the concept of "mainstreaming" to describe the absorption of non-conventional practices into the orthodox domain such that they are "co-opted" rather than accepted. Thus "CAM", including Western herbal medicine, is mainstreamed in the sense that CAM is an umbrella term that asserts control over these non-conventional practices, where CAM becomes an evidence-based method of using natural products. Thus "… the risk is that the integrity of traditional knowledge is eroded through epistemological incursion as these practices are decontextualized and manipulated in order to fit a scientific methodology." Singer and Fisher suggest that co-option leads to divisions within non-conventional practices—an "epistemological bifurcation", seen, for example, in the dichotomies of vitalism versus science and of holism versus reductionism, where traditional herbal knowledge faces being swallowed up by biomedicine.

As Wahlberg[51] points out, these scholars have in common a more-or-less explicit assumption that there is a battle going on between paradigms, where only one paradigm can win or has won, where Western herbal medicine is co-opted or colonised by Western biomedicine, with their differences being, in Kuhnian terms, "incommensurable". Thus Treasure[60] employs Kuhn to suggest that the paradigm of "the herbal" has been replaced by the paradigm of "the monograph". However, a common criticism of Kuhn is that in his view a new paradigm completely replaces the old one, and that this does not reflect actual practices as closely as he portrays. Fuller[114,115] suggests that Kuhn's writing is "syncretistic", combining aspects from different historical periods as if they had always coexisted, thus making it easy to find examples that fit his account of the practice of science. Additionally, Fuller has been unable to find an episode of science that demonstrates the full cycle from normal science through to a new normal science. Despite this, Kuhn's ideas have remained firmly embedded, most powerfully outside historians of science, including in the above scholarly writings on Western herbal medicine.

In line with these limitations of Kuhn, Wahlberg[51] employs Canguilhelm's concept of "normalization" to argue that there has been a more mundane "collaboration" between herbalists and science. Wahlberg argues that the colonisation hypothesis and the other variants of Kuhnian incommensurability cannot account for collaboration between herbalists and chemists regarding the standardisation and industrialising of herbal medicine. His study looks at Vietnam and the UK. The Vietnamese research identified the ten-year cooperation of a Vietnamese herbalist with laboratory chemists to produce Heantos, a herbal medicine to treat addictions. However, in the UK arm of his research Wahlberg does not similarly identify herbalists cooperating with chemists. This is likely to be the case because herbalists in the UK are not seen as an indigenous local resource holding valuable hidden knowledge. Herbalists, many of whom were trained at universities, at least since the late 1990s, are seen to have access to similar knowledge that anyone with access to textbooks and journals would have. They are not regarded as having local knowledge. Wahlberg relies less on ethnography and more on texts to suggest that herbalists in the UK appear to have no difficulty in maintaining different explanations for efficacy in their accounts of how herbal medicines work, drawing from both vitalism and phytochemistry, suggesting that these different paradigms are in fact not incommensurable. This is borne out by the examination of herbal texts recommended in the core curriculum for Western herbal

medicine as described above where texts that occupy different designations in fact draw from each other. Additionally, it is found in the quo-
tation of Kerry Bone above who looks to both science and to Avicenna.
One question, which will be discussed later, is why such differences
are so easily incorporated into the approaches of herbalists. Wahlberg[51]
argues that the "normalization" has occurred through three features.
First, there is an "ethno-scientific taming of the countryside", where
herbalists have worked with botanists and remedy producers in the
Kew Gardens Ethnomedica project to record and archive indigenous
UK herbal medicine usage. The archive functions to provide a resource
for phytochemical and pharmacological research into herbal medicines.
While this is true, and herbalists are generally not opposed to the idea of
working with scientists should they be invited, this is a rare event and
there may be a collaboration of another kind going on in Western herbal
medicine, as we shall see later. Wahlberg's second feature is the "normalization of living laboratories" where phytochemistry is employed
to standardise herbal medicines, replacing organoleptic testing by taste,
smell, touch, and sight. Wahlberg points out that herbalists would likely
prefer to give a sufficient quantity of the native whole plant extract
rather than a defined amount of a particular constituent. While most
companies that supply UK herbalists (e.g., Avicenna Herbs, Rutland
Biodynamics, Herbs in a Bottle, Granary Herbs, the Organic Herb Trad-
ing Company) do not guarantee constituent levels, although some do
use chromatographic techniques to identify species and the qualities
of a batch, a single company, Mediherb, does make such a guarantee
for seventy herbs. They are an Australian company run by Kerry Bone,
introduced above and who was trained in the UK and co-authored the
most "authoritative" textbook in Western herbal medicine.[77,78] His company, which supplies UK and Australian herbalists, has a "Quantified
Activity" programme that ensures the "production of consistent quality
extracts with guaranteed levels of active constituents" without being
"manipulated in any way by non-traditional processes. They are whole
galenical extracts of carefully selected whole herbs."[116] However, this is
the only identified case of such living laboratories. The third feature of
such "normalization" is the "search for plausibility". Wahlberg argues
that St John's wort has become plausible due to the molecular mapping of the pharmacodynamics and pharmacokinetic pathways that
its compounds follow in the body. This would not have been possible
if this herb was simply talked about in terms of vitalism or other

traditional concepts. The concept of synergy, which can be an additive or holistic concept, has been central in the search for explanations of how phytochemicals work together. Wahlberg argues that "synergy" has co-circulated in herbalists' and pharmacological realms, largely because of the different ways that this concept can be understood, and allows interactions between herbal and modern medicine. Additionally, Niemeyer, Bell and Koithan[89], similarly to Conway,[79] suggests that the coevolution of plants and humans allows concepts, such as attractors, emergence, and non-linearity, drawn from complex systems science, to offer a way of bridging the gap between cutting edge science and herbal practice, which may then be seen as increasing the "plausibility" of herbal medicine.

Interestingly, Bitcon, Evans, and Avila,[93] in a study of the Western herbal medicine blogosphere, identified bloggers concerned about the direction that their profession is taking, sharing a conviction that Western herbal medicine should combine both tradition and science, empower individuals and communities, and, most importantly for this book, that this is partly accomplished by sharing basic skills of plant identification. This connection to living plants will be seen to be an important locus for Western herbal medicine.

The above narrative suggests that Western herbal medicine is being co-opted, mainstreamed, or colonised by science with there being minimal collaboration of herbalists with scientists, minimal phytochemical normalisation of "living laboratories", even if diverse knowledges are not incommensurable within Western herbal medicine. Even if diverse knowledges are not incommensurable within Western herbal medicine. However, where there is collaboration is in the relationships between herbalists and plants and medicines made from them, as we will see in the herbalists' cases below, and which suggests that Western herbal medicine is more creative and agentive than has previously been considered.

PART II

METHODOLOGY AND THEORETICAL UNDERPINNINGS

CHAPTER SIX

Methods and methodology

Looking to cases, lists, and walks

Scheid[117] notes that the problem of a debate that uses "traditional" versus "modern" is that "traditional" becomes the "other" of modernity, with no room for seeing anything other than dichotomies. The weight of argument suggesting a trajectory of professionalised Western herbal medicine as engaging more and more with science might not be the whole story. By describing Western herbal medicine as becoming more and more "scientific" and "modern" it is necessarily seen as becoming less and less "traditional". However, this simple inverse relationship would not likely capture the complexities of the knowledge practices of Western herbal medicine. Law[118] argues that human subject matter and human relations are multiple and indefinite, too rich to be caught in total by theories and they are also in a state of continuous flux, with only the possibility of knowing limited moments. This is likely to be even more complex when the nonhuman is considered as part of human relations, as will be seen to be the case in Western herbal medicine. Law and Mol[119] suggest that ways of relating to complexity are needed beyond simply saying that simplification suppresses the complex. They argue

59

that "classificatory systems", "examples", and "maps" are commonly used tools in social science research. Classificatory systems present the possibility of including everything by providing categories that can often be further subdivided; examples claim to be representative of something larger; and maps make totalising overviews. They argue that these tools are not respectful of complexity and instead we are offered some alternatives. Instead of classificatory systems, examples, and maps they offer up lists, cases, and walks. Lists are favoured over classificatory systems, with lists being open in their self-recognition of incompleteness, and not necessarily imposing a single order. They refer to Foucault's[120] admission that Borges's list of animals from a Chinese encyclopaedia "shattered ... all the familiar landmarks of my thought" in that it managed to group together without taming or ordering. The list of animals was "a) belonging to the emperor, b) embalmed, c) tame, d) suckling pigs, e) sirens, f) fabulous, g) stray dogs, h) included in the present classification, i) frenzied, j) innumerable, k) drawn with a very fine camelhair brush, l) et cetera, m) having just broken the water pitcher, n) that from a long way off look like flies". Some list, indeed. While the current research does indeed use some classification, notably in the "entryways" that herbalists follow into the profession, it does not seek to produce a list of herbalists' cases that "add up" to Western herbal medicine, rather it is necessarily incomplete and can be added to, changing what is known about Western herbal medicine. For Law and Mol,[119] cases are favoured over examples, with cases being phenomena in their own right, having the potential to be relevant beyond their own sites, although that cannot be taken for granted. Cases "are able to do all kinds of other work" including sensitising the reader to previously unseen situations, condensing a range of experiences and working allegorically. While the herbalists' cases presented below can be considered discretely they additionally have relevance to what Western herbal medicine may be. And finally, for Law and Mol, walks are favoured over maps, with walks covering space but not giving overviews. In the same way the cases presented here cover space, but do not claim to reflect the entirety of herbalists or of Western herbal medicine. In summary, cases will be used to start a forever incomplete but empirically derived "list" of herbalists' cases that seek to contribute to a growing understanding of Western herbal medicine.

Nuts and bolts

The research was conceived to be extended ethnographic fieldwork with one or two or a few practitioners. However, it soon became evident that this was unlikely to come to fruition. Contributing to this, alongside any personal qualities of the researcher that may have brought about such an outcome, is the absence within Western herbal medicine of institutions where an ethnographer can spend time, move about, develop relationships, not get in the way too much or at all, and shift between being an observer and a participant. The biggest physical institutions in the UK are the training institutions. However, as the focus of this research was practitioners rather than students and lecturers it was decided not to pursue this avenue. Western herbal medicine is practised by herbalists mostly as sole traders, either working from small clinics or from home, making the field-site a rather disparate one, made up of small units variously connected or disconnected with other units, with all the difficulties that that raises for long-term access. While there have been ethnographies of individual practitioners of various disciplines, for example, an Appalachian herbalist,[121] a German Heilpraktika,[122] and a traditional Tanzanian healer,[123] most ethnographies are set within larger physical frameworks that do not exist for Western herbal medicine. Nissen's[102] ethnography of Western herbal medicine may have encountered similar problems in that her main data collection was also via interviews and observation of consultations.

Thus, an extended period of localised immersed research was not possible. Carsten[124] notes that although long immersion is to some extent a romanticised and heroic image of research it is one that is still aspired to within anthropology. Despite these difficulties, the integration of a minimalist biographic narrative interview method with ethnography and disciplinary interests drawn from anthropology, sociology, and science studies has hopefully resulted in a novel and valuable way of understanding Western herbal medicine.

Twenty-six herbalists were involved in the research. Eleven were male and fifteen were female. The gathering of data took place between June 2012 and September 2014. All but one of the herbalists were interviewed at their places of work. The ages of the herbalists ranged from the mid twenties to the late sixties. Geographically, they were located in Yorkshire, Kent, London, Surrey, Norfolk, Herefordshire, Hampshire,

Essex, Lancashire, Sussex, the East Midlands, and Scotland. There was additional ethnographic work involving observation of fifty-eight consultations, for which informed consent was obtained from the patients. Some of these consultations are referred to in the cases that are discussed below. There was also background ethnographic fieldwork at five conferences, eight seminars or workshops, along with numerous conversations and other communications with herbalists and herbal students, as well as participation on three internet-based discussion groups for professional herbalists. All herbalists were members of professional associations of herbalists. All but one of the herbalists were members of either the NIMH or the CPP, which, at the time of the research, had entry requirements of BSc degrees. For those herbalists who qualified before BSc degrees in herbal medicine were offered, all but one of them attained their qualifications at the School of Herbal Medicine or its later incarnations as the College of Herbal Medicine and finally the College of Phytotherapy. Notably, all the herbal medicine degree course leaders were trained via this route, with the university curricula for herbal medicine courses being heavily influenced by the trajectory of the course leaders' own training, along with the input of professional associations and the EHTPA. The reason for selecting twenty-five out of twenty-six herbalists from this background, rather than those who had qualified by different routes and who would be members of different professional associations, was that most new practitioners arriving in practice during the fieldwork did so via degree programmes. However, the author is aware that the stories of alternative educational routes to professional practice have not been included in the current research.

As a starting point herbalists were sought to reflect a variety of approaches to practice. This was achieved with the help of key informants who have extensive knowledge of herbal medicine practice. Subsequently, herbalists made other suggestions of herbalists to contact, thus threading "snowballing" onto "maximum variation" sampling. However, it soon became clear from the interviews and from participant observation that herbalists' stories and their clinical encounters were complex events that should be treated, as much as possible, as cases rather than as examples. So the very idea of sampling for varieties or types was brought into question quite early on in the research process. It seems that herbalists' lives produce narratives with much variation even if some themes may be identified within such complexity.

Some disciplinary influences

The empirical research intersected with various disciplinary streams. Anthropology has provided a strong pull in this regard. The flexibility of anthropology is important, including its methodological approach, borne out of the closeness to its subjects, that allows themes that emerge in fieldwork to guide the research design.[125] Hence, the difficulties in spending extended periods with individual herbalists meant that an interview design that resonates with ethnography was identified as being able to respectfully access herbal biographies. Both ethnography and biographical narrative interviews seek out rich descriptions, experiences, and perceptions and avoid simplification, although ethnography does this through immersed participant observation and narrative biographies do this by allowing the subjects to immerse themselves in reflection. Similarly, Ingold[126] has suggested that "anthropology is not a study *of* at all but a study *with* people … opening us to other possibilities of being". It is hoped that the chosen research methods and the author's insider knowledge of Western herbal medicine as a practitioner have helped to produce a *"with"* approach, where thickness, clarity, and possibilities are evident. Myers[127] has noted that it is often said in teaching that the task of anthropology is to make the strange familiar and the familiar strange, a phrase arising from T. S. Eliot's view of good poetry. However, Myers suggests that over recent decades, while the strange has been made increasingly familiar by anthropologists, making the familiar strange has been less successful "if by that we mean to put the everyday in a broader context, to give our ways a cross-cultural, in some sense, an estranged sensibility". It is hoped that this book contributes to such a sensibility.

In its practice of moving across disciplinary boundaries in the search for new understandings, anthropology has shown that life experiences are relational and develop where histories, people, materialities, and structures meet, and that knowledge of such life experiences can be used to find solutions to problems.[128] The current work will show that herbalists have relational experiences with living plants and material medicines made from them, although this develops within a history and a present where plant agency has been largely made invisible by modernity. From here, anthropological curiosity prompted a partly political search for developments elsewhere that could help explain the enchantment of plants as well as sustain and nourish Western herbal medicine. This led to recent developments in both plant science and the social sciences that, in different but arguably linked ways, move humans away from the centre of everything and raise the profile of plants as nonhuman persons.

Scheid's[4] adoption of science and technology studies as a framework for his ethnography of Chinese medicine in China has relevance in that human knowledge practices are seen to be essentially local, although they can have wider, even global impacts, if these local worlds are recreated such that they retain their key parts. Local practices change how "medicine" or "science" gets done with the result that hybridised knowledge is put into practice.[129] In other words, things get mixed up. The local interactions that herbalists describe in this book may add up to something that can usefully help us to understand Western herbal medicine more fully. However, global impacts are unlikely as Western herbal medicine is still a relatively small knowledge practice, even if it will be suggested that it can strengthen itself by making connections beyond itself. Next, we turn to the question of culture. As Scheid[4] noted in 2002, the anthropological conception of culture had assumed that there was always an identifiable unity in culture that shut down the very possibility of cultural contradictions. However, the very idea of culture has been questioned more recently by the "ontological turn" within anthropology, which has questioned the idea that cultures may differ but nature does not, instead suggesting that both worlds and worldviews vary, favouring an "openness to difference of all kinds".[130] It is hoped that such an openness will be found within this book, with differences found within Western herbal medicine being described but also explained as arising, at least partly, by the inter-species relationships that herbalists have with plants, and with medicines made from them. The final consideration is that of "methodological symmetry", a call to arms that arose within the sociology of scientific knowledge in 1976,[131] and has since been integrated into various social science practices, including the influential actor-network theory. The principle is that all claims to truth, however they may be seen by sociologists, should be handled in the same way, rather than by using rationalist explanations for claims that are viewed as true, and giving social or other external explanations for claims perceived as false. In this book, herbalists' claims are treated symmetrically, which also aligns with biographic narrative methods.

A narrative backbone

Narrative methods are complexity-respecting in their ability to seek out rich description and experiences. Also, they are suited to less well-known phenomena, and can use both inductive and deductive approaches to the generation of explanations. The felt presence of herbalists' narratives and voices is mostly absent from the research that has been conducted into Western herbal medicine. Even in Nissen's[102] feminist ethnography in the UK and in Evans's[112] interviews with Australian herbalists, these herbalists, either through their described actions or written words, are less present in the pages than might be expected, although the structuring of academic work offers an explanation. Furthermore, the author believes that herbalists' narratives are more revealing than his assumptions or researched questions could be. Narrative interview methods allow subjects and areas of concern to arise in the telling rather than in response to pre-formulated asking. This avoids the predetermined assumptions of semi-structured probing, one of the "apparatuses of the interview machine".[132] As a herbalist who is also a researcher investigating herbalists the author wanted to avoid only seeing what he already "knew" or was looking for. The interviewer's initial role as a reflective, receptive participant in the storytelling process was felt to be a necessary precondition for the active retelling of these stories in an authored text. Furthermore, it was felt that the presentation of herbalists' narrative cases would reflect the activities of herbalists in that their consultations involve listening to the illness and other narratives of patients, while herbalists' narratives remain largely untold.

The definition of narrative itself is in dispute.[133] Life stories, stories of events, and personal narratives most broadly conceived of as talk over the course of an interview, are all seen as being narratives. However, narrative is increasingly seen as "performative", functioning to construct and enact identity in relation to the audience. Riessman[134] argues that narrative includes the following functions for the teller: to remember, argue, persuade, engage, justify, entertain, mislead, and mobilise. Riessman[135] also argues that making narratives is a major way that individuals make sense of their past. Each form of narrative helps narrators solve the "teller's problem", that is, convincing the listener of the justification for their perspective.

Some countries have a strong tradition of narrative research, with West, Bron and Merrill[136] pointing back to Max Weber in Germany at the beginning of the last century. Merrill and West[137] suggest that over the last thirty years there has been a biographical or narrative "turn" in academia, largely in response to the historical marginalisation of the human subject in research. This turn is part of wide-ranging challenges to positivism and realism.[134] Langellier[138] locates the beginning of the narrative turn earlier—in the 1960s, with the boom in memoir literature, popular culture, and the rise of new identity movements, therapeutic culture and the turn away from Marxist class analysis in the post-Soviet era, all contributing to the rise of narrative. West[136] adds that, in the 1960s, the influence of oral history movements and psychosocial perspectives resulted in fertile ground for narrative research, seen in the increasing respect for subjects and by the interview as an empowering endeavour for the interviewee. West[136] points out that C. Wright Mills in *The Sociological Imagination* of 1959 observed that biographies represent the meeting point of individual agency, history, and structuring processes. West notes that forty-two years later Bron and West[139] similarly suggest that biographical methods provide insight into the dynamic tensions in people's lives between being "storied" and actively "storying", with degrees of agency being seen in narratives.

While narrative methods had certainly gained academic ground, Loots, Coppens, and Sermijn[140] point out that in the post-war years the eventual acceptance of humanistic narrative methods in sociology resulted in the promotion of the unified singular agentic storyteller, with the subject seen as an evolving story that integrates experiences, actions, and thoughts into a meaningful unity. This linear and singular model of selfhood has been challenged by postmodern and post-structuralist approaches that see narratives as performances in which selfhood is forever constructed. For example, Deleuze and Guattari[141] suggest that thought is not a simple representation of reality but a "rhizomatic" process consisting of an open decentralised network, with branches to all sides, governed by principles of connection, multiplicity, ruptures, and cartography. Thus Loots et al.[142] support the suggestion by Sermijn, Devlieger, and Loots[142] that selfhood be characterised as a rhizomatic story with multiple entryways, where there exists no single correct entry leading to the true self, but rather that the self is open to change. This book suggests that herbalists and their practices, discussed via their narratives, are indeed open to change, and that this occurs in part due to their relationships with plants, with consequences for understanding Western herbal medicine.

Biographic narrative interpretative method for data collection

Biographic narrative interviews were selected partly because autobiographical self-reflection supports research by identifying or clarifying a focus for inquiry.[143] This interview method was also selected because its focus on the story helps to reduce the likelihood of the researcher's own assumptions and background unduly influencing the interview relationship dynamic.

Specifically, the biographic narrative interpretative method (BNIM) as developed by Tom Wengraf,[144,145] was identified and modified as the method for interview data collection. The interview begins with the following "SQUIN" (single question aimed at inducing narrative): "Please tell me the story of your involvement with herbal medicine, that's all the events and experiences that are important to you. Please start your story as far back as you would like. I won't interrupt or ask any questions, but I will take some notes for later."

Using this "minimalist-passive" SQUIN, where the herbalist is not interrupted until he or she has finished, the researcher must be willing to give "control" of the interview to the informant and be willing to be an active listener. This first part of the interview usually ended up with the herbalists saying something like "And that's about it." It was always the subject who brought the interview session to an end. If the herbalist sought help, the researcher responded with a gentle "nudge", for example, saying, "Well, can you tell me a bit more?" Only on one occasion did the researcher "rescue" the herbalist with a further question. It was notable that when this happened it became more difficult to return to the minimalist-passive interview structure.

After this first part of the interview is completed there is a short break if the informant or researcher feels it is necessary. Then the interview continues with the researcher asking questions based on what the informant has said, seeking more descriptive depth on specific topics, using the herbalist's words and phrases, asking questions directly on the subjects that the informant introduced, in the order that they were introduced, without the researcher introducing topics that were not raised by the informant.

However, as the research progressed, the researcher found it useful to ask questions based on what other participants had brought up, either from interviews or based on the ethnographic components of the research. While this broke the "sealed" nature of the interview, these questions were asked at the end so as not to jeopardise the gestalt of the preceding interview parts. However, the price to pay for this additional information was a loss of gestalt towards the end of some of the interviews. To these participants, the researcher can only apologise.

There were two interviews that fell outside the descriptions above. The first was with a herbalist who was also a herbal medicine grower and supplier, where the author sought the story of the journey of the respondent's herbs, from seed to product. The second was with a herbalist who was also a researcher, having recently completed a randomised clinical trial, where it was the narrative about the research process that was sought. Both these interviews were more conventionally dialogic than the BNIM method, largely because they appeared to be less about personal experiences. However, upon reflection it was the method of questioning, in addition to the subject matter, which made the interviews appear to be less personal.

Immediately after the interviews, notes were made on the interviews, with initial impressions and ideas being noted. The interviews were then listened to at least twice. On a third listening further notes were taken. The interviews were then transcribed by the researcher or by a transcription agency. One herbalist chose not to have the interview recorded so handwritten notes were taken during the interview. The interviews plus field notes from the observations of consultations and other ethnographically collected data including printed matter, participant-made DVDs and online videos, emails and other communications with the researcher were then coded, that is, segments of text were identified that had relevance to the research question.

From a happy semantic confusion to a research question

It soon became apparent that the initial question "Please tell me the story of your involvement with herbal medicine ...", was interpreted by some herbalists as simply asking how they came to be interested in herbal medicine, and they spent much time on this before they came to describe later events. Besides the amount of time they spent telling this first part of their narrative, it was the content of these "entryways" to becoming herbalists that eventually led to the question: how do herbalists' entryways relate to the rest of their narratives, to Western herbal medicine and to areas of relevance beyond itself?

Developing an analytical approach

The current project adopted the minimalist-passive interviewing technique of BNIM. Let us now look to how BNIM approaches analysis. Jones[146] describes how the "lived life", meaning the chronological events in the narrative, is analysed sequentially in BNIM by the reflecting teams that have been gathered by the researcher. The teams also address the "told story", or the thematic ordering of the narrative. This is arrived at using "thematic field analysis", which involves the reflecting teams "reconstructing" the informant's system of knowledge and interpretations of experiences into "thematic fields". Finally, the case history is constructed from hypothesising how the lived life informs the told story. There were several reasons for not adopting this approach to analysis. First, accessing reflecting teams would have been problematic. However, the most pressing reason was a desire to include a wider number of herbalists than would be manageable with a BNIM analytic framework. A larger number of herbalists was sought to more reliably consider what Western herbal medicine might be. Although not aiming to generalise from the cases, it was felt that having at least twenty informants would make it more feasible to then select cases and take the discussion towards "Western herbal medicine".

"Thematic" approaches to analysis across cases have been considered by Braun and Clarke.[147,148] However, it was felt that methods that fragment accounts into categories that are then separated from the rest of the individual inhibit the agency of these individuals. Because this book allows for the possibility that plants are agentive, as will be seen, it would have been inconsistent to remove agency from individual herbalists. "Fracturing the data in the service of their interpretation" is a better way of putting what this researcher sought to avoid.[134] This fracturing ignores the sequential elements that are seen in the cases of narrative approaches, which are preserved and treated analytically as units, and which can be used to generate arguments and theoretical positions, as well as forming the basis for other work.

While BNIM has a predefined approach to analysis, Riessman[134] argues that since narrative research varies so widely in terms of kinds of data, epistemology, research questions, and even what narrative is, the method of analysis of narrative data is best tailored to the local particularities of the research. Riessman uses a framework of four questions to look at thematic approaches to narrative analysis that keep cases whole: How is the concept of narrative used? How is the data constructed into text for analysis? What is the "unit of analysis" or focus? What context is paid attention by the researcher—local or societal? Let's take these in turn. "Narrative" in this project refers to the story of the herbalists' involvement in herbal medicine as elicited in the BNIM interviews, along with descriptions from participant observation at consultations and other events attended as well as gathered ethnographic material. Looking to the second question, it is the interview transcriptions, field notes from the observation of consultations and other ethnographically gathered data that form the constructed text for analysis. Turning to the third question, the focus, or "unit of analysis", is the "entryways" of the herbalists, that is, the events and experiences that they value as important in their becoming herbalists, and how they relate to the rest of their narratives. These questions are then later related to what Western herbal medicine may be and what it may be related to. The context that is attended to in this research is thus local as well as anthropological and sociological. The herbalists' narratives are interpreted in light of ideas that have been developed throughout the research. This includes the influence of novel insights from the data themselves, a political commitment to tell the stories of herbalists, and relevant theoretical work, particularly following engagement with the work of Weber, Abram, Szerszynski, Josephson-Storm, and Bennett as will be discussed below. In summary, the aim is to keep the stories "intact", to understand them as whole cases and to theorise from them, as well as to look from cases towards Western herbal medicine and beyond.

Selecting and presenting cases

Not all the cases will be presented. Cases have not been selected to be representative but rather to develop a theoretical argument. The subsample of thirteen herbalists was selected based on the "thickness" of the interview and ethnographic data, that is, the combination of description and context, and the ability to illustrate patterns, particularly what will be called the "push" and "pull" of enchantment, and how both more "traditional" and more "modern" practitioners are open to this process. One herbalist, TE, was included as the case of a relatively "disenchanted" approach to practice, although the possibility of being enchanted by science remains open. Importantly, the herbalists' accounts that are not included as cases in this book contain themes also found within the presented cases.

There were additional reasons for not including some herbalists' accounts as presented cases. These included herbal medicine not being the main treatment that the practitioner used, the difficulty in keeping the herbalist anonymous, and an interview being cut short. Also, as mentioned above, one interview was focused on the narrative of a herbalist's involvement with research and another with the commercial cultivation of herbal medicines, which were not relevant to the question that emerged out of the research. The presentation of the cases is also important. Each case is initially presented in what is hoped to be a "thick description" format, with extended quotes from the narrative, as well as some ethnographic descriptions. Only after this has had the opportunity to "do some kind of other work", to settle into the reader and bring the narrative to life, is there a section reflecting on the herbalist, turning towards analysis of the case after the description has been made. Further analysis is undertaken in the discussion sections of this book.

CHAPTER SEVEN

Entryways

Some entrances are obvious and some are not. Some are so obvious that they are taken for granted, and some are hidden in the undergrowth. "Entryways" suggests a link between the entrance and the way, and as such has been selected to describe herbalists' early beginnings, those events and experiences that lead them to become herbalists. While there is some linearity in the idea of entryways at the start of a "path" to becoming something, it will also be seen that the relationship between herbalists, entryways, and paths is not always predictable and that the agency of herbalists exists in an emergent relationship to the nonhuman, including the plants and herbal medicines themselves.

The subjects of this study are herbalists in the UK who practise Western herbal medicine. Some of their entryways are "visible" in the sense that there is congruence between their beginnings and Western herbal medicine as an increasingly professionalised practice. We will see how personal experience of treatment with herbal medicines, the search for a new career and spending time in nature are visible entryways, providing routes into the profession. These entryways are unremarkable in that empirical experiences of the activities of the profession, the desire for a career, and contact with the tools of a profession are common routes for entry into any profession.

But other entryways are "hidden", meaning that they relate to plants themselves in ways that challenge boundaries between humans and nonhumans. Almost by definition they have not been seen in the political history of the profession or in the profession's engagement with science, even if they have been pointed to in Nissen's[102] ethnographic account of Cathy and Emn. The visible entryways will be discussed first, before we root around in the undergrowth to look at the hidden entryways. The entryways were elicited in the biographic narrative interviews with herbalists.

Barnes[149] has described how anthropology has looked to "shamanic traditions and to experiential entryways such as dreams, visions, spirit journeys, pivotal illness experiences, and family traditions", with much of this literature being concerned with "traditional" healers outside Europe and North America. Barnes also points out how parallels between such entryways and the practice of psychotherapy were sought between the 1960s and 1980s in North America. Barnes notes that while there has been a research interest in how different groups pursue professional status, there has been little interest in the experiences that motivate or move people to take up training and practice as a CAM practitioner, with questions of vocation quickly turning into questions of professionalism. The adoption of a biographic narrative interview methodology, with its single initial question, avoids this problem, preferring to let the respondents reveal their narratives themselves. The entryways, both visible and hidden, will now be briefly discussed, most of which we will return to later in the cases. Direct quotes providing "thick" descriptions will be reserved for the subsequent cases. For now, the intention is simply to highlight the difference between visible and hidden entryways.

Visible entryways

FW describes how the successful treatment of her own children with herbal medicines, along with her German mother-in-law's experience of receiving herbal medicine within orthodox health care, contributed to her decision to study herbal medicine in the UK. She was also looking for a safe alternative to orthodox medicine. Also important for her was having her own profession.

TE describes the importance of growing up with a mother who was passionate about gardens for his eventually becoming a herbalist. He was also searching for a second career after his law practice lost its appeal.

CP comes from a very medical family. Her mother was a private GP who worked from home, whose clinic phone CP used to answer on her behalf. Now CP also works from home and her own son answers her clinic phone for her. Later she became interested in the clinical encounter and decided to study acupuncture. She then had difficulty becoming pregnant. She was prescribed Chinese herbs from one of the most respected Chinese medicine practitioners in the UK, as well as from a top gynaecologist in Fujian province in China. Neither treatment helped. After hearing about a Western herb for fertility she visited a herbalist and became pregnant.

FD ran a smallholding, keeping goats, chickens, and pigs. She read a book by Juliet de Bairacli Levy about treating animals with herbal medicines and eventually studied to be a professional herbalist after initially doing a one-year introductory course.

EP's father was a surgeon, her mother a nurse and her stepmother a pharmacist, and EP herself went into nursing. She remembers a patient who was taking steroid suppositories for an anal fissure without success and saw a herbalist who treated her successfully. This impressed EP because she thought that if you were taking steroids there was no alternative.

SB traces his involvement with herbs back to when he was three or four years old when he used to spend time with his grandmother at weekends in her herb garden. He loved chemistry at school and became interested in plant chemistry. He grew about 150 herbs in his parents' garden, knowing them throughout their life cycle. He dried the herbs and stored them but didn't know what to do with them. When he studied for a chemistry degree he left herbs behind him. Much later, when looking for an alternative to his lecturing career he discovered a textbook on herbal medicine.

GA grew up on a tough housing estate and getting out into the countryside was an attractive refuge for him. Spending his time walking and bike riding he developed an interest in identifying and tasting herbs. Later on, a girlfriend of his was treated by an acupuncturist, who prescribed herbs, including yarrow, and GA realised he could just go out and pick it instead.

MN started medical school but only lasted one year, becoming disillusioned with the training, where the "human being was nowhere to be seen". He then became interested in the organic food movement and started growing herbs. He found the work of the French herbalist Maurice Messegue, which he said "sang to me".

DP came from a family where his grandfather, father, and brothers were all doctors. He qualified as a doctor but during his studies became ill with an undiagnosed condition. He wrote in to a doctors' magazine seeking help. He received advice from doctors, suggesting nutrition, herbs, homeopathy, and "being happy". Eventually he studied homeopathy and later, Western herbal medicine.

CJ looks back to her childhood, where her gran looked after her wounded husband after WWII, using folk remedies. CJ also sought a second career beyond accounts and was drawn to the quantifiable nature of herbal medicines.

PT's husband had experienced Western herbal medicine at a training clinic for his hay fever and found that it helped him. PT loved gardening and looked for a new career after her children were at school. She read about the herbal medicine course at the College of Phytotherapy and went down to have a look at the college, where she met one of the staff who appeared to be trying to put her off, saying that "You'll never make a living as a herbalist," but she was already hooked at that stage.

NE's wife grew sick with severe diarrhoea in an Ecuadorian frontier town on a trip into the rainforest. After trying all the drug medications available without success, they were directed to a guest house run by a woman who gave NE's wife some herbal medicine and within an hour her cramps disappeared. The next morning, she told NE, "I'm really hungry."

From these brief summaries, the majority of which will later be connected, in the case studies, with their later lives and with Western herbal medicine, it is possible to see the importance of the empirical experience of the treatment of self, family, and others with herbs in deciding to study herbal medicine formally. Also important is the search for an alternative career or profession. And the third focus is the experience of herbs as part of nature, in gardens and the countryside. The direct experience of herbal treatment, familiarity with nature and living herbs and the search for a career are unsurprising and visible routes to Western herbal medicine. This is consistent with Nissen's[102] survey of herbalists and her ethnography which found that personal positive experiences of Western herbal medicine, a desire to help others, and a "love of plants" were important motivators for a herbal career.

Hidden entryways

Let us now turn to the hidden entryways that individuals found to becoming herbalists. CT grew up in a mining village and describes himself as having, since childhood, a "naturphilic" predisposition, simply through spending time in nature, particularly in broadleaved woodland. He found nature to be a refuge and safe place. He was influenced by Native American culture. He would listen to the wind passing through the trees and try to understand what they were saying. He also had a spiritual orientation that he developed through his engagement with and questioning of Roman Catholicism. He found "something transcendent" in nature rather than in organised religion.

VH says that "My vocation was established at four years of age." He goes on to say that he, of course, "didn't realise it at the time". He remembers "running, playing He" on a farm which had a gypsy caravan on a warm sunny day. He was running and fell over and smelt yarrow while lying on the ground face down. "I didn't know its name then. I kept my face in the grass … I was involved with plants without being involved at all." Also he found that he knew things about the body at school without having ever learnt them, and children approached him for help. He also knew as a child that the herbs in his Letts diary were medicinal, he just knew.

RM remembers being in her pram and having a sense of wanting to do something of value and that later this became "doing something of service". She also remembers, at about the age of fourteen, having "an epiphany" while living on a loch in Scotland. She remembers "looking at this absolute glory of nature" and thinking "What am I, what do I do with this knowledge or this appreciation?"

AF's father was interested in natural history and would take AF out on walks, identifying birds and trees and seeing meadows covered with butterflies. At the age of five the spirits of the plants called him. He remembers sitting and looking at the plants and becoming aware of the differences between all the plants. He became aware of red dead-nettle, "as a separate entity with a separate spirit … that's when the spirits of the plants called me."

BC remembers being called by grass when she was still in nappies. She was surrounded by grass taller than she was and experienced a "still, beautiful, complete world". When she was about five years old she noticed grass growing through paving stones and experienced a similar "sense of enormity" that she describes as "a calling".

And finally, we have KA. She remembers that trees started talking to her as a kid. They stopped and then started again. The noisiest trees were yew trees. She had conversations with these trees, listening and tuning into what they were telling her about themselves.

Meetings

Visible entryways, in addition to the empirical experience of the efficacy of herbs as medicines and the desire to enter a profession, include the experience of spending time with living plants, either in gardens or in wider nature. However, the cases of the hidden entryways highlight more closely the connection between people and nonhuman living nature. It becomes not simply about a person being *in* nature, surrounded by it, but the blurring of boundaries between a person and nature, between subject and object.

CT talks of "naturphilia", in fact he spells it out, "N-A-T-U-R philia", even dropping a letter, merging the words, where he listens to trees and sees god as speaking from nature, finding something transcendent in nature. This may not be as acceptable to some as simply stating that those who enjoy nature are more likely to end up as herbalists than those who don't. However, the link between spending time with nature and meeting it may turn out to be more blurred and important than is thought.

VH identifies as important the smell of yarrow, while lying on the ground after having fallen, at the age of four, in his genesis as a herbalist. VH also simply "knew things", about health and about the herbs in his Letts diary, without having been taught them. These again point to something hidden from view, something learnt from or about plants. VH also identified a personal and pivotal illness experience on his route to becoming a herbalist.

RM's experience of a sense of service at such a young age that she was in a pram, and her concern as a teenager with wanting to do something with her appreciation of nature, also suggest something outside the visible entryways of simply liking plants.

AF being called by red dead-nettle at the age of five, like BC being called by grass while still in nappies, and KA's conversations with trees, are arguably the most powerful examples of boundary-blurring entryways and meetings between the herbalists and plants. This has not been significantly explored previously, although Nissen[102] reports that a herbalist describes herself as having been "called" by plants, and another describes her "deep affinity" with nature.

Barnes,[149] identifies dreams, visions, spirit journeys, pivotal illness experiences, and family traditions as being important steps on the road to becoming shamans. Similarly, with the herbalists in this study, key factors in their genesis as herbalists include being called by plants, illness experiences, and family traditions of medicine, if not herbalism. DuBois[150] identifies the importance of being called by spirits, the volition or acquiescence to spirits, compulsion with the threat of terrible consequences if the call is refused, and transformative spiritual ordeals as being important factors in the lives of those who were to become shamans. In the cases of the herbalists discussed there are some similarities with the experiences of shamans. There is calling in the entryways of BC and AF; there is illness experience in VH's account; there is volition, rather than compulsion with threat, in these narratives, for example, in RM's wanting to know how she could be of service with her appreciation of nature, and in CT's listening to trees. While there are no experiences that can easily be labelled as transformative spiritual ordeals in the entryways, there are such ordeals in their later narratives, which will be discussed in the individual cases, notably those of FD, VH, and BC. These similarities suggest that healing traditions from the heart of modernity and the localism of shamanism likely have more in common than was thought.

A question

Participants' narratives reveal both visible and hidden entryways to becoming herbalists. The former speak of the importance of personal experience of successful outcomes to taking herbal medicines, the search for new careers and spending time in nature. The latter, hidden entryways, bring into relief contact with nature, such that the boundaries between the human and nonhuman arguably touch. Indeed, the entryways of herbalists are not that far removed from the entryways of shamans. However, as we have seen, much existing social science research into Western herbal medicine suggests that there is a clash of paradigms between tradition and science, with the latter either dominating, co-opting or colonising the former, or with some minor degree of collaboration on the part of herbalists in the "normalization" of Western herbal medicine. Yet both these perspectives, either implicitly or explicitly, view traditional knowledge as being eclipsed by science. This argument is given weight by the historical development of the profession, which has been shown, in its fight for survival and political recognition, to have promoted a scientific conception of Western herbal medicine.

The existence of meetings as described in the hidden entryways of contemporary herbalists, and the apparent dominant influence of science is an interesting tension that may be explored by asking the question: what is the relationship between the herbalists' entryways, the rest of their narratives, and Western herbal medicine? It is this question, and where it leads, that this book explores. The cases presented will explore the first part of this question, while its relationship to Western herbal medicine and beyond will be considered later. Now we will turn to a consideration of the key authors that have helped provide orientations for the data.

CHAPTER EIGHT

Conceptual orientations

To address the question of how and why some entryways are more visible than others and how herbalists' beginnings relate to the rest of their narratives and to Western herbal medicine we will soon turn to those authors who provide conceptual orientations for this work. These writings can broadly be positioned within debates on the place of enchantment in modernity. While these terms are at times slippery, the enchantment found within Western herbal medicine will later be described and defined. Looking to the concept of modernity, Michael Saler[151] points out that although the term is often defined in divergent and even contradictory ways there is a working consensus that diverse factors merged synergistically in the West during the period from the sixteenth to the nineteenth centuries and which generated what we have come to understand as modernity. These factors include the ascendency of the rational, autonomous individual, the emergence of democratic liberal states, the development of self-reflexivity and the rise of the "isms", particularly secularism, consumerism, capitalism, nationalism, and scientism. Max Weber (1864–1920) and his observations on the displacement of enchantment by rationalisation in the modern world provide a starting point that will lead us to the contemporary thinking of Bruno Latour, David Abram, Jason Josephson-Storm, Bronislaw

Szerszynski, and Jane Bennett and how they relate to Western herbal medicine.

However, before we look at these specific contributions, it will be useful to consider that prior to and alongside Weber, other social theorists also developed conceptual landscapes that articulate in different ways with (dis)enchantment and may have been necessary for Weber's thinking. For Thomas Hobbes (1588–1679), the state of man can only be improved upon. He wrote "… during the time men live without a common power to keep them all in awe, they are in that condition which is called war; and such a war as is of every man against every man."[152] For Hobbes, this necessitated mutual contracts in order to lay the foundations for political society and government, important institutions of liberal states within what would become modernity. "Awe" comes not from nature, religion, or from the past but from political institutions which have the power to enchant and pull men away from conflict. While Hobbes was enamoured with the development of modern political institutions, Weber's sense of the loss of something in the face of modernity is found amongst other social theorists. For some, like Weber, it is a price worth paying and for others the cost is too high, with various solutions being proposed, some conservative and some revolutionary. For Rousseau (1712–1778), loss is powerfully present, which can be seen in the famous opening sentence of *The Social Contract*, "Man is born free, and everywhere he is in chains."[153] While natural man lives free and happy in the forest, the modern condition is defined by inequality and unhappiness, even if families, cities, and technology provide some solace. Something has been lost, even if something has been gained. As such, the task is to build political institutions that allow compassion to be at the heart of legislation. For Marx (1818–1883), the history of the world is a history of class struggle, where "alienation" describes the estrangement of people from their nature that arises due to living in a class society.[154] In the disenchanting process of alienation people become foreign to their world. And at the root of alienation is the selling of one's labour. The products produced are not an expression of the essence of the worker; workers do not see themselves in their products and consumers do not see workers in products. This alienation through labour exploitation was the foundation for the revolutionary thinking of Marx. The capitalist world as seen by Marx was certainly disenchanted with only the possibility of revolution offering enchantment. Looking forward to Durkheim (1858–1917), a contemporary of

Weber's, modern society, having lost traditional social and religious ties, provides little moral guidance. This loss results in "anomie",[155] or derangement, arising from a dissonance between individual actions and social ideals and practices. Anomie could have devastating effects on individuals, including suicide, which had previously been examined as a purely internal human matter. Finally, turning to another contemporary of Weber, Sigmund Freud (1856–1939) viewed civilisation as broadly suppressing human desire. However, despite the often negatively conceived effects of suppression, Freud mostly favoured disenchanted science and the secular, which enabled modern man to rationally master the unconscious-instinctual life.[156] While Rousseau and Durkheim look back to an age when things were purer and simpler, and Marx holds out for post-capitalist enchantment, Hobbes and Freud are mostly drawn to the power of modernity to master life.

What coheres most between Weber and these social theorists is the existence of dichotomies—between the state of war and the civilising effect of political institutions (Hobbes); between the forest and the modern condition (Rousseau); between individual actions and social practices (Durkheim); between alienation and revolution (Marx); and between civilisation and human desire (Freud). These theorists helped to lay the foundation for the dichotomy between enchantment and disenchantment that Weber will be seen to describe. Michael Saler calls this a "binary" approach to enchantment, where enchantment is a "residual, subordinate 'other' to modernity".[151] Modernity, by this definition, separates itself from enchantment. However, Saler suggests that an "antinomial" approach is a closer description of empirical reality, where "fruitful tensions" are seen to exist.

Max Weber, and his observations on the displacement of enchantment by rationalisation, will provide a starting point. However, the hidden entryways, which raise the possibility of nonhuman agency, question Weber's position of the lack of enchantment in modernity. We will turn to David Abram to suggest that the sensuality of plants may play a role, not only in the beginnings of herbalists, but elsewhere along their narratives and in Western herbal medicine. However, while Abram sees few opportunities for enchantment outside indigenous cultures, Josephson-Storm argues against the very fact of disenchantment and includes the argument that Weber himself may have had enchanting experiences. We then turn to Bronislaw Szerszynski, who sees new forms of enchantment powerfully present in (post)modernity, and is drawn upon to argue for the continued influence of the "sacred" in nature, including in Western herbal medicine. Finally, Jane Bennett will be arrived at to suggest a definition of the enchanting power of herbs and to argue that both the traditional and scientific realms of Western herbal medicine provide opportunities for such enchantment.

Max Weber, disenchantment of the world, and the profession of Western herbal medicine

Weber famously lectured in 1917, and was later published in 1919,[157,158] stating that

> The fate of our times is characterized by rationalization and intellectualization and, above all, by the disenchantment of the world. Precisely the ultimate and most sublime values have retreated from public life either into the transcendental realm of mystic life or into the brotherliness of direct and personal human relations. It is no accident that our greatest art is intimate rather than monumental.[157]

"Disenchantment of the world" is a phrase that Weber borrowed from the poet, philosopher, and playwright Friedrich Schiller, who described how modern fragmentation follows from the specialisation of knowledge and experience.[159] Sherry[160] points out that "disenchantment" is a poor translation of "Entzauberung", and that a better translation is "losing its magic". Notwithstanding translation difficulties, the sense behind the phrase as used by Weber is that the world seems to have lost some of its attraction and seems somehow dull and lifeless. The "disenchantment of the world" describes a mass of social, intellectual, and other forces, which have their origins in the Protestant Reformation, the industrial revolution and the development of scientific knowledge, driving and being driven by rationalisation and its bureaucratic tools. The result is the undermining and decline of religion. Weber's words are best referred to directly here, when he argued in a lecture given in 1917, that rationalisation via science means:

> the knowledge or the conviction that if *only we wished* to understand [the conditions in which we live] we *could* do so at any time. It means that in principle, then, we are not ruled by mysterious, unpredictable forces, but that, on the contrary, we can in principle *control everything*

by means of calculation. That in turn means the disenchantment of the world. Unlike the savage for whom such forces existed, we need no longer have recourse to magic in order to control the spirits or pray to them. Instead, technology and calculation achieve our ends.[157]

Weber is split as to his feelings towards this disenchantment process. While he refers to this as a loss, he is not nostalgic because it is the loss of an illusion, so is broadly welcomed in humanity's search to become master of its own destiny. Yet, at the same time, he describes this process of rationalisation as being an "iron cage". The cause of this sense of constriction for Weber is that scientists are not concerned with answering Tolstoy's questions, namely "What should we do? How should we live?" Religion has lost out to science, and in this victory meanings are replaced by scientific knowledge and the means-ends pursuit of material interests.[161] Thus, scientific progress and human progress are not necessarily seen as being one and the same. Sherry[160] points out that Weber brushes aside Baconian and Newtonian thought, which prefigured Einstein's position that the task of a scientist is to trace out the signs of God's wisdom in the laws of nature. Instead Weber appears to separate out mystic experiences with their concomitant emotions from processes of rational thought.

Looking beyond enchantment, Ritzer[162] points out that Weber also contributed to debates on the professions, particularly in his recognition that professionalisation, like bureaucratisation, is an aspect of the rationalisation of society. Although Weber suggests that it was particularly Calvinism that was instrumental in the genesis of the professions, he also suggested that professionalism was important in the development of rationalism in the Occident: "This worldly asceticism as a whole favours the breeding and exaltation of the professionalism needed by capitalism and bureaucracy. Life is focused not on persons but on impersonal rational goals."[162] Weber sees bureaucracy as being a necessary (if life-suppressing) requirement for the efficient implementation of rationality by professionals. He says: "The bureaucratization of all domination very strongly furthers the development of 'rational-matter-of-factness' and the personality type of the professional expert."[162] The understanding that rationalism can be seen in the development of professions allows the argument that rational goal-oriented behaviour may be seen in the actions of the professions. Furthermore, when professions engage positively with science, as the arch-rational sphere of life, and with bureaucracy, as the social practice of rationalisation, they are more likely to achieve their goals.

The case of the profession of Western herbal medicine will be considered in this context. We have already seen how the profession, from the mid nineteenth century, has been tenaciously determined in its objective to gain political recognition by statute, and that this was promised by the government in 2011, although this is unlikely to be delivered within the foreseeable future. The profession's engagement with science, as another element of rationalisation, has also been described above in the training, journals, and pharmacopoeias of the profession. While individual herbalists do not have to engage with particularly high levels of bureaucracy, other than completing annual CPD forms, tax returns, and data protection practices, there is certainly much bureaucracy present within the profession as a whole—seen, for example, in the exam boards and course reviews for the university delivery of degrees; in the various committees of the NIMH and other professional bodies; in the work of umbrella organisations like the EHTPA that liaises between government organisations and individual professional bodies; and in those suppliers of herbal products to herbalists that have chosen to seek good manufacturing practice (GMP) accreditation.

Let us examine how Weber looked at the case of the profession of the priesthood. This will be useful in that the profession of Western herbal medicine has always sought to separate itself from the label of the "quack", "witch", "charlatan", or unqualified practitioner, just like religious authorities have always sought to distinguish themselves from "magicians" or "sorcerers". For Weber, it is the rational and theoretical training of the priest that does the most to distinguish him from the sorcerer. Ritzer[162] sees eleven characteristics of the priest given by Weber that could be applied to professions generally. These include: power, or monopoly over work tasks; doctrine, or specific ring-fenced knowledge; rational training; vocational qualification; specialisation; a full-time occupation; the existence of a clientele; salaries; promotions; professional duties; and a distinctive way of life.

Of these characteristics, it is the lack of the first one—the power to have an exclusionary closure around its activities, that has driven Western herbal medicine, in the face of constant threats to its existence, to move via professionalisation and engagement with science towards the establishment of a profession that has a room of its own in modernity.

From this perspective, the profession seems to be engaging with Weber's modernising force of disenchantment, which has rationalisation at its core. However, as mentioned, Weber also senses that these processes cause isolation. Braun[163] argues, drawing on Berman, that this isolation stems from an unmet human need for ontology, which is also described as being a spiritual need to have a "felt sense of the sacred". It is this sense of ontology—of closely knowing existence, which is found in the hidden entryways of herbalists, and which may be called "enchanting". And it is this that may be further found in the later narratives of herbalists and hence, to some degree, in Western herbal medicine.

David Abram and the senses of Western herbal medicine

Although David Abram does not use the word "disenchantment" he can be seen to be telling a similar tale to Weber's in that they both identify a loss in modernity. Abram[164] highlights the importance of the senses in understanding the relationship between humans and the natural world and it will be seen in this book that it is the senses that are central to understanding the enchantment present in the hidden entryways and later narratives of some herbalists. Abram explores shamanic traditions. He argues that the shaman's communication with spirits is better seen as communication with other-than-human consciousness in the natural world and not communication with some transcendent world "out there". The shaman's role is to serve as an intermediary between the human and nonhuman. "It is not by sending his awareness out beyond the natural world that the shaman makes contact with the purveyors of life and health, nor by journeying into his personal psyche; rather, it is by propelling his awareness laterally outward into the depths of the landscape at once both sensuous and psychological ..." It is this that will be further explored in three of the case studies below. Three herbalists will be seen to know herbs in different ways, including by tasting them, inhaling aromas while herbs are being decocted in water, and by working with them physically. Their sensual ways of knowing can be seen as somewhat aligned with such a view of what a shaman might be. Abram further argues that it is anthropology's inability to see the shaman's allegiance to nonhuman nature that has led to the situation where it is possible to enrol in "shamanic" workshops as an alternative form of therapy, where in fact the primary role of the indigenous shaman is to keep the human community and the natural landscape in balance, and that this requires sustained exposure to nature. While herbalists may be less exposed to nature than shamans, in different ways they do spend much time with their plants, with the importance of taste, smell, and physical labour being explored in the cases below.

Abram's work is situated in the phenomenology of Edmund Husserl and Maurice Merleau-Ponty, particularly in its recognition of the importance of direct experience, and the reciprocity of perception. Husserl brings to attention the real world, or "life-world", as being a collective field of experience, while Merleau-Ponty asserts that the self is not independent of the body. At the core of Abram's writing is the ability to become aware through the senses, with this perception being a "reciprocal interplay" between perceiver and perceived. Were such "interplays" brought to awareness in the early, enchanting, hidden entryways of the herbalists discussed above? Being "called" by plants needs such reciprocity.

Abram suggests that we should simply let things be alive, "Just allow that things have their own agency, their own influence upon us, whether it be a slab of granite, storm clouds, a stream, a raven, a spider."[165] Or a living plant or a medicine made from it. If the agency of herbs is seen in the entryways of herbalists, it will also be visible later in some of the narratives.

Abram argues that our separation from nature began with the invention of the alphabet. For Abram, it was writing that led language to become separated from the world. Abram tells a story from Plato's *Phaedrus*, where Socrates informs a friend that "I'm a lover of learning, and trees and open country won't teach me anything, whereas men in the town do." Abram suggests that the alphabet can separate humans from experiential relationships with the natural world. He compares the sensuous relationship that indigenous oral cultures have with nature with the separation from nature that is found in alphabetic cultures. While oral cultures use all their senses, the written word needs only eyes and ears. While pictographs initially maintained a visual connection with nature, by the time the Hebrew alphabet became the Greek alphabet the letters had lost any visual meaning and separated the human from the natural. Abram says that "With the phonetic *aleph-beth*, the written character no longer refers to any sensible phenomenon out in the world ... but solely to a gesture made by the human mouth".

For Abram, the "animating interplay of the senses has been transferred" from the animate earth "to another medium … the written text". He suggests that "The participatory proclivity of the senses was simply transferred from the depths of the surrounding life world to the visible letters of the alphabet … our senses are now coupled synaesthetically to those printed shapes as profoundly as they were once to cedar trees, ravens, and the moon." Trees and texts alike can be enchanting.

Abram's work resonates with Michel Serres's[166] book *The Five Senses: A Philosophy of Mingled Bodies*, published in 1985 although not in English until 2008. Serres sees language as blinding vision, numbing touch, distorting hearing, and overpowering taste and smell. He argues that language has taken the place of our connection with what is all around us. Chimisso[167] notes that Serres turns Descartes on his head, with the senses, rather than the thinking mind, guaranteeing existence, with the individual never separated from the objects that are perceived. The senses cannot and should not be separated from each other, for this would result in their destruction. Connor[168] notes that the senses are knotted together, with each sense being a "nodal cluster, a clump, confection or bouquet of all the other senses".

Reading Abram and Serres raises the question as to whether it is purely coincidental that some of the herbalists' hidden entryways occurred when they were very young, while "still in nappies", and as a five year old, and while "in a pram", before they would have their senses fully distracted by written words? Maybe enchantment with nature is easier without texts. Another possibility is that the contact with nature seen in the narratives of the herbalists could explain why allegiance to particular written texts seems to be less emphasised in Western herbal medicine than in other traditions that also use herbs, such as Chinese medicine or Ayurveda, where systematic written-down theories of cure are more readily found. If knowing plants sensually and directly, particularly through taste, smell, and touch, and temporally, through simply spending time with them, is important for herbalists, then there may be less need to locate "the animating interplay of the senses" in texts. Western herbal medicine may be less textual and less positioned within a theoretical framework than other practices that employ herbs.

While Weber and Abram can both be seen to be telling disenchantment tales with their concomitant senses of loss, we now turn to Jason

Josephson-Storm, Bronislaw Szerszynski, and Jane Bennett, who suggest that there are plenty of opportunities to trace the more visceral presence of enchantment in modern life, including those found in cross-species encounters as well as in science, and which will be seen to resonate with, and help understand, herbalists' narratives.

Josephson-Storm, the myth of disenchantment, and Western herbal medicine

Josephson-Storm[169] provides a convincing argument against the fact or event of disenchantment, even if the story retains power. He reviews sociological surveys revealing that in contemporary Europe three in four people believe in the supernatural, with the British, for example, having attachments to belief in ghosts, telepathy, premonitions, and faeries. Importantly, he shows that the very idea of a disenchanted modernity was born at the same time as Germany, France, and Britain were enjoying occult and spiritualist revivals. He argues that Weber is most likely to have arrived at his concept of disenchantment while holidaying at the neo-pagan Monte Verita commune in Switzerland, with disenchantment "likely born of an excess of enchantment not its lack". Also, Weber was not alone. The lives of other theorists of modernity, including Muller, Adorno, and Carnap, intersected with magic and spiritualist contexts and panpsychism can be seen in the philosophy of Spinoza, Goethe, Henry David Thoreau, William James, Henri Bergson, and Gregory Bateson, to name but a few; and looking further afield, Marie Curie was interested in parapsychology and Alan Turing believed in psychical powers. Josephson-Storm raises the possibility that Weber may have had a mystical experience: in answering the question as to whether he could imagine himself as a mystic, Weber says, "It might be that I am one … It is as if I could (and would) just as well withdraw myself entirely from everything." Josephson-Storm argues that it is better to rephrase disenchantment as "disenchanting", indicating that it is an ongoing process rather than an historical event. The existence of enchantment within modernity and within rational thinkers will be seen to resonate with the herbalists' cases later, where enchantment with living plants and medicines made from them may be found in the narratives of herbalists who draw both on science and on traditional knowledge. Additionally, this enchantment facilitates diversities of practices that can comfortably sit side by side within and between herbalists rather than simple dichotomies that cannot.

Bronislaw Szerszynski, enchantment, and the axes of Western herbal medicine

Bronislaw Szerszynski,[170] like Josephson-Storm and unlike Weber and Abram, sees enchantment as being powerfully present today. At the beginning of his argument Szerszynski suggests that the very act of rendering the world devoid of spiritual significance actually entices new forms of enchantment. He asks us to consider some examples:

> A young protestor locks himself to the top of a swaying tree in order to prevent the construction of a new road and the consequent destruction of an area of native woodland. A middle-aged woman sees an acupuncturist to unblock the natural "healing powers" of the human body. A farmer walks out into his fields with a canister of herbicide, determined to eradicate the weeds that are "invading" his crops. A woman, still smarting after an argument with her partner, stops her car at the roadside on a deserted mountainside to take in the view, and feels able to get things back in proportion. A botanist collates all the data from his experiments, and tries to discover the law that underlies the different patterns of growth he observes in his plants. How does nature appear in these examples—as "dead matter" of a mechanized world-view …? Or is it sometimes an object of absolute intrinsic value, a healing energy, an evil to be subdued, a calming presence, or an obeyer of laws? and if so, what does this say about ideas of nature's disenchantment?

While this book starts at the entryways of herbalists and traces connections with the rest of their narratives, then into Western herbal medicine and beyond, Szerszynski's main focus is to address the sense that contemporary attitudes to nature and technology have religious qualities to them. Religious meanings do not simply evaporate over time but they change. Both this book and Szerszynski follow threads, with the former being concerned with individual narratives and the latter with historical narratives. The Gaia hypothesis and the internet, for example, possess religious meanings. And both cutting edge science and experiential knowledge of plants will be presented as enchanting in Western herbal medicine. Szerszynski suggests that:

> As Weber himself put it in a different context, under conditions of modernity "the many gods of old, without their magic and therefore in the form of impersonal forces, rise up from their graves, strive for power over our lives and begin once more their eternal struggle amongst themselves" ... I have been similarly suggesting in this book that in contemporary society we can see not a decline but a profusion of the sacred; dispersed across the social, natural and technological landscape, the sacred becomes feral.

Szerszynski traces the "long arc of transcendental religion" and argues that in the "primal sacred" of historically indigenous cultures (and arguably in indigenous contemporary cultures) an archaic form of the sacred emerges, with sacred power located in things, places, and people—a horizontal axis. However, with the arrival of Judaism and Christianity there comes the transcendental axis of the "monotheistic sacred", which is located outside this world—a vertical axis. Supernatural power is banished from this world, which is left purely empirical. With the arrival of the "Protestant sacred" God becomes both infinite and involved with individuals and nature such that life itself became the location of the sacred. And with the "modern sacred", the transcendental axis is "pulled" into the empirical world, producing an immanent ordering of the sacred, seen in the sacred nature of life itself grasped via Enlightenment reason. The most recent manifestation of the sacred is the "postmodern sacred", where multiple orderings (a "multiplex reality") of the previously discrete "sacreds" are possible and are grounded in very individual subjectivities. Szerszynski follows the trajectory of the sacred through different epochs and this book follows the trajectory of enchantment through narratives and into Western herbal medicine. The sacred and enchantment have in common that they are not limited to either nature or culture, science or society, but they spread out along trajectories that can be followed. Thinking about medicine, Szerszynski argues that in the Christian era there are two models of healing, a vertical one based in dependence on saints and sacraments, and a horizontal one with pre-Christian origins, founded on the maintained connections with the natural and social environment. With the Protestant sacred there came a more cognitive approach to the self and health, including rational self-care and the validation of inner life stories.

In the hidden entryways of herbalists a horizontal axis is visible where power is located in the plants and nature. Such horizontal axes of relationships with the natural environment will also be seen in the subsequent narratives of herbalists. On the other hand, a vertical axis of dependence may be seen in Western herbal medicine in, for example, the growing power of "evidence-based medicine" that is argued to inform clinical decisions and the requirements that legislation, such as data protection, and professional bodies, through CPD, ask of their members. The location of the sacred in individual subjectivities in the postmodern sacred can also be seen in the importance that all herbalists in this book attribute to facilitating the patients to be able to "tell their story" as a therapeutic endeavour, and which will be borne out in several of the cases below.

Just as religious meanings don't simply evaporate over time but change, the enchanted early experiences of herbalists do not simply evaporate, but are still present in their later narratives, and hence in Western herbal medicine.

Jane Bennett, modern enchantment, and the sensual affective energy of Western herbal medicine

We now turn to Jane Bennett[50,171] who, like Szerszynski[170] and Josephson-Storm,[169] sees modernity as providing multiple opportunities for enchantment. Bennett writes with infectious and backed-up optimism, in opposition to the pessimism of writers such as Berman[172] who yearn for re-enchantment.

For Bennett,[171] "Encounters with lively matter can chasten my fantasies of human mastery, highlight the common materiality of all that is, expose a wider distribution of agency, and reshape the self and its interests." Bennett[151] summarises Weber's notion of rationalisation, pointing out firstly that the suffix "ion" indicates that it is never complete. Rationalisation is seen to promote accuracy, consistency, and reliability over the vague, the novel, and the extreme, alongside which there is a concern with a theoretical mastery of reality. Thinking becomes instrumental in that calculations lead to a practical end. With rationalisation, tradition is replaced by calculation. In this process, it is largely science that reduces the world to materiality, which in the "disenchantment tale" is the opposite both to spirit and to meaning. Bennett describes how the disenchantment tale of Weber shares six elements with many other versions of the tale that continue to hold cultural currency: there is a bygone era when God lived in nature, agency was widely distributed among living animals, humans, and plants; there is a desire to rediscover this cosmology; there are only two binary incompatible options, namely an enchanting cosmology or a disenchanted materialism; the processes inherent to disenchantment, namely rationalisation, secularisation, materialisation, scientisation, and bureaucratisation are said to have speeded up; loss of meaning causes human suffering; and rational selves look outwards towards mysticism and in other directions for true satisfaction.

Indeed the "disenchantment tale" is told within Western herbal medicine. Thus the bygone era of herbal medicine was when less time was spent studying curricula and more time in contact with plants; the desire to rediscover this cosmology has led more herbalists to look to experiential methods of knowing plants; the dichotomy of science and tradition suggests that each of these paradigms is incommensurable; recent changes in education, the dominance of the scientific investigation of herbs in research studies and the regulatory framework for herbalists have snowballed over the past fifteen years; herbalists possibly understand less about herbs than they used to; rational herbalists search for deeper historical roots within their own tradition or look to other traditions such as Chinese medicine or Ayurveda for satisfaction. In talking to herbalists all these elements of the tale are present somewhere in Western herbal medicine today, and most of them will be seen to be present somewhere in the cases below. However, it is also true that there is another side to this story, one that involves enchantment being found in unexpected areas of Western herbal medicine, not just by looking "back" to a bygone era. Bennett,[50] like Josephson-Storm,[169] suggests that enchantment and disenchantment can exist side by side. For Bennett enchantment offers opportunities for a new ethics and a new understanding of materiality. To be enchanted, for Bennett, is to "be struck and shaken by the extraordinary that lies amid the everyday". This "includes a temporary suspension of chronological time and bodily movement". It is "to be simultaneously transfixed in wonder and transported by sense, to be caught up and carried away". It is a "surprising encounter" and a feeling of being "simultaneously charmed and disrupted".

The hidden entryways of herbalists reveal moments of enchantment that gel with these definitions. Although the narratives did not capture long descriptions of these moments, if the reader puts herself in the position of these herbalists, they are likely to point to powerful feelings, possibly now lodged in the herbalists' amygdalae. Trying to understand what trees have to reveal by listening to the wind pass through them, being involved with plants without being involved at all, the smell of yarrow, knowing things without having been taught them, being in a pram and wanting to do something of value, being called by red dead-nettle, being called by grass while still in nappies and being talked to by trees are likely to stay with you, at the very least.

In an interview, Bennett[173] argues that enchantment may be indispensable to ethical action and that it does this through providing a fuel or spark of "aesthetic-affective energy". The enchantment that this book seeks to investigate and follow in Western herbal medicine should be regarded as more "sensual" than "aesthetic" to emphasise the primacy of all the senses. It is also "affective" in that this sensuality influences what is felt and that this has consequences for herbalists. The sensual is affective and is also energetic—it spreads outwards. Not in all directions but in some, which the cases below will describe. As Seigworth and Gregg[174] argue, "Affect arises in the midst of *in-between-ness*: in the capacities to act and be acted upon ... affect is found in those intensities that pass body to body (human, nonhuman, part-body, and otherwise), ... Affect, at its most anthropomorphic, is the name we give to those forces .... that can serve to drive us toward movement, toward thought and extension ... Affect is in many ways synonymous with *force* or *forces of encounter*". However, they point out that affect "need not be especially forceful ... In fact, it is quite likely that affect more often transpires within and across the subtlest of shuttling intensities: all of the molecular events of the unnoticed." Grossberg[175] sees the concept of affect as a "magical way of bringing in the body". Affect can be regarded as "pre-personal", being "a moment of unformed and unstructured potential", unlike feelings, which are personal and biographical, and emotions, which are social.[176] On the other hand Wetherell[177] suggests that affect is not limited to the unconscious and the automatic, and is not separated from discourse that is characterised as conscious and deliberate. Rather, affect is a dynamic blend of bodily responses, feelings, and thought processes as well as verbal and other communications. Affective life is a crossing of all of these.

Whether affect, in the sensual affective energy of enchantment of herbalists by plants and herbal medicines is pre-personal or not, it is argued that it is a force within Western herbal medicine. Affect is passed on, "forming what can seem like pulses of energetic relation".[177]

Enchantment, as a "sensual-affective energy", on an individual level, is what matters most to people. While it is not the focus of this book to understand how enchantment "works" in individuals, Milton[178] has developed a framework for how individuals relate to nature, showing how emotions may operate in ecological relations rather than simply in social ones, with emotions being brought forth by interactions with nature. In opposition to conventional Western assumptions, Milton, like David Hume and William James, does not see thoughts and feelings as separate processes. Rather, emotions may be a learning mechanism, and hence perfectly compatible with rationality. While Milton's focus is purely on the human, this book aims to look beyond the human— with living plants and herbal medicines possessing more agency than is allowed by taking a purely human-centric approach.

For Bennett, enchantment may be found in multiple sites, including modes of communication among nonhumans and complex systems, in the teleological world of Paracelsus as well as in the amazing world of interior reason invented by Kant. Drawing on both Haraway's cyborgs[179] and Latour's nature/culture hybrids,[47] Bennett discusses cases of cross-species encounters that provoke wonder in herself. Bennett prefers "crossings" to "hybrids" to reinforce the notion that new things are brought into being. She considers metamorphosing creatures such as Catwoman, the interests of the small creatures in the film *Microcosmos*, the pig star in *Babe*, the machine that beat Kasparov at chess, Deleuze and Guattari's "organless body", and children playing animal games. Bennett argues that these crossings act as sites of enchantment and provide an opportunity to cultivate an "ethical sensibility" towards animals, vegetables, and minerals.

Where Bennett speaks to Western herbal medicine is in her recognition that while enchantment may be found in the life of Renaissance physician Paracelsus, where the world was seen as divine prose, it is also found in the Kantian faculties of the mind. Bennett describes Paracelsus as being a Christian animist who combined the idea of a heavenly creator with that of plants being powerful agents whose virtue was visible in the plant. This may sometimes be seen in Western herbal medicine today, although with less Christian overtones. For Kant, however, the reading of signs leads to errors, and he prefers to engage interior reason, which Bennett sees as the first wonder of the Kantian world, with the second wonder being nature itself. Rather than modernity embracing apparent contraries such as rationality and wonder, Bennett argues that rationality itself can be full of wonder and enchantment. And certainly, the world of Western herbal medicine is one that has engaged with the rationality of science, both in its Herbalism 2.0 form and in its various interfaces with trajectories of cutting edge science, as will also be seen in some of the cases below.

Jane Bennett is not alone. Historians are now suggesting that modernity is not disenchanted. Michael Saler[151] suggests that postmodernism's acceptance of the messiness of reality and the demise of grand narratives have helped avoid the binaries of the past such that enchantment and disenchantment can be found together. Saler takes an "antinomial" approach to enchantment, where modernity is seen to be "Janus-faced", full of "unresolved contradictions and oppositions".

If we look back to those social theorists who predated Weber or who were his contemporaries and who separated a disenchanted modernity, or hope of one, from what came before, it is possible to discern in their work the coexistence of exactly what they sought to separate. Thus, as Saler[151] notes, Marx's writings are peppered with "metaphors and similes of enchantment" such as spectres, ghosts, and commodity fetishisation, thus maintaining the presence of the religious and even the pagan in modern thinking. Turning to the question of how modern society can remain moral in the face of the loss of tradition, Durkheim developed the concepts of "collective consciousness" and of the state as an organ of social thought. The idea of a shared consciousness with a political institution as its reflective centre can be seen to resonate with the enchantment of the pre-modern world, although it is now politics that is deified. Turning to Freud, while he championed the power of modern civilised and rational man to master human desire, he also worked with what may arguably be viewed as the enchanting concepts of transference and the unconscious. These are powerful agents that evade easily verifiable disenchanted explanations. Thus, as both Jane Bennett and Bronislaw Szerszynski suggest, the past is powerfully present. It is difficult to get away from enchantment. Turning to science, Saler[151] argues that modern science has become a "central locus of modern enchantment". Although science may not provide the transcendent meanings that religion used to offer, it still provides wonder, by "embracing the enchanting possibilities inherent within contingent and provisional meanings". The absolute enchantment of religion may have gone, but imagination becomes a "source of multiple yet finite meanings that enchant in their own way". They "delight but do not delude".

Another writer who sees wonder in science is Philip Fisher.[180] In his examination of the history of attempts to explain rainbows, he follows Descartes's explanation of why the bands of the rainbow need to be around 40 degrees, suggesting that scientific explanation can induce the wonder of seeing a rainbow for the first time. Geometric shapes with their lines and arcs may be enchanting. He argues that the experience of observing a rainbow is always new and wonderful despite science having explained the phenomenon. In fact, it is "unreflective and immediate" wonder that motivates the search for explanations. The surprise of wonder easily leads to thinking. What is potentially even more wonderful about rainbows than the rainbows themselves is his observation that they exist only in the way that we see them due to the four-way relationship between human anatomy and physiology and weather patterns and light. It is human eyes, made and positioned as they are, that allows humans to see rainbows as we know them. An enchanting thought that is not possible without a scientific explanation. A contemporary scientist who published at the same time as Fisher is Richard Dawkins, who also considers rainbows. He argues that "The feeling of awed wonder that science can give us is one of the highest experiences of which the human psyche is capable."[181] He seeks to oppose Keats's view that Newton had destroyed all the poetry of the rainbow by "reducing it to the prismatic colours". For Dawkins, science is inspiration. Wonder inspires science. He points out that Newton's "unweaving of the rainbow" led to spectroscopy, a key technological development without which our understanding of cosmology would not have happened. It is the work of Einstein and Hawking that causes his heart to leap.

Another author who sees the disenchantment of science as being a tall story is Peter Watson. For Watson[182] the timing of Weber's remarks is crucial. Weber gave his lecture during the smoke and devastation of WWI. Watson points out that within two years of the cessation of hostilities Eddington confirmed the existence of relativity that started the road to quantum mechanics and wave particle duality. The big bang theory also has its origins in the 1920s. Watson suggests that had Weber lived beyond 1920 he would have changed his mind on the bond between modernity and disenchantment.

Pels[183] suggests that pre-modern enchantment and the modern rationalist are myths that require empirical scrutiny and that such research can explore the magic that is peculiar to modernity. Pels argues that while early pioneering anthropologists such as Ruth Benedict and Bronislaw Malinowski suggest that political oratory, advertising, and property are modern forms of magic, a closer investigation is required into how magic "belongs" to modernity. Looking to Weber himself, the architect of the disenchantment thesis, Pels suggests that Weber's disenchanted modernity is in fact itself "haunted by two magicalities"—the reification (even deification) of national institutions and the enchanted freedom promised by charisma.

Thus, Jane Bennett, along with Saler, Fisher, Dawkins, Watson, and Pels, suggest that things are more complex than a simple following of the disenchantment tale might tell. And that is certainly the case in Western herbal medicine, as we shall see.

The implication of these authors for Western herbal medicine is that enchantment, a sensual-affective energy that herbalists draw from, as well as being present in the hidden entryways of herbalists' meetings with plants, may also be found elsewhere, both where you expect to find it and where you do not, both within more traditional and more scientific approaches, which can easily occur within the same herbalist. How these meetings relate to later aspects of the narratives of herbalists may change how we come to see Western herbal medicine.

PART III

CASES

CHAPTER NINE

Visible entryway herbalists

Thirteen cases of individual herbalists will be discussed. These cases will look at the entryways of the herbalists and how they relate to the rest of their narratives as well as to the ethnographic and other data collected relevant to their practices. The first eight herbalists are those who can be defined as having visible entryways to becoming herbalists, while the last five had hidden entryways. The question of how these thirteen cases relate to Western herbal medicine and beyond will be left for the subsequent discussion.

This section will look at eight herbalists who had visible entryways, meaning that there is no tension between their beginnings and Western herbal medicine as an increasingly professionalised and disenchanted practice. We will start with a herbalist who appears to be most clearly aligned with a disenchanted way of engaging with herbal medicines, although he may be enchanted with the science, a subject that we have discussed above and will discuss again. Then we will move on to three other herbalists who reveal glimmers of enchantment in their relationship to herbal medicines, theory, and nature. None of these first four cases highlights enchanting relationships to living plants that are important for them as herbalists, although one of them is arguably enchanted by particular herbal medicines. However, the second group of four visible entryway herbalists reveal how knowing living plants in various ways is important for their practices and points to another way of understanding aspects of Western herbal medicine.

TE

Entryways

TE's mother was a keen gardener:

> I suppose when I was younger I was always very involved with gardens because my mother was quite a big gardener and she also, she's Irish, southern Irish, she had quite a, a bit of folksiness in her so she was reasonably interested in things like you can use this for such and such, didn't know a lot about it but was quite interested in what plants did and what kind of plants and she got me very involved with gardens. So I suppose that's where my interest in plants …

TE had first wanted to be a surgeon:

> … my earliest recollection of wanting to have a career was I wanted to be a surgeon and I think that lasted until I was about eleven or twelve, at that stage I decided I wanted to be a lawyer and that stayed with me and I went to university and studied history with the intention of doing a law conversion course afterwards, a post-graduate diploma, and that all worked out.

TE qualified as a lawyer but didn't enjoy practising law. As a distraction, he looked for an adult education evening class and found one in herbal medicine:

> … at the end of the three months I thought, actually I really, really like this, so I just started having a look into degrees in herbal medicine and seeing what I could do.

Like a GP, but more so

He studied herbal medicine while working full-time as a lawyer. Since qualifying in herbal medicine he has published academic papers on herbal medicine, supervises herbal medicine students in a training clinic, and lectures on clinical medicine, clinical examination, and pathology to herbal medicine students. Soon after qualifying he sat in with a herbalist and osteopath who worked in an NHS integrated medicine practice as well as sitting in on GPs' consultations. The practice manager approached him about working in the practice:

> ... she asked me would I be interested in pitching to the GPs basically and saying this is what I offer, would they be interested? So I said, definitely, and I put together a paper which I started off thinking was going to be all the merits of herbal medicine, what I can treat, all of this ... but actually turned out to be basically talking about costs and saying to them, at the moment you probably refer this many people for gastrointestinal medicine through to secondary care. The cost of this to you is such and such. The cost of the prescriptions to you is this much. This is your success rate there, and she helped me put together some of the figures and then I superimposed on that what a herbal medical practice might be able to offer. I showed them how health cuts could be made and costings could be sorted out and they were happy enough to take it on, so they said yes. So I started working there for two half days a week.

TE sees both NHS and private patients at the NHS practice. The NHS patients are only charged for the medicines, not for the consultations. He initially ran workshops for the GPs looking at the treatment of the patients that they had referred on to him. The GPs refer particular patient groups to TE:

> ... they became more invested in it and now I think they're pretty convinced that if there's a gastrointestinal complaint they will more or less refer to me. So most of the gastrointestinal medicine comes through to me because the results are probably 95% positive for it and probably I think they find it, apart from giving blanket prescriptions of Omeprazole, PPIs and things, they find it quite a difficult, quite, gastrointestinal quite difficult to treat whereas we find it a much, probably one of the easier ones. They also send through a bit of respiratory, some dermatology, quite a lot of older patients who have, who just have quite a lot of complications and need somebody to spend enough time with them to understand what's going on and it, I was, I'm quite pleased that some of them have enough confidence now that they will send through people who

have congestive heart failure and complex conditions that they seem to feel happy with me prescribing alongside the existing medications and they're a couple of patients I'm treating for congestive heart failure and it's going reasonably well ...

He explains to patients that herbal medicines are drugs:

> ... I see quite a lot of patients who aren't interested in taking conventional medications whether I think that reasonable or not. I'm quite prepared to take them myself but some patients just don't want to take drugs and I'm quite careful to explain to them that this is a drug as well but they seem to be much happier taking something that has a natural origin.

While TE has access to his patients' NHS medical records, he takes the cases from scratch and adopts a very orthodox medical approach:

> ... this is one of the nice things, they don't expect me to rely on their previous diagnoses. I'm expected to do a separate triage with each patient I see. So diagnostically, although rarely do I differ from what they've come up with but quite often I get sent patients that they're not quite sure what, what's going on with them so I do a whole, I start off, I take the presenting complaint, go through a whole normal case history and do my examinations at the end if they're needed and then I write down all of that into the medical records ... It will put mine up there and it would also go, seen by herbalist, at the top so that when the GP goes in you can just see, OK he's seen by the herbalist on 16th March, said blah, blah, blah, blah, blah, on examination, auscultation of lungs unremarkable, some crackling at bases or whatever. So it's all the, exactly as they would. So I'm expected to adhere to a very orthodox medical model and it's the one I feel more comfortable in and I would, I'm very shy of writing any terms that I don't think that they would understand and by understand I also mean they wouldn't appreciate. So I'd never write down that somebody has a damp condition or a hot condition. I don't really understand how that works myself but I'd keep it very much to clinical language, medical language.

He only includes details of his herbal prescriptions on the NHS system if they might have an impact on the patient's drug medication:

> ... only if they, if I think that they might have a crossover. So if I prescribe *Datura* or something that's a bronchodilator and I didn't want them to be potentially doubling up on dosages, I'd write that down. If I prescribe *Hypericum* I will write that in as well and I also check whenever I prescribe one of these that they're not being given it and next time I see them I'll make sure that they haven't been prescribed something in the interim that would mix with anything but otherwise they're not really that interested in what goes into the patient.

TE takes a full case history, but only transfers onto the NHS system what is relevant to the patient's presenting condition. His NHS notes are more extensive than the GPs' notes:

> ... normally my notes are that much on the screen (indicating a large size) whereas their notes are that much on the screen (indicating a small size). So I do do a lot more and I go into a lot more detail. So if somebody comes in, they'll say, the typical GP, somebody comes in with IBS or something, he'll go, patient with history of IBS, says acute symptoms over last two days, no blood or mucus, suggests Omeprazole by four, come and see again four days or something, whereas mine will go, patient had, complains of IBS, onset maybe seven years ago with blah, blah, blah, blah, blah, recently more acute attacks have presented with blah, blah and blah, patient says feels limits daily activities by blah and blah, priorities are, and then I'll go, on examination increased bowel sounds to ileocaecal valve, blah, blah, blah, blah, blah. So mine will be much more like that. So mine will actually be more medical than theirs probably in what I write down ...

This has led to suggestions by the GPs that he qualifies as a medical doctor:

> Because I remember one of the GPs coming to see me because two of the GPs keep going, go back to medical school and qualify fully,

and they call it "fully" ... go back to medical school and qualify fully because the way you work, you'll have so much more freedom because you work like us but you don't have the freedom to prescribe the stuff that we can prescribe and you don't have the freedom to refer and you don't have the freedom to move within the profession. You can't go into secondary care, you can't go into blah, and I do see a lot of that and I thought really, really hard about going to medical school afterwards but I'm not, I don't think I'm going to ...

TE does more physical examinations than the GPs:

> ... they've got seven minutes. If they, their clinical examination consists of shining a light into the mouth or very occasionally they might listen to lungs or heart sounds and things but they don't, I, especially if they do a musculoskeletal examination. They will ask the patient to lift to here and then they go, OK that's fine, and you're going, where's the end range of movements ... so it's just not something they do and that's why they love having the osteopaths. The osteopaths are booked up for months in advance because GPs run a mile from any musculoskeletal or neurological problem because they just, it's not their comfort zone at all and similarly I think they're quite like it with the gastrointestinal as well.

Like a GP, but less than

He doesn't see himself as an equal to the GPs in the practice as he is dependent on their goodwill:

> I think one has to tread carefully and make sure that you don't ever assume a position that's, that puts you on a, as a peer. I don't know if they would like that or not. I, regardless of what I think in how they relate value wise, I would always, I suppose I'm relatively new to it as well but I always think of it as their territory and I'm very respectful because I'm working in an NHS practice and I'm there by their grace really. So I wouldn't push my luck too far but then I will go and speak to, I had a complicated patient the other day who one of the GPs had seen the day before and when I was speaking to him I asked, is your lower lip normally that shade? And he said,

why, what? And he wanted to have a look in the mirror. He said, yeah, it's fine. I said, are you sure? And he said, oh maybe it is a bit bluer than it normally is. And I … he had this cough and I carried on chatting to him and he previously had a triple bypass … there were lots of indications that there might be a cardiac problem going on so after I had a chat with him I went through and found the GP and said, you saw this guy yesterday. I read through the notes and I hadn't picked up that you'd seen anything like this, but I just wanted to mention it because I can't refer him through to a cardiologist because I'd have to refer back to the GP but I just said, I, because he's under your care I'd just like you to know that these are the things I observed and I've written them up on his medical notes. So that's as far as I go …

Relying on (a lack of) evidence

TE says that getting to the point of writing a prescription is difficult due to the lack of good information available on herbal medicines:

> I find it a slightly frustrating process I have to say because there are so many herbs that we don't understand.

The main book he uses, by Kerry Bone (2003), is ten years old, which he sees as being out of date. Although TE has a more recent book (Fisher, 2009), which has lots of research references, he finds it difficult to apply to writing prescriptions. He uses his knowledge of the physiological effects of plant constituents to select herbs:

> There's very little decent guidance out there. I try to stick to about five because I think if I dilute them too much, if I put in ten or twenty herbs I just wonder if there's any therapeutic value in what I'm doing and I try to make it, I just look at the actions and I try to make it as specific as I can from what we understand about the herbs. So, if I'm treating gastrointestinal, I'm looking at antispasmodic, anti-inflammatory, anything that has an antacid or whatever. So, I work on what constituents I understand are in them and what the physiological effect of those is. I have very little outside influence like, is it a certain type herb or does it potentiate this or whatever? It's very, it's quite down the line and I'm sure that's

a good thing in some ways but I recognise in other ways it's not such a great thing because it, it's not, it steps slightly outside of the whole traditional healer thing where there's a lot more taken into account but I don't see people as certain types of, people look and say "That's a kind of verbena person" or something, that's what will benefit them. I don't get that …

He sees himself as working within a very orthodox approach to herbal medicine, and does not include traditional energetic herbal knowledge in his decision making:

One hundred per cent pharmacological. I, partly because I don't, I never really studied that as well so I don't really understand it so I don't know what I'd be doing. I'd probably be throwing some-body's energetics in the wrong direction if I tried.

TE prefers to use herbs based on scientific evidence rather than reputa-tion or traditional use:

I don't use *Calendula* very much at all and I think of it more for what I think we know about it, which is it is antibacterial. We do know it's anti-inflammatory but I think less for the gut and I think more possibly topically and then it has a reputation for lymphatic things which if somebody came to me and they wanted help with lym-phatic stuff I might put it in because the choice of herbs is somewhat limited. I'd do what I could but I wouldn't have a huge amount of faith in whether it would work or not because I'd either need to see it written down for me or I'd need to have seen it from somebody or seen it myself to work in order to have confidence in it but I don't, I wouldn't discount something on the grounds that I haven't read it or seen it work. I'm not a complete doubting Thomas …

In selecting herbs, he uses his knowledge of physiology. In his deci-sion making he uses drug pharmacology to identify particular effects that he requires and then searches scientific papers to identify appro-priate herbs:

So I generally, if I'm making a decision I tend to, the herbs are the last things I'd look at. The first thing I look at is what I need physiologically to sort it out. So say I didn't understand what was happening with breast cancer, I'd then research the drugs that they use like tamoxifen and go, OK, so that's having that physiological effect. Can I mimic that looking at herbs if I didn't know another way of dealing with it? So then I'd be going, OK, so I do need to be looking at something that has an effect like a selective oestrogen receptor modulator. So I'd use those and then I use things like PubMed and results from Cochrane reviews, all kinds of stuff. So I use quite a lot of internet stuff.

TE worries that there is not that much to differentiate him from the GPs:

I feel like I, "emulate's" an unfortunate word, I mimic their practice so much that I'm more likely to be redundant in that respect unless the patient asks for me. From the GP's point of view, I'm probably more redundant than somebody who does work in energetics and that adds something that is completely different, something a GP doesn't step into …

Reflection on TE

TE's case locates two entryways to his becoming a herbalist—his mother as a keen gardener, and his childhood desire to be a surgeon. These visible entryways form a thread with the rest of his narrative: in the end, he combined plants with medicine in studying herbal medicine and then in practising and teaching herbal medicine.

This thread, that started with gardens and medical aspirations and continues with practising herbal medicine in an integrated medicine GP practice, is one that is congruent with the fragmented history of Western herbal medicine. That history showed that while orthodox medicine has said a long goodbye to herbal medicine, herbal medicine is still attached to orthodox medicine. And from TE we see that his practice of herbal medicine is still wedded tightly to orthodox medicine. So tightly that he, like his particular training, chooses not to engage with more traditional or energetic understandings of herbal medicine. There is no talk of "hot" or "cold", of "trophorestoration" or "tissue states". Just as at the end of the nineteenth century the profession sought to exclude particular elements of its traditional image, such as the astrology of "Culpeperism", so TE avoids anything except a scientific approach to herbal medicine. He uses the principles of orthodox medicine and of evidence to identify herbs that may be useful to his patients. He takes drug pharmacology as a starting point in seeking to identify herbal medicines that might be useful for a patient. He starts with physiology and drugs rather than with herbs.

The case of TE suggests that science is dominant in his practice. He turns to pharmacology, monographs, and databases rather than traditional use or "herbals". However, this does not mean that his practice has been "colonised", "co-opted", or "mainstreamed" in a Kuhnian takeover of one paradigm by another. TE is very happy to practise this way and he is not doing anything in his integrated medical practice that he would do differently elsewhere. TE's engagement with physiology, pharmacology, and phytochemistry as starting points can be seen to be part of the "search for plausibility" that Wahlberg[51] identified as being one aspect of this "normalization" of herbal medicine. TE seeks to know, through being shown evidence, that a herb works and how it works. He needs to know the pharmacodynamics and pharmacokinetics of herbs as they travel round the body. For this he turns to science.

However, his position also reflects his training at an institution whose curriculum was influenced by Hein Zeylstra and the desire to put herbal medicine on a firm evidence-based footing, one that replaced physiomedicalism with phytochemistry. At the level of the individual there is little to suggest the co-option of TE's practice, and at the structural level, the engagement with science was something that came out of the profession, rather than was forced upon it, even if not all herbalists agree with the direction that was taken and prefer to forge their own way.

TE has found acceptance as a herbalist in an integrated medical practice. He admits that in some ways he "mimics" the medical practices of the GPs, and that his NHS case notes are "more medical" than the GPs'. In some ways this is beneficial. Wahlberg[42] identified that the "ethical field of battle" for who is a recognised CAM practitioner is today based on qualifications, competency, responsibility, conduct, and development, almost irrespective of the particular therapy. Similarly, the GPs are not interested in knowing the tools of TE's trade, namely the herbs in the prescription. And TE only passes on details of herbs if there is any potential interaction with drug medication. The GPs were happy to take him on based on a presentation that focused on cost-effectiveness in treating gastrointestinal conditions. No herbs were mentioned. Similarly, and subsequently, the GPs are not interested in TE's prescriptions, "in what goes into the patient", but are happy simply to see that his approach is similar to their approach. He is qualified, competent, and responsible and that is enough for them, even if some of them have suggested that he should train to be a medical doctor, just like them.

While TE's medical approach is useful in gaining acceptance, the fact that herbs are barely mentioned in his NHS case notes and that he sees them as drug medicines, explaining to patients that "this is a drug as well", means that the herbs are rather hidden. Additionally, they do not have a physical presence at the GP practice. They are kept at his home. This combination of taking an orthodox medical approach and the hidden nature of the tools of his trade, namely the herbal medicines themselves, makes it difficult for him to define his practice against what the GPs do. Besides prescribing his hidden herbal medicines, what he does is very similar to what a GP does. And this makes his professional identity less secure in that he is not apparently offering something significantly different from what a doctor offers, with the exception of the (hidden) herbal medicines themselves.

We now turn from TE, who relates to herbal medicine through the lens of orthodox medicine and science, to CP, who relates to a particular herb through her empirical experience of it as a medicine.

CP

Entryways

CP comes from a medical family. Her mother was a private GP.

> My mother qualified pre antibiotics. She's got extraordinary stories from her war years in the infirmary, seeing people cough their lungs into tin buckets in the consumption wards, you know it being the Forties. And stories about doing domiciliary work ... in tenements off the Royal Mile, when people had no running water. She spent the first year of her medical degree doing botany, I mean obviously not every day, but they used to go to the Botanic's once a week.

Her mother worked from home and had a clinic phone that CP used to answer. Now CP also works from home and her own son Sam answers her clinic phone for her. She uses her mother's desk, which had previously belonged to a relative who had been an eminent physician in the early nineteenth century, and which contains hemispherical pockets for the guineas that he would have received as medical fees. She became interested in the clinical encounter and decided to study acupuncture.

After graduating with a degree in acupuncture she sought clinical experience and worked for free in GPs' practices for two years, seeing about sixteen patients a week.

> I wasn't being paid, so I felt I could be assertive about my terms, and suitable referrals. I said, I don't want your heart-sinks, and I don't terribly want complex long-standing musculo-skeletal, you can send me acute musculo-skeletal; but what I'm really interested in is gynae, headaches and psychological stuff.

CP had difficulty becoming pregnant. During a study trip to China she visited a Chinese medicine doctor:

> The doctor I was training with took me to see a wonderful and much revered old lady. I was told she was the top gynaecologist in Fujian province, which has a population of 80 million people or something. She took my pulse and looked at my tongue and talked to me through interpreters. And I was given this prescription that felt like the Holy Grail, and I got it straight out of the hospital pharmacy. And I took that, for several months, but noticed no change, nothing.

She also saw an acupuncturist in the UK who took her to see her own supervisor. They disagreed on her diagnosis, with her acupuncturist seeing her as "kidney yin deficient" and the supervisor saying she had "phlegm fire harassing the heart". This disagreement was difficult for CP:

> Jacqui's diagnosis was of a deficient condition, and his was a full, excess condition. There was no, or very little, overlap. His condition was up here in my chest, and her condition was down here in my pelvis … It was very dismaying to have these two very experienced practitioners have such a fundamental disagreement.

After hearing about a Western herb for fertility she visited a practitioner of Western herbal medicine.

> She gave me herbs, which included *Chamaelirium* and *Vitex*, and I started taking them in September and I took them until December. And then I got fed up with the whole thing. By this time I'd been trying to become pregnant for about five years. I stopped the herbs, and then I got pregnant in the next, the next few cycles. There was a very key physiological change taking the Western herbs, but I'd never noticed any difference with the Chinese herbs.

The physiological sign was stretchy cervical mucus:

> But it, the stretchy mucus, which I now absolutely attribute to *Chamaelirium*, I hadn't had that for years, I hadn't had it for years. I saw it one morning, Brian was about to go to work, I said, come back! And that was it—that was Sam!

After this experience, and despite already having studied acupuncture, which is part of Chinese medicine, CP studied for a degree in Western herbal medicine. Her personal experience of Western herbal medicine that resulted in her becoming a mother had led her this way.

Chinese medicine: the triumph of theory

Early on in her career CP began to treat women who were having difficulty becoming pregnant. In one year she had a 100% success rate with her fertility patients, with twelve women under forty-five years old becoming pregnant. She was then getting two or three new fertility patients a week and thereafter found that she had to start a waiting list. By this time she had completed her herbal medicine degree and was treating some patients with herbs. In her acupuncture practice, which is firmly rooted in yin yang theory, her fertility patients come to see her four times a cycle:

> Ideally I like to see them at the start of their period. What we're thinking about is getting a nice clean bleed. A clean start and stop, few, or no clots, no pain, red blood. We do the sort of points you would use if you were inducing labour. And then the next time

they come back which is a few days later, we're wanting to nourish the blood and the yin. So that's a much more nurturing, containing, supporting treatment, and it's much stiller, and you don't want to move. Unless there's someone with a lot of blood stasis and pain, in which case you might want to move in a sort of residual way. And then the next time we see them which is when they get their stretchy mucus, just before ovulation, you want to move, because you want everything moving in the fallopian tubes, and you want the ovaries to release the eggs smoothly, and you want all the cilia in the tubes to be moving. And you want the sperm to come up, you want things nice and mobile, so it's all about moving. And then the fourth treatment, which is when you are hoping there's a conception, and you want to hold and contain it, is all about nurturing yang, which is the warmth of the second half of the cycle. So in a way, very crudely, we sort of do the same thing with each woman.

A similar approach is taken with herbs that are used within Chinese medicine:

> When I was taking Chinese herbs I had I think four different prescriptions within each menstrual cycle, or at least two different prescriptions.

Vitex and Chamaelirium: the triumph of empiricism

While CP uses theory as the foundation for treatment with her acupuncture patients, it is her own personal experience of taking Western herbs, notably *Chamaelirium luteum* and *Vitex agnus-castus*, and her subsequent training in Western herbal medicine, that is crucially important for how she uses herbs in her herbal practice.

> When patients first come to see me, I generally ask, do you get fertile mucus? "Oh, I don't know." And I describe it and they say, "Oh, I don't know." Sometimes after a few cycles of treatment they'll notice fertile mucus: "I've just got it, I've seen it!" They're so excited and very often they're pregnant within a cycle or two. I was on *Chamaelirium* and black cohosh, and various other things. I was on *Vitex* separately in the morning.

Because Chinese herbal medicine didn't work for me, I don't do it. I'm very fascinated by how individual physicians may be scientifically trained, may know the importance of controlled clinical trials, and yet what actually affects their clinical thinking is their own clinical experience. David Taylor Reilly did fascinating work on this in the Nineties. And one's own personal clinical experience is even more salient than one's patients'. So the fact that I had one prescription for three months, and I don't think Sarah saw me once during that time, and then I got pregnant, is a powerful influence on my thinking. So when I prescribe herbs, I tend to wait until I've seen them through at least one menstrual cycle and I see the basal body temperature, and then I prescribe on the basis of what I see on the basal body temperature chart, and of course on other signs and symptoms and the conventional medical diagnosis, if there is one. I work very much within the context of a conventional medical model. However, there is a wonderful richness of information that we glean from the BBT, and it is hugely empowering to patients because they get to see what is happening with their ovulation, with their luteal phase—and they also, hopefully, get to see the fruits of treatment. I would say that within the context of gynaecology, yin yang theory and conventional medicine, which are separated by thousands of years, work together seamlessly, and beautifully. But on the whole the prescriptions look quite similar. Women get peony and liquorice if there's a problem with ovulation, they very often get dong quai and *Chamaelirium*, and very often *Rehmannia*. Sometimes *Vitex* goes in the main prescription and sometimes the *Vitex* is separate. They almost always get *Vitex*. Sometimes they just get *Vitex*.

Side by side: Chinese herbs and Western herbs

CP describes the case of a patient who had had several failed IVFs. Subsequently it was found, after a hysteroscopy, that she had uterine adhesions and scarring and was not building up her endometrium, explaining why she wasn't getting pregnant. One of the herbal medicines that CP gave was a liquid tincture formula focused on her endometrial health.

So she started coming to me nearly a year ago. She was just embarking on IVF, knowing that the endometrium was problematic, and what I needed to do was prescribe her a herbal medicine to help her build her endometrium. I'm very simple minded when I write herbal prescriptions. I tend to think about one thing, I'm not very holistic, I don't tend to think about the whole person. Or I think about the whole person through the lens of this one problem. I want to stay focused. So with this particular woman, I gave her three Chinese herbs and three Western herbs. I want to build blood, which is a Chinese idea.

This patient's herbal medicine included three "blood building" Chinese herbs—Chinese angelica, peony, and also *Rehmannia*. This last herb has two common preparations in Chinese medicine—the "raw" herb, sheng di huang, and a "prepared" preparation, shu di huang, the second of which is warmer and more of a blood tonic, so this was included. However, the Chinese angelica was also selected because it is a "uterine tonic" and "oestrogenic", which are both terms from Western herbal medicine rather than TCM. Similarly, the *Rehmannia* was selected for its "adrenal tonic" action. The next three herbs, *Centella*, dandelion (*Taraxacum officinalis*) and liquorice, were included in this formula for mainly "Western" reasons:

> I gave her *Centella*, because of the scarring and adhesions. I always use it whenever there is any endometrial damage, or any risk of endometrial damage. And then I gave her *Tarax* because she's going to be having loads of drugs over many cycles. Normally I don't get terribly fussed about the liver, I always think that actually the liver is an organ with a huge amount of capacity. And most IVF drugs look like human endogenous hormones. I mean you know, some of the FSH used in IVF actually is sourced from menopausal ladies' urine, it's not as if it's some toxic substance unknown to human physiology, do you know what I mean? ... It's follicular stimulating hormone, and in menopause we have buckets of the stuff. So I don't get very excited about needing to support the liver in IVF but this woman was going to have many cycles over a long period. It was such a palaver and over such a long period, I thought that the liver could do with some support. And *Tarax* regulates oestrogen. It's said to up the expression of oestrogens and obviously that's really important for her. And it's eliminative, so she had quite a bit of *Tarax* in her prescription. And then she's got liquorice, because from a Chinese

point of view it takes things down into the lower jiao, and it's anti-inflammatory. I always think all herbs are anti-inflammatory but liquorice is also for adrenal support, and also she was going to be on aspirin quite a lot of the time. And at her first IVF cycle, her endometrium had got up to over 6mm, which it had never done before.

Thus, while CP uses Chinese terms such as "blood builder" and "blood tonic" for the Chinese herbs angelica, *Rehmannia*, and peony, she also applies the Western terms of "uterine tonic" and "oestrogenic" to angelica. Furthermore, drawing on Western herbal medicine's knowledge of *Centella*, *Tarax*, and liquorice, she uses mainly "Western" reasons for including them, for instance to treat "adhesions", to "support" the liver, and for anti-inflammatory activity, although liquorice is also included to "take things down to the lower jiao". Chinese and Western herbs are included in the same formulae, with Chinese herbs having Chinese and Western justifications, and Western herbs having both Western and Chinese justifications. It all gets mixed up in the bottle.

Reflection on CP

CP came from an orthodox medical family background but ended up practising acupuncture and Western herbal medicine. She had significant fertility problems herself, and attributes her own motherhood to Western herbal medicine. This experience forged the path into her now practising Western herbal medicine and working almost exclusively with women trying to conceive.

Although CP did not have any enchanting, and therefore hidden, human-nonhuman entryways into Western herbal medicine that involved meetings between herself and living plants, there was an enchantment of another sort. This involved her own experience of taking Western herbal medicine. This experience was "sensual" in that it involved the physical manifestation in her body of cervical mucus changes, which became stretchy and resembled raw egg white. And she understands this change to have been caused by the *Chamaelirium*. It was also "affective" in that, beyond her own joy in becoming pregnant with Sam, it is now something that CP and her patients look for. And when it is found, it is experienced as a welcome sign, understood within her close monitoring of the cycle as a whole, which includes attention paid to basal body temperature and other markers.

These cervical mucus changes act as a clear indication that a patient's fertility is improving, providing a sign that is a sustaining "energy" in her practice, helping to encourage perseverance in what can be a long and stressful process from reduced fertility to the birth of a child. There is a sensual-affective energy, or enchantment, in her practice that started with her taking a liquid medicine containing *Chamaelirium*. It starts with a material medicine made from a plant, rather than with the plant itself. CP's empiricism can be seen in her approach to formulating herbal medicines, in that Western and Chinese herbs, and Western and Chinese knowledge of Western and Chinese herbs, are easily placed together in a focused prescription that addresses the clinical needs of the patient. This may be contrasted to the use of herbs within Chinese medicine, where the overall balance of the prescription is likely to be more important than in Western herbal medicine.

While CP embraced the enchantment of empiricism in her herbal medicine practice, we now look at a practitioner of Western herbal medicine who turned away from the empiricism of Western herbal medicine towards the enchantment of theory that she found in Chinese medicine.

EP

Entryways

EP came from a family background of conventional medicine:

> I grew up in a terribly orthodox family, my father's a surgeon and then he became an anaesthetist later on, and my mother was a nurse, and my stepmother a pharmacist and I went into nursing ...

EP's experience of seeing herbal medicine help a patient successfully withdraw from steroids was important for her becoming a herbalist:

> Well, I suppose I became a herbalist when my children were quite small and I met somebody who had a birth trauma which ended up being an anal fissure and she took herself to, she was taking steroid suppositories ... But the more she used them, the more she had to use them and she took herself to a herbalist who sorted the whole thing out and got her off the steroids, and I was mind-blown because I started out in nursing and I thought if you had to have

steroids, it was serious and there wasn't an alternative, so I thought, hang on a minute, this is a bit, it really took me by surprise.

After this experience, EP eventually studied herbal medicine at the School of Herbal Medicine.

Learning through challenging patients

One of EP's first patients as a qualified herbalist challenged her to come up with a solution where orthodox medicine couldn't.

> One of my first … the thirteen, fourteen year old with osteochondrosis, where the metacarpal couldn't keep up with the growth spurt and it just started to disintegrate. And, yes, that was fantastic, she'd been, for, she'd taken ages to get to see an orthopaedic guy and eventually she did and he basically said, we'll give you anti-inflammatories, and then we'll operate and we'll remove the bone and you'll be crippled for life. And so I did a foot soak with comfrey, arnica and wintergreen, and gave her internal anti-inflammatories, with quite a lot of comfrey as well, and within two weeks, she favoured that foot, it was amazing. It really was amazing, which is why now, the "duck poo", as it's called, the comfrey, arnica and wintergreen ointment, which looks like duck poo, is so, is one of my most popular things, I've just made it, ever since then, into an ointment, to make it more user friendly …

EP likes to treat local problems locally:

> And that is a very Western approach, because wintergreen is 98% aspirin, and then comfrey and arnica, it just makes sense. And you just put it where it's needed, so it's really good.

Green medicine—the triumph of empiricism

After qualifying in herbal medicine she started to provide first aid and acute herbal medicine at green festivals. EP remembers being challenged by an acute case to come up with an immediate solution:

> He was about nine, he had had a piece of hay in his eye, and his eye swelled up like a ping pong ball, it was right out of the socket,

he could not blink. It was very frightening. I said, "Hospital now!" And the father said, "I don't believe in hospitals, this happened last year, it wasn't so bad, you can do something. We don't need hospitals or orthodox medicine." And it's horribly surprising how often you hear that. And I said, "No, no, please, he can't blink, he'll get an ulcer on his cornea, it will cause blindness. Let me take him, somebody has to take him." They refused. So I said, we'll see what we can do, if it's not substantially better in half an hour I want you to take him to hospital. So I cut a slice of cucumber and stuck that on his eye immediately, made him a pot of eyebright tea and gave him a STAT dose—take now. He was nine or ten. I was so frightened by it, it was 10ml of *Ephedra* and 10ml of FE of *Urtica*. And he quaffed that back and by the time the kettle was boiled and the tea was made the eye had gone straight back into the socket. It was phenomenal, it works well, but you do get put on the spot far too often with people who don't want to go anywhere near orthodox medicine.

EP developed formulae for particular conditions:

> … the formulas definitely came as a result of my wanting people to use things that I knew were going to be effective, and I'm very happy for people to take the formulas away with them and just, if I've learned something I think it's my duty to pass on the information, rather than hold it to myself, I think that's just an appalling thing to do, really it's, why would you do that, you want herbal medicine to be known for its excellence, not known for people not quite getting it right …

On a visit to a festival where EP was organising and providing first aid and acute herbal medicine, there was a team of five supervisors, seven experienced herbalists, seven newly qualified herbalists, and five students. I was one of these volunteers. In the dispensing caravan, tinctures of single herbs were lined up alphabetically by Latin binomial name on shelves along a wall. Tinctures of herbal formulae were on shelves along another wall. They included "constipation mix", "allergy mix", "UTI", "stop panic mix", "asthma mix", "cough syrup", "GE cough syrup", "acute infection mix", "hay fever mix", "allergy mix", and "hangover mix". The "acute infection mix" contained the herbs *Echinacea, Baptisia,* and *Phytolacca* (pokeweed). EP describes their inclusion:

> [These herbs] are specifically for respiratory, upper respiratory or lower respiratory chest infection and I just found them to be so effective year after year that I just knew that, that if you've got an acute thing, I mean we were told pokeweed is when you really need to "poke it out" and it's really stubborn, why wait until it's really stubborn before you use it, if you use it in an acute situation, when it's brand new, you won't end up with a chronic problem, so I just picked those herbs because I'd seen them work so effectively so many times. And then you can tailor the rest of the prescription to sinusitis or otitis or whatever it is …

The empirical use of herbs for particular conditions is further demonstrated by the following case of a patient at a festival: I was in the caravan dispensing a medicine when a young man in his twenties knocked on the door asking if we had the prescription forms from last year. I replied that they were not here. He said that he had put his back out last year and had been given some herbal medicine that had really helped. "I really just want the same thing," he said. "I have done it again." I took him into the damp first aid tent, as it had been raining heavily, where I introduced him to the supervisor who said that she had also been there last year. They recognised each other. She said that she could remember what she used last year. "I use a fairly standard approach for acute back problems. Did it taste of liquorice?" "Yes, and it cost about £20, you gave me enough for a few weeks." She replied, "I think it was devil's claw, vib op, and liquorice."

Chinese medicine—the triumph of theory

While the above examples show a concern with using particular herbs, or particular herbal formulae, for particular medical conditions, EP found that she was not having the success she wanted with dermatology patients.

> I suppose about two or three years in, after qualifying as a Western herbalist, I realised that I didn't have a clue what I was doing with

dermatology and sometimes I got it right and things healed beautifully, and sometimes I got it wrong, and nothing worked, and I didn't know why I'd got it right and I didn't know why I'd got it wrong, and I just knew I didn't know what I was doing. And so I decided to learn Chinese herbal medicine, because they have a reputation for being good at dermatology.

Initially she was resistant to learning the theory of Chinese medicine, but then became enamoured by its understanding of patterns:

... when I first started studying it, I just thought, this is a load of bunkum, absolute rubbish, how can it be that simple that wind brings diseases, and you get hot or cold or, I really thought I'd lost the plot when I first started studying it, but then it takes, you have to really understand Chinese medicine at some depth to realise how complex and how fantastically simple and complex it all is. It is, it's really amazing. So, because I'd learned the herbs, I started using them, and because they diagnose, they put all sorts of symptoms together that Western medical people wouldn't do, like things like floaters in the eyes and restless legs, or leg cramp, foot cramp, that kind of stuff, with low energy, and they'd say it's a blood deficiency, and you kind of think, Western people wouldn't connect any of those things together, let alone have a diagnosis, so if you know that, and people say, oh I get so much leg cramp and you say, and do you get restless legs, and do you get floaters in the eyes, and do you feel really rather tired in, just energy crashes. And they'll say, "Well, how did you know that?" And it's just, it's, so lots of people who come with symptoms you can hone them in to a pattern, a diagnostic pattern that Western medicine just wouldn't recognise, so it just makes another toolkit really for getting people well.

After qualifying in Chinese herbal medicine she later qualified in acupuncture and now combines Western herbal medicine, Chinese herbal medicine, and acupuncture in her practice. She finds that Chinese medicine helps her to talk to patients about their conditions in ways that make sense to them:

Chinese medicine's very poetical and very, it's very based on nature, so they'll talk about qi stagnation as if you've got a river that's got debris in it, that'll be, causes the qi to stagnate, or the river doesn't have enough qi in, then it'll stagnate because it's just not flowing properly, or if it's too hot then it'll dry up and it'll stagnate, or too cold and it'll congeal and turn into ice cubes, so it'll stagnate or, so they have all these different ways of talking about it and you can tell somebody if you've broken your arm, of course that's local stagnation, it's like a branch went across the river. So they like hearing their diagnosis in those sort of terms and it just makes it much easier to explain … yes I much prefer to talk to patients in terms of Chinese medicine, than I do in terms of the Western medicine, but quite often I'll say, well Western medicine will say this, that and the other thing …

She finds that Chinese medicine's approach to diagnosis leads easily to a treatment approach:

Take a lipoma or something like that, that would be considered as "phlegm" in Chinese medicine, and phlegm comes from dampness that lingers around too long and you get dampness from certain dietary things, so you can go into, these are the damp forming foods, and if you cut them out, it will go a long way to sorting out your damp, and then if you put these foods in, that'll also help. So, they like to hear things, self-help things, eat a lot of seaweed, and put, pungent things like horseradish [into your diet] … you know that if you eat horseradish, you're going to start streaming aren't you, so it cuts through phlegm, it makes sense and people just get it. And aromatic things are moving, they make the phlegm move or the mucus move, so they encourage dispersing and movement, and they'll break up stagnation of that sort, so it makes sense.

She compares Chinese medicine with that of a Western approach in Western herbal medicine:

I mean, what would you do about it, a lipoma in Western terms, you'd probably say, well you're stuck with it, have it cut out. Yeah. So the Chinese would have ways of trying to explain to you how that happened and therefore hopefully you won't end up with ten of them, which people do, obviously get more and more, if they don't alter their diet and their lifestyle.

The safety of Western herbal medicine, the attraction of Chinese medicine

While Chinese medicine has added a more poetic, theoretical approach to EP's practice that allows treatments to logically and consistently follow on from diagnosis, EP still values Western herbal medicine and finds that Chinese medicine and Western herbal medicine go well together:

> ... because I've been doing it so long, I integrate them very comfortably, and for a while, if people came with, let's say indigestion, I know that the Western herbs work so well for that, that I wouldn't really bother with Chinese herbs for indigestion, because why would I, when I know what works so well in Western herbs, but then, if somebody doesn't get better with the Western herbs, then I switch to Chinese, that's quite often the way I'll do it. But if someone presents with something that's very obviously going to fit into a Chinese box, then I'll just go hone in to that. But I, most of my prescriptions are a mixture of Chinese and Western herbs, so I'll pick the best from each discipline and put them together.

EP gives the example of treating different Chinese medicine presentations of infections with both Chinese and Western herbs:

> If you think of Chinese medicine and the wind-cold and the wind-heat ... wind-cold means that you feel cold and achy even though you have a fever and so I would make sure that 50% of the prescription is that acute infection mix and then peony, cinnamon, *Eupatorium perfoliatum*—fantastic herb for aching bones, really really useful ... And when you're feeling hot and have a sore throat Chinese would call that wind-heat. So I would use the acute infection mix and then *Lonicera*—honeysuckle, or *Forsythia*, and obviously *Achillea* or *Sambucus* are fantastic, we would use those. *Mentha* is used in both Chinese and Western herbal medicine.

The herbs from the different traditions sit easily together in her prescriptions. However, when it comes to case history taking she doesn't mix up the different elements from the two approaches. She prefers to follow a Western herbal medicine case history, only introducing the Chinese medicine questions at the end. She sees safety as coming from her Western training:

The Chinese case history taking ... I mean, honestly it's so super-ficial and just, it's just not good enough, I'm sorry, it's really not good enough, I mean they ask, they'll ask you to tell, tell me what's the problem, to go through your stuff, and then they'll say, do you sweat normally, do you sleep normally, do you eat, how's your appetite, how are your bowels, ... sweating, and thirst is another one, they want to know thirst and whether your body temperature, do you feel hotter than anyone else, or are you feeling cold, chilly ...

... very little, very, very little, I couldn't do it that superficially ... but I suppose I'm steeped in the Western stuff enough to need to feel safe in my practice with that. I don't think I'd feel very safe in my practice without it, I really don't.

Reflection on EP

EP's entryway of seeing herbal medicine working more effectively than orthodox medicine, in the case of a patient taking steroids for an anal fissure, is also visible in one of her first cases as a qualified herb-alist, when she successfully treated osteochondrosis of the foot, thus preventing the need for the patient to have surgery. The influence of an orthodox family medical background that led to her initially adopt-ing a nursing career can be seen in her interest in first aid and acute herbal medicine, something that is not normally covered in herbal medicine training courses. The empirical nature of the formulae that she developed in her acute Western herbal medicine practice, with for-mulae treating particular medical conditions, reflects the empirical side of Western herbal medicine more generally. Experience has led to the development of knowledge of particular herbs used for particular con-ditions, even if these have been more and more influenced by rational scientific thought as well as diverse approaches that practitioners have brought into their practices.

While taking an empirical approach had led to notable successes, EP's engagement with Western herbal medicine had been without what a later herbalist will call a "theory of cure" that could help her to understand the root causes of illnesses, as well as their solutions. Reflecting on her lack of consistent success with skin conditions, EP even says that "... and I didn't know why I'd got it right and I didn't know why I'd got it wrong ..." It was this lack of clarity that led EP to study Chinese medi-cine. While the success of much of her empirical approach to patients may have provided the energy necessary to maintain her practice, it is her engagement with Chinese medicine that is arguably more enchanting for her. Although it took EP a while to be drawn into Chinese medicine, she eventually found the simultaneous simplicity and complexity of Chinese medicine to be "amazing", with its references to nature and patterns making sense to her and her patients. While synthesising the traditional with the modern in specific practices is the hallmark of Chinese medicine in contemporary China[4], EP synthesises Chinese medicine and Western herbal medicine in her UK practice, producing further plurality. In particular, EP found that Chinese medicine theory meant that diagnosis easily led to treatment. Rather than living herbs being enchanting for EP, it is Chinese medicine's theory of cure, with its direct link between diagnosis and treatment, its respect of patterns and language that engages with metaphors drawn from nature, as being enchanting. The sensual nature of Chinese medicine can be seen in any discussion of its theory or practice. For example, EP talks of "wind-cold" and "wind-heat" and of "phlegm". These are phrases that one feels as much as one thinks about. A look at any discussion on the yin and yang of Chinese medicine also reveals the primacy of the senses: yin has the qualities, for example, of being docile, dark, earthy, cloudy, soft, moist, slow, and cold, while yang is seen as dominant, bright, sunny, hard, dry, fast, and hot. It is not possible to study or practise Chinese medicine without engaging the senses. Its theory necessarily engages with empirical experience. It is this meeting of sensual empiricism with theory that may be seen as the logical end of EP's narrative trajectory that started with the empiricism of developing her own Western herbal medicine formulae. This was followed by the identification of her own lack of theoretical knowledge, with EP eventually studying Chinese medicine and then easily integrating the chalk and cheese of Chinese medicine and Western herbal medicine in her practice.

JK

Entryways

JK's introduction to herbs came from her family:

> Well, I suppose it all started with my mother and grandmother, both Italian and always using simple herbs like elder and chamomile, marshmallow, those are the herbs that my grandmother used to know and pick, although she didn't know anything about herbal

medicine, but it's still used in Italy, in a very simple way. So we always had elderflower tea made in hot milk when we were, when we had colds and had to sweat it out and so I'd always had that in the background.

Visiting an exhibition on indigenous North Americans was also important:

> ... I suppose when I was about eighteen, I went to an exhibition on North American Indians and was fascinated by the medicinal side of it, and actually bought a herbal, on the Chippewa Indian tribe, who treated again, very simply, with herbs. I was just fascinated to know that actually there was more to it than that ...

Hein Zeylstra and training: the rise of science and decline of physiomedicalism

JK went for an interview to study herbal medicine at the School of Herbal Medicine:

> ... then I started the course, went for an interview at Leicester with Fred Fletcher-Hyde, and at the time we really, we didn't really have any smart clothes or, we lived in utter poverty, me and my friend, so we had to buy tights and dresses up on the way, and make sure our nails were clean and everything, because we heard that was what he was interested in, personal appearance, and just talking to you. And he was quite taken by both of us and allowed us on the course, so that was the interview process ...

JK started her studies in 1979 and finished in 1985, having two children during the course. Hein Zeylstra was the principal of the School of Herbal Medicine and brought in a more science-based approach:

> And yeah we did a lot of pharmacognosy actually, a lot of examination skills later on as well, so and Hein's wonderful *materia medica* lectures, I mean we just, that was the, probably the best thing actually and everyone hung on to his every word, because he's such a good speaker, and such a good, he convinced, certainly convinced

you that what scientific knowledge there was, he could bring it over and actually convince us that we needed scientific basis where we could. So he discounted quite a few herbs actually that were traditionally used because there's no science behind them so, I remember he was, he wasn't really into *Hypericum*, "Oh, *Hypericum* doesn't work," because at the time there was no, there was nothing on it really ...

Hein disapproved of "polypharmacy", where many herbs were used in each prescription:

He was trying two things, to get people out of polypharmacy, using simples, and knowing where they were with the medicines, what action they would have. He said, how can you tell, if there's thirty herbs in a bottle, you can't tell what's going on. And to some extent it's true, you can't, it's very difficult and so he was very much into using simples ...

Hein anticipated that understanding herbs as pharmacological agents would be required:

... he'd obviously use three or four herbs in a mix, but he'd say, this is your nervine, this is your, and then see if that nervine works. So you can understand the principle ... But he was just trying to re-educate people into thinking, look, try and look what's going on scientifically, rather than have a mishmash of, you know, you don't really know, because I think he foresaw that we were going to have to prove to Europe that our herbs worked scientifically ... in Europe, they, the pharmacists were, the pharmaceutical industry were the ones who governed herbs in Europe, and they were already looking at a herb, on its own, and what the action would be, so the first herbal pharmacopoeia came out in the late Seventies, early Eighties.

Before the School of Herbal Medicine established its own teaching clinic JK trained with a physiomedical practitioner:

... I used to go to her clinic ... every week and she was fantastic actually, she was really, really good ... She was incredibly interesting because she operated on a polypharmacy basis and although

I didn't, I never did the dispensing, she had a dispenser, we were just seeing patients, but looking at some of her stock bottles, they were mixtures of maybe three or four herbs together, for ease of dispensing, because she always used those together, so I know somebody, I remember she used to use *Vitex* with, and this is *Vitex* tincture, with *Chamaelirium* and, *Vitex and Chamaelirium* together, yeah, that's it, those two … Other ones she did were, always, always used *Echinacea, Baptisia, Phytolacca*, so strong immune mix really, that she'd then add other things to, and actually they do go well together, really, yeah. There were lots of others, she'd never use just one astringent, say you were treating the stomach, she'd use tiny amounts of lots of different ones, so my reasoning, my reckoning on the reasoning there was that you'd be using similar groups of herbs with slightly different actions, but if you wanted astringency, you'd get maybe 25% astringency from different ways and that sort of thing, so nervines would be mixed as well and I still tend to think in that way, although I don't use thirty herbs in my bottle, but I do tend to amalgamate certain actions that I want to bring out, rather than using a simple nervine, I'd use a group of them, so maybe two or three, yes.

After completing her studies JK worked as a clinical supervisor for Hein. She continued to use herbs that Hein considered didn't have sufficient scientific evidence behind them:

If, I suppose if it hadn't been for Hein, well he was, probably wasn't the only one, but he was so fervently against it, he used to say to me, oh, when I was teaching for him, he used to say, and I'd come up with this herb, and he'd say, why are you using that, and I'd say, well because it works, and he'd say, oh I forget, you were taught by ST, you poor thing, so, jokingly say that but …

The continuing influence of physiomedicalism on JK

Despite the waxing of science and the waning of physiomedicalism in her training, thirty years on, JK still finds physiomedicalism useful to her:

We'd been taught on a fairly pharmacological basis really, and not an awful, not a great deal of philosophy behind it, except for the physiomedical philosophy, which was kind of going out of fashion at the time, so they were half-heartedly teaching us, because it was the only thing that we had, but it was, I found it quite interesting actually and still consider it in my choice of herbs and when I'm looking at a person, not just purely from a pathological, clinical medicine point of view, I'll look laterally at them and try and figure out what they, what the balance of their tissue states are. So I look very much along the line of tissue states, so when I'm prescribing I think of herbs which are going to alter those tissue states, so alteratives, nervines, I mean everything does it to a certain extent, but triggering that change that's going to then help the body to regenerate and recuperate ... So the physiomedical thing was quite an influence, but we always took it with a pinch of salt, because some things have been disproved, that funny idea of the circulation and that, but I think some of the things still stand ...

JK gives some examples of how the physiomedical approach to tissue states influences her practice today:

So it's looking at whether you need to improve the circulation to an area to actually help relieve inflammation or, if you take basic inflammation, if it's very acute then you need to just calm it down a little bit, so you'd be using counterirritants, all of the counterirritants, you'd be using something cooling and there's enough circulation there to help, so you wouldn't particularly give anything that would dry the circulation out. And if it becomes sub-acute, or chronic, then obviously you need to think about getting that, almost challenge the body to react again, so that it can clear it. So that's the basis of really, of whether you're going to stimulate or relax, and I suppose you can use that term, in terms of nervines, or you can use it in terms of movement in the body, so that's basically it. And each type of tissue, whether it's a mucous membrane or the outer part of the skin, or a solid organ, has its own method of working in a sense, so mucous membranes, they like to produce mucus, what is it for? It's for protection, it's for lots of things, so you're looking at that, if that is breached in any way, then you're going to get the wrong kind of, if you like, toxins getting through, affecting tissues which aren't supposed to be affected, so whether it's the stomach, you need to think along the lines of, is the, are the tissue states conducive to getting things better?

Proper diagnosis

Some herbalists feel that Western herbal medicine is lacking a discipline-specific philosophy behind its approach to diagnosis. However, JK prefers the "proper diagnosis" of orthodox medicine:

> The Chinese is Chinese, it's rigid, it's this and that's it. With ours, we come from different strands, so our philosophy has kind of been a little bit watered down and a little bit elusive, and so elusive to some that they hanker for perhaps the Chinese way or the Ayurvedic way, and so they'll amalgamate that to help them perhaps diagnose, because they haven't really got involved in proper diagnosis. I like the proper diagnosis, I just love that, the actual physiological diagnosis and seeing things laterally ...

JK uses an orthodox medical approach to diagnosis, obtained by taking the case history and by physical examination:

> So when I see a patient now, I think case histories is by far the most important thing, I do like to examine the patient, and where necessary obviously send them for tests or, but I find the whole idea of diagnosis just such, such a pleasure. It's like being Columbo or somebody, it's just great. And I don't know if you play bridge or cards but you get dealt a pack of cards, a hand and when you pick it up you've no idea what's going to be in it but it's, but you can make something of it, and you can, and it's, and then playing out that hand is very exciting because you're making the most of what you've been given. So a patient comes and they've been handed, basically, a hand of cards, and it's, in their complex lives, things that, there are things that maybe they have to live with, maybe they've been dealt a lucky hand and just, so it's helping them really play it out to their best advantage. And obviously if someone comes with a particular condition or pathology, then you have to decide whether or not you can actually reverse that, or quite, and actually whether

they're able to reverse it themselves, because I find that they do tend to get themselves better, with a little bit of our help.

While she sees her approach as "orthodox" she also looks "laterally", beyond orthodox diagnosis, to identify what may be contributing to a patient's condition:

> ... you may come to the conclusion that they've got hardening of the arteries or something, arteriosclerosis, but you're also looking at the way they respond to stress, and the way they process their food, and so, yeah, it is, it's not just then giving them anti-lipids or whatever, it's actually looking at the whole digestive process, and stress levels and the stress brings up cholesterol ...

Three patients: "proper diagnosis" and physiomedicalism

JK describes a patient with digestive symptoms that she identified as being of nervous origin, mediated by the autonomic nervous system:

> ... she had a whole series of setbacks during childhood, psychologically, had actually come out of it quite well, but in some ways somatised some of the psychological problems ... digestive problems, so getting very, very bogged down in taking supplements, being told by this and that person that she had parasites, that she had candida, that, and that she needed, so this supplement and that supplement. And then in talking to her, I'd, I realised that actually, if she just let, if you could break in somewhere, that if she felt all right with herself, she was quite depressed, if she felt better in herself, then actually her physical problems would improve as well, without her getting too obsessive about the little bits and pieces, because the body does that, it's, and so I explained to her how it was linked with the autonomic nervous system, she understood everything I was telling her. I find it's partly an education, that you educate your patient, to understand what they're going through really. And she actually, she agreed that tackling predominately the nervous system, and a few simple measures with the diet and digestion, that that was the way forward. She gave me a big hug when she left and I think you quite often get that, you get just such a release

of the patients', actually just being listened to and has had actually a therapeutic boost, just by the consultation, I can't stress the importance enough really. And also making sure that you've got enough details, I'm quite thorough, but only what they want to tell me. I don't interrogate them.

Before he arrives, JK describes another patient to me. He is retired with a twenty-year history of sinusitis, frequent upper respiratory tract infections, and monthly chest infections. He takes antibiotics regularly. He also has hay fever, nasal polyps, a history of ear discharge, and is prescribed two types of inhalers. He is diabetic—he takes the drug metformin. He had prostate cancer three years ago, which was successfully treated by radiotherapy and his PSA tests are now normal.

During the consultation, he asked about saw palmetto for prostate health but JK suggests that for now, because his PSA levels are fine, it would be "better to take turmeric, it's very good for the prostate, anti-inflammatory, anti-growth". They talk about the herbal medicine he had been taking. She says that "It takes a little while to tone the mucous membranes," and that the herbs included are "to help with the airways, deal with inflammation, and breathe more easily. Making phlegm more liquid so it can come up more easily." JK then tests his lungs with a peak flow meter, testing three times. She listens to his chest with a stethoscope, asking him to breathe in and out with his mouth open. She then uses an otoscope to look in his ear, saying that "That must be a healed perforation." Next, she gets a tuning fork to test his hearing. She makes the tuning fork vibrate by squeezing and then releasing its two long ends simultaneously. She first tests his good side and then his bad side: she positions its base behind his ear on the mastoid process, asks him when he can hear it stop and then holds it in front of his ear and asks if he can hear it now. She then makes another tuning fork vibrate and places the base firmly against the top of his head and asks him if it sounds the same on both sides.

JK's prescription for him is made up of eleven herbs: *Grindelia camporum, Myrica cerifera*, the fruit and flowers of *Sambucus nigra, Echinacea angustifolia, Baptisia tinctoria, Hydrastis canadensis, Glechoma hederacea, Plantago sp, Ephedra sinica, Glycyrrhiza glabra, and Inula helenium*. She describes the prescription as including "some doubling up of actions but slightly different effects. *Glechoma* and *Plantago* are similar in action—tonics to the mucous membranes and for catarrh ..." The other herbs are included for their effect on the immune system, mucous membranes, for pain, for inflammation, for cough and for loosening a cough.

Considering another patient, who is here for the first time, JK asks him how she can help. He replies: "Something for depression really. Look at it holistically. Previously had felt melancholic for eighteen months. But I have accepted within myself that it is more than melancholy." He is taking antidepressants but is reducing the dosage. He had lost a business that employed twelve people. He then retrained as a paramedic, during which he was assaulted several times, since when he has had regular nightmares and has seen a counsellor. He is now working as a builder.

JK says, "You are in need of some sort of tonic?" He replies that "Yes, if there is a gentler, more rounded way of treating this, that is why I am here." JK replies that "Stress can affect the adrenal glands … we have uplifting herbs—nervous restoratives—help you with stress and concentration and energy."

She later suggests that as well as depression he has "PTSD really". He says that "Talking to you here I can put a front on, but inside there is not enough enthusiasm."

JK: "It sounds as if you have been quite hurt and you need to recover from that."

She measures his height and weight, then takes his pulse and blood pressure, which is a "bit high" before asking, "Would you like a bottle of medicine?"

He says yes and then she tells him about the herbs she will give him: *Schisandra* "works on adrenals and concentration", "some vervain and wood betony, a nervous restorative, traditional for fears and nightmares and pain but basically a nervous restorative, and some lime flowers, which have a calming effect on the heart and brings the blood pressure down a little bit, and also some Siberian ginseng to help with stamina. *Schisandra* is also an immune tonic, vervain also works through the digestive tract for detoxification. They have more than one action." He replies, "Like most things."

These three patients, the first one talked about, and the second two observed, suggest that orthodox medical knowledge and the influence of physiomedicalism sit well together in JK's practice. While a concern with the mediating power of the autonomic nervous system in human physiology is now basic medical knowledge, such a focus was central to physiomedicalism, which arose at the time when this system was being seriously investigated. Although both orthodox medicine and JK take this system seriously, JK's treatment of the digestive system by giving a range of medicinal agents that affect the nervous system is something that is generally not available to orthodox medicine. JK's comments on this patient also show the importance of the "therapeutic boost" of the consultation, a concern that was important in physiomedical practice. The second patient shows how orthodox diagnostic techniques of auscultation with a stethoscope, visualisation of the middle ear with an otoscope, and cranial nerve testing using tuning forks sit neatly next to a physiomedical approach seen in the use of polypharmacy, including in the "doubling up" of herbal actions. The second and third patients show how the medicines are chosen for particular tissues, organs or systems, for example, mucous membranes, the immune system, adrenals, and digestive tract. Although JK does mention bringing blood pressure down and treating inflammation, there is generally more attention paid to tissues, organs, and systems than there is directly to pathologies. It is the state of the various tissues that is addressed.

JK's wood

JK spends a lot of time in woodland with her family and dog, saying, "I just always wanted to pretend I lived there." She collects some herbs from woodland:

> … rosehips and hawthorn, yeah, mushrooms, I met John there once and he took me mushrooming, just by chance, he was actually picking rosehips, because I didn't know a thing about mushrooms so, yeah, so we used to go and get oyster mushrooms and, so yeah, it was more for the therapeutic nature of the woods, rather than for the herbs that you get out of it, I just really felt it was just beneficial to health, woodlands …

She explains its attraction:

> … walking through trees, just the variations in it as well, where you might get an open bit that is rather meadow-like … very grassy and thick, thick, trees, where you can get lost in them and bluebells and all the sort of different layers that you get in woodland, it's just, it's endless, endless really charm and interest. And little brook that

goes through it, and all the different plants that you get growing in different areas. So yeah, so I thought, I might get a wood.

Eventually she did buy a wood, where she spends time with her family and friends, often camping overnight:

> ... we're actually going to go birch-sapping there soon, it'll have to be soon because otherwise it'll be too late, I'm just waiting for some weather really to be able to go down there ... So I've got two plots, and put a little, or quite a big shed actually, probably about, nearly the size of this room, but it looks really small there, just storage and shelter. And, yeah, I just go there and do all sorts of things, it's ancient woodland and a lot of it ... chestnut coppice and oak and hazel, and then some areas are plantation, so I've got some planta- tion as well, Scots pine, so it's just really lovely ... I did some brash- ing, that's why I took the photos, so I had a reference magazine and showed how I'd done the deer fencing with the brash ... To protect it from, the coppice, so they're a bit naughty, the deer, and when they get hungry they'll eat anything, even chestnut ... we did do a, with Flo and another herbalist, we did a plant survey and I aim to do that every year ...

However, although she loves her wood, for JK it is not easier to be a herbalist with a wood than without one:

> No, I'd be able to, no, I'd be able to be a herbalist, you don't need a wood to be a herbalist, and in a sense I didn't buy it because I'm a herbalist, I bought it because I love woodlands and I like to play in woods, so it's more, that's why I'm finding it hard, I should be con- necting it more, and I could, but it's pure diversion, yeah.

She also loves making things from wood:

> And wood, I just love wood, working with wood, so I'm learning all these woodland skills, so I'm going, on Sunday actually, to a bodgers' meeting ... bodgers are chair makers and they gener- ally turn, so they have, traditionally they have these hand turning lathes and I've made myself a shave horse, which is, it's a bit like a vice, which you sit on, so you have the thing that traps the wood in

there, and you sit astride it and you operate it with pedals, so it's on a pivot and then you use a shave, a spoke shave or a drawer knife and you can carve wood, and it's so easy and so beautiful and you can carve, you can sort of make, well I made a swill, you know one of those baskets made out of chestnut and, shown how to do that, and it's such fun just doing, I just love making things really.

She also loves to make herbal medicines:

> … if I had the time I'd make tinctures as well but I love making the creams, making tablets, and that kind of thing, I think it's the hands on jobs, and all herbalists love to do it … so I just sit there, listening to the radio, making slippery elm tablets, when I have, and just relaxing. And the patients love them, because they're just pure slippery elm and they're, they suck them and they melt in their mouth, but that, that's quite laborious but I don't mind taking time over things like that. I make my own creams, apart from *calendula* cream, which I can't, I just can't get on with the resins in calendula …

JK discusses her favourite herb, which is a tree. Like her herbal prescriptions, that combine more herbs than other herbalists might use, she selects a medicinal plant which offers up many parts as medicine:

> I think I'd have the elder tree, yeah. Because it's, you can use any part of it, I, it's useful for a whole range of different things, from constipation to arthritis, to immune function, to catarrh, to, so that one is quite useful …

Reflection on JK

The knowing and picking of herbs and their use as medicine by JK's family members was an important step on her way to becoming a herbalist. Now JK spends time in woodland with her own family. The entryway of visiting an exhibition on indigenous North Americans and reading a book on Chippewa medicine and traditions[184] has continuing relevance for JK, partly because she enjoys the sensual pleasures of woodwork and medicine making, but also because she has adopted a clinical approach that includes an appreciation of physiomedicalism, which was conceived in North America and, as previously described, grew out of Thomsonianism, which borrowed from indigenous North American *materia medica* and knowledge. In fact, the armorial ensign of the NIMH includes an indigenous North American figure holding herbs used in ritual purification, with the NIMH in the UK being a professional body of physiomedical practitioners up until the 1980s.

While physiomedicalism is an influence on JK, she has shed much of its theoretical considerations, for example, of sthenic and asthenic constitutions, and of pulse and tongue diagnosis, but has kept a concern for tissue states, with her prescriptions mostly addressing organs and tissues rather than diseases. There is less theory in her practice than past physiomedicalists might have drawn on. This may be due to the influence of her training, particularly in the primacy accorded to science by Hein Zeylstra and other teachers, and by the pleasure that she gets from the "proper diagnosis" of the case history and physical examination that is drawn directly from orthodox medicine.

The material body, with its organs and tissues, is the object of her treatment. The other materiality that she is involved with, besides the materiality of her patients' bodies, is that of her wood. She says that she doesn't need a wood to be a herbalist. She bought it for the pure pleasure of playing in woods. This suggests that spending time in nature may be a powerful sensual experience for JK, maybe even enchanting, but that it is not necessary for her to be the herbalist that she is. The wood does not obviously cross over into practice, even if it does cross over into her. Practice and living plants run side by side for JK, although she does say that "I should be connecting it more, and I could, but it's pure diversion, yeah."

Reflection on TE, CP, EP, and JK

The entryways of these four herbalists highlight the influence of family, childhood aspirations and the experience of seeing the benefit of taking herbal medicines for themselves and others. The narrative of TE comes closest to Weber's idea that rational thought can "master everything through calculation". Thus databases, randomised controlled trials (RCTs), and peer-reviewed articles rather than traditional knowledge and energetics are central to TE's practice, even if the lack of scientific knowledge of herbs means that arriving at a prescription can be a "slightly frustrating process". However, the lack of evidence of enchantment by plants does not mean that enchantment is not present in herbalists' engagements with orthodox science. Bennett's[50] position that rationality itself is the first wonder of the Kantian world and may be full of enchantment can be seen in the case of randomised controlled trials. While existing as the "gold standard" of evidence, RCTs may be seen as alchemical in that control and randomisation are invoked as devices to transmute the complexities of human subjects and an intervention into certainties.[185] Such a structure may be enchanting even if reduced uncertainty is inversely proportional to the ability to reproduce trial results in real world medical practices.[186] Additionally, science has a relatively recent history of looking to the enchanting and "wondrous" processes of life, while avoiding sentimentalising, as located in the work of E. O. Wilson, James Lovelock, and Carl Sagan.[187] TE's case also demonstrates how his engagement with science is a political act, making him acceptable to the GPs, with whom he exists in a dependent relationship. However, the case shows that the congruence of TE's way of doing herbal medicine with the GPs' way of doing orthodox medicine fits so well that TE calls his own professional identity into question.

Similarly, the remaining three cases do not reveal enchanted meetings between humans and living plants in their entryways or in the rest of their narratives. However, hints of enchantment are seen in relationship to the personal experience of taking herbal medicines, in the attraction of theory and in the pleasure of woodland. Thus, CP particularly relates to *Chamaelirium luteum* through her experience of taking it as a medicine and through prescribing it to patients. Her knowledge of this herb is largely based on her experience of taking it and prescribing it, even though her training in Chinese medicine encourages her to think more theoretically. EP, on the other hand, moves in the other direction, away from the empiricism of her Western herbal medicine training and towards the sensual theory of Chinese medicine that provides easier correspondences between diagnosis and treatment than she found in Western herbal medicine. And JK keeps her practice, and the "pure diversion" of spending time in her wood, as separate entities, although she hints at some connection.

We will now look to those visible entryway herbalists who identify, in their narratives, the importance of knowing their herbal medicines as living plants. This ranges from simply knowing living herbs through spending time with them in various ways, to the development of more formal methodologies.

SB

Entryways

SB traces his involvement with herbs back to when he was three or four years old and used to spend time with his grandmother at weekends.

> So I think from that age I can remember every weekend being told about all the different uses of plants, weeds and things and go for a walk in the hedgerows and things. So I was always absolutely in awe of plants and what they could do. And the scents and the smells and thinking about it now, talking about it to you all the scents of the lemon balm has come flooding back when I think of my grandmother in the garden and what she was doing there.

At school, he loved chemistry and became interested in plant chemistry. He grew about 150 herbs in his parents' garden, knowing them through-out their life cycles. He dried the herbs and stored them but didn't know what to do with them. When he studied for a chemistry degree, and later a PhD, and took on a lecturing and research career, he left herbs behind him. Much later, when looking for an alternative career, he discovered Simon Mills and Kerry Bone's *Principles and Practice of Phytotherapy* and said to himself, "OK, I'm going to be a phytotherapist!"

While studying for his degree in herbal medicine SB also worked for a cancer consultancy that gave patients access to complementary medicine. In his role he interviewed cancer patients about their health. When he graduated he set up practice, with about 70% of his patients being cancer patients. He gets referrals from other practitioners, includ-ing herbalists, nutritionists, naturopaths, and medical doctors.

Orthodox, but beyond

SB spends up to two hours on a first consultation to get a full case history. He covers the presenting complaint, past medical history—"because that's essential for me to understand what's led to where we are today", before looking at drug history, family history, social history, and diet.

> And then I'll say because I work as a holistic practitioner I'll then spend the last ten or fifteen minutes of the consultation asking

questions about different body systems such as the heart, lungs, digestion, nervous system, just so I can get an overall picture of how you're working as a whole person and to identify any weaknesses or imbalances in the body.

Most of his cancer patients have already been "prodded and poked so much by people who are far more qualified than me" that he doesn't often do physical examinations. However he will:

> … check the blood pressure, look in their eyes if they've got any problems with high blood pressure … but obviously if I've got someone who's got a pain in their tummy I'll do a full abdominal examination or if somebody's dizzy I'll do a full neurological examination.

While this suggests an orthodox medical approach, SB finds that this has limitations:

> … I think the conventional diagnosis is absolutely brilliant because it's a tool but it's only a tool. It's not the only tool. And I think it's an important, an integral part of my practice but it's not enough on its own because I think then again you just get, you get a symptom. You're not getting beneath that to see what the cause is so any medicine you give is only going to treat the symptom. It's not going to treat the cause. It's like if you've got someone with eczema you wouldn't just give a cream for it. You'd give something internally as well. I would, that's where the conventional medicine fails. It only does topical presentation, which doesn't do much but you need to actually get to the imbalances below in the biochemistry in the body. So yeah, it's definitely an important part of my practice the biomedical model but I think also as well understanding more holistically what's going on and analysing where homeostasis has broken down in the body, where there's an imbalance, where something isn't working as it should be. And also as well a little bit of energetics as well working out if the patient is hot or cold or very astringent or whatever just helps sometimes to get a feel for what herbs are going to work perhaps slightly better for them than others.

He sees his patients as people rather than as diseases:

> I treat the person. I think if you try and treat just the cancer it's such a reductionist thing to do. You're not going to have good successes and that's one of the reasons I think why conventional medicine fails so much because it's only treating one symptom rather than the whole cause beneath that. So anyway I see, when I see a cancer patient ... so I do a full case history and go through all the different body systems and often identify weaknesses. A lot of my breast cancer patients I think have thyroid problems, which has a link there with the cancer, so definitely see that. I would say my approach is, because of my training in chemistry and biochemistry and working in a hospital, it's, some of my point of views are very medical based. So I will diagnose people in the orthodox sense so if a patient came to me for this and had polycystic ovarian syndrome with hypothyroidism as well so I would see it in that term rather than in energetic terms or anything like that. So very much a conventional diagnosis but I would go beyond that and with other, this patient came in obviously problems with their endocrine system, problems with their immune system and everything like that. So I'd go through the whole person and I wouldn't just treat the polycystic ovarian syndrome or just the thyroid. I would treat other things that were going on as well in my general prescription as well.

SB sees his patients as all being very different in terms of what they need phytochemically and constitutionally. He works his prescriptions out for each patient rather than using pre-existing formulae.

> ... I think people's energetics, their constitutions are different. Now I always say to my patients, non-cancer patients particularly I've got ten patients with the same cancer in the same place, exactly the same presentation, treat them (with the same prescription) and I'll get different results for all of them. And I think that's been the epigenetics. I think the way that people deal with pharmacological compounds differs so greatly because we're all genetically, tend to be different. So I, that's why I tend to really work my prescriptions from first principles if I can, just try and work on what I think will work for that particular patient ...

Root causes—onions, triggers, and kernels

SB seeks to look at the whole body and treat the different layers of the problem:

> ... I also think that, I would say that, to people when I'm treating them, treating you is like, it's like peeling an onion. In fact you treat one layer then there's something else underneath and you keep on going down until you get to the nugget of the problem.

SB needs a long case history in order to get enough depth of understanding of the patient, often identifying stressors in his cancer patients:

> ... if I don't look into enough depth at what's going on I can't possibly work out what's going on, particularly with past medical history which is often very convoluted in cancer patients, well lots of stresses and lots of strains. It's not until you dig into that you find out that's the reason. With all my cancer patients I'll say definitely there's been a major stress in two years prior to diagnosis that's led to the cancer developing, well maybe the cancer taking off and growing. So I find it's very key to find the cause of all that trigger so it's very much quite a Sherlock Holmes way of going, delving through the past medical history trying to work out what's been going on and the causes and things.

He then seeks to treat the stressor:

> Well I think I find it, well it depends what the stressor is. If there's a viral infection or something like that I might use antivirals just to try and get rid of the trigger that might have led to the cancer from growing, for example. Or if they're very stressed then that will show to me their immune system is down and work on their immune system. Or if that stress was terrible at work because their boss was awful and still going on, say to them, well you need to try to change your lifestyle, work out if actually if staying with that job is the best thing for you or not and consider if getting a transfer or a new job elsewhere. So I think it's very, again it's, it's not just in my herbal prescription it's in the whole lifestyle thing as well I think it's important to realise that.

Identifying triggers for illness is useful for SB because it allows him to seek to reverse the process that led to the illness:

> It's a, that system's been used for a long time with autoimmune diseases working out the two or three triggers for autoimmune diseases, then working to go backwards in time and reverse the process of that. So I feel that's quite useful. At least we've identified them. Sometimes I can't. There's nothing I can do. I can't think of any way of doing anything with them. But at least I know they're there and at least I've talked about it with a patient and often I find patients will come back to me the next consultation and they'll say, I've been really thinking about this and I realise what effect it's having on my life. And I've gone and talked to so and so about this and I feel that's cleared …

This also applies to his cancer patients:

> I like to work out what is going on, mentally, physically and spiritually … [the cancer] is just something that is going on there and there is reasons why the cancer is there but I see them as a whole person and work out, I dig very carefully to try and work out, because particularly with cancer there are five or six triggers for a normal cell to become a cancerous cell, a lot of those are environmental or psychological events, if you can work out what they are, work to reverse them, then there is a chance you can make the cancer less aggressive … certainly you can make things better.

He looks to Ayurvedic medicine for support for his approach of "going back to the kernel":

> But I think, I do think a lot of medical conditions are due to unresolved issues from the past. There's been emotional traumas and things and it has an effect and looking at [Ayurvedic] medicine they say that there's six or seven stages to disease … then gradually it builds up to the macro world sort of thing then. So I think if you can reverse that and look, go backwards then you can actually reverse things, far better, far more long-term than otherwise so I think it's the opposite of Western medicine where you can, you're

just touching the outer layer, not going back to the kernel of what actually triggered this in the first place.

In an observed consultation SB treats a male patient, P, who has ME and whose symptoms are moving more and more towards fibromyalgia, and who also has prostatitis. SB says to the patient:

> Let's go back to when you originally had your illness triggered … when your immune system was activated.

He identifies two episodes of gastrointestinal infection as being triggers for the ME and says:

> … as the bowel is a problem … I do wonder if things like prostatitis are linked with that because of the sheer proximity of the bowel, having some sort of leaky gut, having some transference around the gut through the gut and out the other side, leaky urothelium … epidymitis fits in with that picture … the bowel has obviously set off some sort of immune reaction.

He talks about the patient's appendectomy that he had ten years before developing ME:

> … the appendix is a good reservoir for bowel bacteria so prone to bowel problems if have appendix removed, bowel bacteria an essential part of the body, without it the enterocytes can't function properly, they die …, they are as much a part of our body as any of our cells are …. That is very key, having your appendix out.

Thus, in addition to prescribing herbs that act as nerve tonics and treat pain and fatigue, he also includes the Ayurvedic herb *Andrographis* as a tonic for the gut, even though the gut symptoms have long passed. He says to the patient:

> There is a lot going on, trying to hit everything at once is almost impossible, it's like the old onion idea, work on one layer and gradually get down to the nugget. To mix my analogies it's trying to find that grain that has caused the pearl to grow around it.

SB gets a tub of herbal tablets made of *Andrographis*, *Echinacea*, and holy basil and lets P smell them. "Wow," responds P. "Yes," says SB, "that's the holy basil." They sit silently for a long moment, breathing in the aroma.

Feelings for people and plants

A lot of SB's patients have stage 4 cancers. He feels that his treatments help with their quality of life:

> ... and yes they will die at some point but they'll die at a time when they're a bit more ready for it ..., they've got to the journey where they've actually got to a stage where they can actually accept the death rather than it being inflicted on them.

However, remissions do occur:

> ... there's been a few cases, probably about ten, fifteen over the years where there's been a complete remission. The cancer's gone. And that's, that happens anyway so whether it's actually anything to do with me and the herbs who knows? I wouldn't claim that. But certainly it's done something, the process, they've changed their lifestyle, got rid of the stress, done something that's changed the environment that let the cancer grow and it's gone. I wish there were more of those but there are some and there are, they are abso-lute real wow, amazing. It makes me feel really good about what I do then.

SB loves plants and feels that knowing living plants through their life cycles helps develop intuition that benefits his patients:

> I love plants. I love all plants. I think they're amazing beings. I see them as fellow beings, I just, I mean all of them. I really am. They're living factories. They're just absolutely wonderful what they can do. They can do, they're a lower life form supposedly. They can do much more than a lot of higher life forms can do quite frankly. So yeah, I, before I use herbs, most of my herbs where I can I've grown them so it's like I've bought the seed where I can, grown them as the seedlings and the plants into other plants, harvested them so

I know them. I feel in order to know a herb properly you have to have really gone through the stages with it to understand what it's about which is very, totally against what you might think from a scientific point of view. But I think you need to do that and I feel if you know that herb then you know how it's going, who it's going to be useful with in a person … So there is a huge intuition and I think that does come from knowing the herb. I don't, people who treat herbs just as the phytochemicals in a bottle I think that's just so very, a dead way of looking at it because I think herbs are more than that. There is something else as well. There is some, there is a life force, a vitality in there as well that's, that you need to know about, to understand what the herb's good for.

SB is in awe of the herbs in his garden:

It's one of the most magical things I can do is to go in my herb garden. It's so grounding and no pun intended but it's that sense of majesty, of awe, of being around them. There's a certain, per-haps I'm imagining it just because I want to imagine it but there's a sense of magnificence there. There's something about them that's just absolutely, it's absolutely awe inspiring. I can't think of any other way of putting it. I just, I'm in awe of the herbs. I just, I bow down to them. I feel very humbling in being able to use them, how to help people.

He dries some of the herbs from his garden for his patients, loving how his senses appreciate them:

I do dry them so I will use them for herb, for teas for people and it's nice. I love things like marshmallow leaf so you're, you dry it yourself and it will be a beautiful silvery colour which you buy and it tends to be a bit dull browny, yellowy colour and not particularly very nice but you dry it yourself and it's beautifully aromatic. And raspberry leaf when you dry it yourself you just open the bag and it smells of fresh raspberries. It's beautiful. So it's the whole, all the senses get involved in it, which I think it's essential, so yeah. So I couldn't be without my herb garden. I would never be able to not have a garden.

He needs this contact with plants to be able to practise:

> I think it's so important to be around I think living herbs. I don't think I could practise without that connection. I think it's essential for my practice.

He also has contact with plants through dispensing his medicines:

> I think that it is the life that is in the herbs that keeps me going. I love handling them, fresh herbs, dried herbs, even the tinctures, I am passionate about the tablets even though they are tablets, smelling them, it is a very sensual experience. A lot of people get bored dispensing, but I just love it 'cos I just love looking at them, checking the quality of them, that sort of thing. It's rewarding. I don't think I could be a doctor in a hospital prescribing, it would be too soulless …

One of his favourite herbs is *Echinacea angustifolia*:

> I love it and it's an obvious one. I love *Echinacea*. I think it's a beautiful plant. I love everything about it and I love it as a medicinal herb actually. It's so, so useful. It has so many different activities. It's not the herb I use the most at all but it's one that I know if I use it, it will work. And I love *Echinacea* and I love growing it. I love the *Echinacea angustifolia*. I think it's beautiful. I love it more and more. The more vibrant and showy *purpurea*, actually, and its beautiful sword-like leaves and the softness of the silver leaves and the purple flowers and the beautiful seed heads, the spiky seed heads and the lovely snaky roots. So I just think it's beautiful. It has to be *Echinacea angustifolia*.

Reflection on SB

As a boy who was interested in chemistry and then plant chemistry it is not surprising that SB should find a home amongst a profession that has increasingly engaged with science. This can be seen in his clinical approach that includes orthodox medicine rather than leaves it behind.

SB's entryway experience of spending time with his grandmother in her garden is not one that talks of being "called" by plants or of having conversations with plants. But spending time in his grandmother's garden is a beginning that engaged his senses over time, particularly seen in the beauty, scents, and touch of plants. This entryway "continues" into his practice in that knowing plants throughout their life cycle generates a familiarity with living herbs that helps him to select the most useful herbs for his patients.

As a child he was "in awe" of the herbs in his grandmother's garden, and as an adult he is "in awe" of the "magnificence" of the herbs in his own garden. Importantly, he needs the experience of this contact with plants in order to practise herbal medicine. It sustains him: "I don't think I could practise without that connection." This sustaining energy may be seen as a sensual-affective energy that helps him to treat patients who are often seriously ill. While he does have other strategies in place, such as meditation and monthly sessions with a psychotherapist who also offers talking help to medical doctors, the inseparability of SB from his herbs—"I don't think I could be a doctor in a hospital prescribing, it would be soulless"—points to a meeting of sorts.

For SB it is essential to look for "root causes", for "triggers", to peel back "the layers of the onion", to get to the "kernel" of the problem. He seeks to go beyond symptomatic management, to find the "nugget" and treat that, even if that involves going back in time.

How could this desire be related to plants? Deleuze and Guattari[141] suggest that "arborescent" thinking, the "tree model", is the model on which Western thought is grounded. The tree grows from a seed, with a trunk, which branches out, growing and spreading upwards. The phenomenon of the tree is always traceable back to the seed. This thinking, where an origin is always sought, has the consequence of setting up oppositions: what is the cause of the patient's illness? What is not? One position is favoured over another. This thinking is, of course, not particular to Western herbal medicine, or to SB, but is it a coincidence that herbalists, who use plants, often seem to look further "back" than those practising orthodox medicine? SB looks beyond the diagnosis of cancer or eczema or ME/fibromyalgia, even travelling back through time to treat the trigger.

SB is not the only herbalist who spends time with living plants. Herbalists, as we shall see, experience them through time, touch, work, smell, and beauty. Being in contact with herbs, which may be followed from flowers to leaves to branches to trunks and roots and seeds, may partly explain the desire to get to the origin of conditions for their patients.

FD

Entryways

FD ran a smallholding.

> ... right from when the children were very little, we'd had animals
> ... We had zero-grazed goats, we had chickens, we had pigs. And it
> was all really so that we could provide cheap food for the children,
> and food that we knew what had been fed to it, and where it had
> been, and what had happened with it. We weren't vegetarian, so the
> animals were part of that. I had one son, who was allergic to cow's
> milk, so we had the goats, and of course goats are universal foster
> mothers, and you can use goat's milk to feed almost anything. The
> other problem with goats is they're either dead or alive, there's not
> really any in-between, they don't do ill. So what would happen is,
> if there was a problem with the goats, it would be very expensive
> because you'd have to call the vet in, and in the end, I started off by
> reading a herbal handbook, *The Farm and Stable*, by the French lady,
> Juliet de Bairacli Levy, who is now dead. I understand she died,
> I think she died about eight, ten years ago. And I read her book, and
> the way she talked about rearing animals, and, by inference, rearing
> children made a lot of sense. So that was the sort of introduction.

While continuing to have an interest in animal welfare FD initially studied a one-year introductory course in herbal medicine. While studying
this course, which had a biomedical orientation, she became "bogged
down in DNA", fascinated by the work of Watson and Crick and eventually decided not to study to be a veterinarian but to complete her
professional herbal medicine studies.

"Up against authority"—professional life and statutory regulation

During FD's career in herbal medicine, she has felt "up against authority" in her professional life. This started during her training where she
observed that some students were favoured over others:

> ... you became very aware that you didn't upset people, because
> if you did, you might not pass your exams. It was that bad, and I
> wasn't, it wasn't me being paranoid, I know from talking to a lot of
> colleagues over the years, that actually that was their experience as

well. If you weren't in, you weren't in, and you were likely to not pass your exams ...

FD, along with five others, made a formal complaint:

> So my political career started quite early, and it wasn't particularly pleasant.

She viewed the university delivery of herbal medicine training as a progressive move, because she saw it as "taking away the personalities".

Later she worked at a CAM clinic where she identified poor management practices and also found that some conditions were not being adequately diagnosed:

> I like to see things done right, or how I perceive right. I like to see things done in particular ways with particular processes. I like to see processes in place, so that if the people change, the processes are still there ... But basically, what I discovered was that there were things not in place, which meant that actually this whole set-up was dodgy. Not necessarily intentionally, it just hadn't been done properly ... So that, one of the consequences of that was that it made me very unpopular, and the herbal medicine was fine, but I started to find that patients were being sidelined to other practitioners, not herbalists, but other practitioners, so they were being diverted away from, which was a bit disconcerting. And the other thing was, I was getting patients coming the other way who were turning out to be seriously ill, because other practitioners were not picking up, they weren't doing the diagnosis that we'd been trained to do. So patients were coming, this approach hasn't worked. This hasn't, and then I'd be saying, no it won't work because actually this patient needs to be having medical treatment because there's a real medical problem here.

Later she worked at another clinic, where she identified conflicts of interest:

> ... none of the people on the board of directors could actually claim to be completely impartial. Every single person had a vested interest in what was going on. And the documentation simply had not been put in place properly.

FD also trained in another therapeutic discipline, one that is often used to support cancer patients.

> I then came back and worked for a while ... but again, the bloody politics, oh it was awful. I had something like eighty patients, in the end, over a period of two years, and you were working with people with cancer. And because [this therapy] tends to be the last resort, it ought to be the first, it ought to be the first thing that anybody does ... If a person with cancer at the very first indication of having cancer does intensive dietary intervention, and intensive therapy and sustains that, it, you can bring the body to the point where it can turn the cancer around. That, without a doubt, that is true. The problem was the people that I had come to me were terminal.

She found that patients were coming to her from other practitioners who were wrongly diagnosed, or poorly treated or not under the care of an oncologist.

> ... and then realised that I was getting people coming to me who had been under other practitioners, and I was doing their assessments, and they were coming to me in crisis, a lot of them. And it was, OK, but why are you doing this? And why are you doing that? You've got this going on, that going on, why are you doing those things? That was what the practitioner said I could do. Well, not sure that that's actually appropriate, and there were all sorts of things, again as a medical herbalist, people that had been working with them before were nutritionists. Nutritionists are not expected to do diagnostics, so they were putting people on a therapy and there was no obligation on them to check some of the diagnostic stuff. So I had patients coming to me, and there is an obligation on me, to check the diagnostics. And I was finding that, just as an example, there was one woman, who had been told she had myeloma, and when I went through all the details, she didn't have myeloma at all, she didn't even have cancer. And she'd been put on the [this treatment], which involves using thyroid and Lugol's, which ups your metabolic rate. When she came to me she had hyperthyroidism. And she was really, really, really ill and she was being told by the practitioner, it's all in your mind, it's psychological. And she'd lost huge

amounts of weight, she was in a terrible state. And we did turn it round, we turned it round, I wrote a long letter, a long report, a long summary to her GP, said this is what's going on, this is why she's like this. She's not paranoid, she's, this is why she's like it, this is what needs to happen. And with the GP and a herbalist who was more local to her than I was, we turned it full round. But she was very sick for a very long while. And I was getting people ringing me up, they'd been to the [overseas] clinic, and the doctors are supposed to be supervising them. And one phone call, the chap, I could hear his wife screaming in the background, and he was telling me, and he said, "I'm with, we can't get hold of the clinic, they won't give us any help." "And I said, is that, what is the noise?" He said, "It's my wife, she's in agony," and I said, "How long's that been going on?" "For, a day." "I said, "I'm sorry, but even if it's a healing crisis, if your wife is in that much pain, there's no healing going on, you have to get the medics in," and they got the A&E in. I got into trouble for that. I said, "Well, I'm sorry but you cannot allow, there's no way that that woman is doing any healing work at all, she's in too much pain." [A man] rang me, and wanted a herbalist to look after him, he was staying in London. And I said, "Well, OK, fine, who, because again, you have to have an oncologist on board, who are you seeing?" "I'm not seeing." "OK, I can't take you on unless you are. How are you monitoring what's going on?" I didn't hear any more for a little while, and he came back again, it was about 18 months, and he said, "Well, I've done the therapy, and I'm cured." And I said, "OK, so did you see an oncologist?" "No." "How do you know you're cured?" "Well, I've done the therapy."

Her concerns eventually led FD to withdraw from practising this therapy.

As well as the above institutional and political conflicts, a larger authority was also problematic for her. This was the possibility of the statutory regulation of herbalists:

Very early on, almost within a year, a couple of years of qualifying, I remember going to one of the conferences and Philip saying it was like the Sword of Damocles hanging over our heads, and actually he was quite right, that is exactly how it feels, that is exactly how this whole registration process feels, that at some point, this sword is going to drop down and that's going to be it. And I think that's been my whole experience of the political thing.

In particular, FD was concerned that statutory regulation might lead to the scrutiny of her practice:

Is somebody going to turn up with a clipboard, and start tick boxing? How I'm working, my, how I operate my dispensary, whether I'm doing my CPD ...

FD reflects that her involvement with politics has dominated much of her career as a practitioner:

Yeah, I know, it's what I do. It's what I've done all my life, stood up and said, no this isn't right, and then get shot down. And I'm just, even just talking to you now, I'm thinking to myself, where's the herbal medicine in all this, because actually it's all politics, and that's been my career.

Finding home in a community

FD lives with her husband near a Christian religious community, having moved there when their children grew up. FD goes to most of the services—four prayer sessions per day plus meditation. FD looks after the library, prunes the apple trees, and makes curtains and some clothes.

FD has had a religious awareness from a young age:

There's always been an awareness of other, right from being very small. I come from, I had a very dysfunctional family, very violent early life. And I think there was always this awareness that there had to be something else other than this.

FD's religious relationship is with Jesus rather than with the Church:

I know that I have a personal relationship with the man that died on the cross 2,000 years ago. That's my personal belief, it isn't anything more elaborate than that, because anything more elaborate than that is man-made. All the theology that's gone on for 2,000 years has just created total confusion, people don't understand and they get, they then get to the point where they're fighting over what the interpretation of this word or that word is. And that's not, that defeats the whole object. Defeats the whole point of it. So for me, and if you talk to somebody about that, and you say to them, well this is my personal belief, but I can't say to you, go to that church or that church, because whatever church you go to, it's flawed. It's a flawed system.

She had visited the religious community many years ago when Jesus spoke to her:

And what is even more astonishing, and which I didn't say at the time, was in 1992 when we came here as a parish group, originally, a very first visit here I sat in the church over there in tears because a voice in my head was saying this is your home, and I'm thinking, don't be, and I literally said to this little voice in my head, don't be so bloody stupid ... how can I be at home here? And then I thought about it and I thought, oh you silly thing, what the voice actually meant was it's your spiritual home, in other words, you come back here and touch base every so often. No that wasn't what the voice meant, the voice actually did mean *this* is my home, and that's been, that voice has been something that's been constant from the age of about three onwards, I've been aware of that.

A near-death accident, and knowing herbs differently

During a holiday to the Isle of Skye, on an Easter Sunday, FD had a serious accident, leading to a meeting with Jesus who told her that it was not her time to die and that she had more lessons to learn:

I fell down a mountain, I fell 200 odd feet, bounced apparently. But I actually, I slid down like that, and then tipped, and that initial tip is the only thing I can remember. Because from that point onwards, I went through the tunnel, I had a life review, as far as I was concerned I was dying, I wasn't going to, I wasn't going to survive, falling that far, I really wasn't anticipating coming to, basically.

And I don't know how, I think it took about three, four minutes, but it seemed like a very long time, but I don't, my husband, Arthur, says, you just literally bounced like this down the thing, which I'm laughing at but I don't suppose it was funny. And this great feeling of peace and light, and this voice that there was a life review. And this voice saying, it isn't your time and you have to go back and the lesson is to learn to love ...

Yeah, it was [Jesus] that I met when I fell down the mountain, because I had this near-death experience, and sent me back. Much to my disgust, because it sent me back and told me I'd got to learn to love, and I thought I did. I've got a family, what more do you want? I've got children. Yeah, that's not what I'm talking about. That's easy, it's easy to love your family, well no, it's not that easy, actually, because I don't speak to my mother. But theoretically, it's easy to, easier to love your family ... The difficulty is loving the people that come here who can be thoroughly obnoxious. And who are coming with so many, so much baggage, that you think I don't want your baggage, go away. But the thing is here, that we're supposed to treat them as though they were Christ. We are supposed to treat them as a, if He were to walk in the room, how would I treat Him?

Since the accident and "life review" FD has developed insight into patients that she didn't have beforehand:

And I can look at somebody, who I can see, somebody can walk in the room and I keep thinking, oh yeah, OK, they've got so and so, and so and so. The chap that's staying here at the moment, I knew he had something seriously wrong, I knew it was something that was involving his whole body and was serious. I didn't know that it was diabetes, but I knew that there was something not right, and that it was something that was going to cause real problems. And sometimes, I can say, yes it's, they've got a tumour here or there or wherever, and I just think I really didn't want to know this.

Since her accident and life review, FD has become uncomfortable with using herbal medicines that she hasn't had direct experience of as living plants:

And ones that I've, and things like ginseng and ginkgo, which I have actually experienced in their home, when I went to Korea last year, I ate my ginseng and ginkgo berries, and I, they feel like old friends. So I would use those quite comfortably, but things like *Corydalis* and stuff like that, I think, no this is not, and even *Bupleurum*, stuff like that, I would look at it and say, no I'm not comfortable, I don't know these as, I don't know them as plants, I don't know them as, and therefore I'm not comfortable … I need to know the plant, I need to have an image in my head, of what the plant looks like, and what it looks like growing.

FD compares how she saw herbs before and after her accident:

They were just medicine, I was a tincture herbalist. Quite happily prescribe stuff without really, I didn't know what *Cimicifuga* looked like, I didn't know what *Caulophyllum* looked like, I didn't. Now, I really couldn't, it's almost, putting the integrity back, this is, if you don't know the plant what are you doing using it? If you don't know what it looks like and you don't know how it grows, and so I can quite happily use *Atropa* because we've got *Atropa* down the garden, in the meadow, and *Solanum dulcamara*—bittersweet, because they're down in that, and meadowsweet we have down here, and I can use, even quite serious stuff, if I've got the image in my head of the plant, and know what it looks like, but not, and interestingly that's articulated itself just this afternoon as we've been talking, thinking, yeah, that is what it is.

She also finds that she understands the trees that she cares for:

Well, the trees tell me what I'm supposed to do with them, because I prune them, and they tell me when I'm standing in front of them. Say OK, I've just done some yew trees, and I'm standing there, and it gets easier, each time, because the communication is easier each time, so OK, it's that time of the year again, you have to have a haircut. it's all intuitive, it's all instinct. Nobody's ever taught me to do these things, I've read the principles, looked on the internet and said, well, what am I trying to achieve here, but at the end of the day, the tree's a living thing. So, I won't be doing any more after the end of this month because they'll all be growing, and that hurts them, if you do that.

A helpful tree

Two years after her accident FD had only 10% shoulder movement. Her doctors said that an artificial shoulder was required and an operation was scheduled. During the interim FD travelled abroad to undertake some further therapeutic training, where she experienced a "healing crisis":

> I went out in the May, knowing that when I came back I was going to have to have this surgery. But, I thought, well, I'll go and do that initial training … And you'd do the therapy for a week. On day three I had a huge healing crisis … I'd gone for a walk, and there was a tree, and this voice in my head was saying, go and talk to the tree. Oh don't be stupid, this is ridiculous. Go and stand in front of the tree, OK, stand in front, now put your arm on that branch there, OK, fine, OK. So I put my hand, I lifted this arm up on to the branch, got the hand hooked on to the branch. And then couldn't move, because I couldn't lift it up to get it off, and my weight started to pull on it, and there was the most horrendous cracking and crunching and God knows what else going on. I'm thinking, oh I really did swear, I thought, I've dislocated my shoulder, I've really done damage here, this is frightening what's going on. Eventually I managed to disengage myself from the tree, went back to the cabin, and actually it didn't feel too bad. But I was very concerned, and that night, I went into this healing crisis, which I didn't recognise that that's what it was. My shoulder was on fire, it was absolute, I was in agony. Absolute agony. I just wanted to go home, I was running a temperature, I was in a terrible state, had roaring headache, felt really, really ill.

The next morning she found that she had more mobility in her arm:

> I went to do a coffee enema the next morning and I'm lying there having this coffee enema, and quite without thinking, I started scratching my arse, it was really, with the hand that was damaged

... my butt! So I was sort of lying on the floor and I'm going like this and I'm thinking, I suddenly realised what I was doing, because that arm could not reach, and because I went into the next workshop, "I can scratch my butt!, and they all, "What? What the hell's this woman talking about?" And basically, that's what had happened.

She went to visit the tree that had helped her the previous day:

And I then went, that was that day, the next day, I walked up back where the tree had been, and the tree had been cut down. Wasn't there any more, and I just stood there absolutely in pieces, the tree had gone! They'd cut a number of trees going up the track and it was one of the trees that had gone. And I just, I thought I don't believe this, I really don't believe this.

She came back to the UK. She was terrified at the thought of the surgery:

I was absolutely in a state, and I went for my pre-meds, and I was literally shaking, every single muscle in my body was shaking, and they said what's the matter, and I said, "Well, I just am absolutely terrified, I just don't know whether I want to have this done or not." And really just to convince me that I needed to have it done, they sent me down for an X-ray, basically to prove to me that nothing had changed. Except that it had changed. And when they put the, there was a long delay, I was sitting there thinking, what's going on, and he called me back in and he showed me the two pictures, and in the November, the shoulder was dislocated and right down here somewhere. I'd come back ... the shoulder was in the socket, and the movement that I had, he then, he showed me that, and I said, "Oh, it's relocated." He said, "Yes," he said, "we don't know how that's happened," and I told him about the tree ...

The consultant told her that a shoulder replacement wouldn't improve her range of movement any more than it had increased since she had gone abroad. There was no need for her to have the surgery any more:

... and apparently according to the consultant, I'm the only person in the country where that's ever happened. Everybody else that's had that sort of injury has ended up with the shoulder replacement, because it's the only way you get any mobility back …

Wise woman versus professional herbalist

FD remembers, in the early Nineties, attending a herbal conference of her professional association when the dress code had been relaxed. She saw a tension between the "traditional" and "professional" herbalist.

> It was the first conference where they didn't have a dinner and dance where everybody was dressed in formal evening wear, and they did the foxtrot and the waltz, and all this sort of thing, and they had a ceilidh. But it didn't go down too well with the older people who felt that it should be much more formal … and I think there still is this tension between the traditional role of the herbalist, rooted in village life, which is the medieval wise woman … somebody slightly up from self-help, but not in the ranks of being a professional physician. And these professional men who had fought … who had fought to establish herbal medicine as a profession. And as a profession on a par with doctors, and there was this definite dichotomy between the two …

Rather than seeing herself now as a professional consulting herbalist, as she had in the past, she sees "patients" on a much more informal basis:

> Somebody came to Mass here a couple of weeks, not that long ago, two, three weeks ago, and she came in, she was in Mass and part way through Mass she came out, and at the end of Mass which was about an hour later, Arthur came across to find me and said would you go and see this lady. He said, "She's sitting in the loos, in tears." "Why?" "She burned herself before she came out." She'd actually poured boiling water on her knee, from the kettle, straight onto her knee. And she didn't stop, she just came out, so I grabbed my lavender oil, and my, and a bandage, and the nearest thing I could get hold of which was just a clean hanky and my marigold cream and went across, and put lavender oil on it, and stuff. And as I'm doing this, I'm trying to do it very surreptitiously because there's two nurses, well there's two nurses in the congregation, there's two

nurses in the community. I'm just, OK, well we'll do this quietly, nobody'll notice and the, and I put this, I put the lavender oil on and I put the marigold, slathered marigold oil on, because I'd treated Arthur with steam burns, so I knew it was perfectly OK. Covered it all up, said to her, "Just don't do anything with it, just take it home and sit quietly," and of course one of the nurses just happened to come in. "What have you put on it? What have you? You shouldn't have put anything on it." I just said, "I've done what I've done, and it's fine. I've done it in my professional capacity, it's not a problem." And she got the message, the woman rang me up later on and said, "Actually the pain went almost as soon as I got in the car," and she, it was a blistered burn, and she was fine. She said she's got a lovely butterfly now, she says it looks like a tattoo of a butterfly.

FD's informal practice of herbal medicine often takes place within the religious community where she lives:

And that's the sort of herbal medicine I'm now practising. Stuff like that, I say to people, "Why don't you try a pot of this, or a pot of that?" And I will make people up mixes, because I do know quite a lot about people's backgrounds here, like you do when you're in a community, you know some of their backgrounds. And I will make up, but I will make up stuff that I know isn't going to be any problem in terms of stuff they might or might not be taking. I had a gentleman with, who was having really, really bad problems with IBS, and I just said to him, you need to take chamomile tea. Six weeks later, he said that's amazing, I can't believe that, and he's fine. And then the same chap sitting in church, and he had a funny turn, and you look at him and you could see straight away that he was cold. So I grabbed a coat, somebody had left a coat, like you'd left that there. Grabbed it and put it round him. Said, "Right, you need to get warm," and then sitting at the end, talking to him, and one of the nurses, who works, no she's a physio, not a nurse, works in cardiac rehab: "Oh we'll reassess you next time we're at cardiac rehab." And I said to him very quietly, I said, "What dose of your heart medicine are you on?" And he told me and I said, "I think you need to go back to your GP and ask for that to be reassessed, I think you're on too high a dose, and your blood pressure and your pulse and everything are too low."

And also within her broader social village community:

> I've got one lady that, yeah, another lady that was absolutely hysterical: it was actually Arthur. Arthur met her in the supermarket, she was in a terrible state, and he said, "I think you need to ring her." He said she really is desperate. I rang her, I went round and talked to her, and it's taken a long time, because she was mentally, she was in a really bad way, with what had been going on. And we just gradually, gradually, gradually over a period of about a year, without any, there's no, not been any formal stuff at all. Very, I've been making notes, but she's not seen me making the notes, very, very gradually brought her round to the point where, actually she's now 100% better than she was, and actually it was to do with the medication she was being given and the runaround that she was getting with the NHS. And we just sat, and have taken it a bit at a time, and talked her through it and worked through it to the point that she's now working perfectly normally and she's fine ... Stuff like that really. Yeah. That's up to date, really.

This move to a more informal, community-based herbalism is something that she has seen other herbalists also being drawn to, including herbalists who had previously been vocal in advocating increasingly professionalised practice. She remembers attending a herbal seminar:

> It was inspirational what people were thinking about but I'm thinking, these are the people that when I first qualified were telling us we need to go down the registration route. And now the things that they are talking about are community herbal projects and the village herbalist stuff ... These are the people that having pushed, and pushed, and pushed registration to everybody else, they've now decided in their practices to go back to working, and I just think, OK, so where are we with it all now?

She remembers having a conversation with a herbalist who was involved in the politics of statutory regulation:

> She'd come back from yet another interminable meeting ... and she just, I asked her how she was, I said, "I'm not interested in the politics, I'm not interested in any of that. How are you as a person?"

And she looked and she stood there, and her eyes all welled up, and she just said, "I have realised that it's all a waste of time, because actually the most important thing is love. And we just stood quietly, and we just stood with that, there wasn't anything else to say. And I look at it and think, this is the problem, we've got so bogged down in all of the politics and people telling us how we should be doing it, that actually what it's really about is sitting with people over their kitchen table even, and listening and then offering whatever happens to be around in the kitchen or around in the dispensary as a love offering for the person to try to see if it helps. And yes, you can put that into a more complicated therapeutic setting, but at the end of the day it's very simple.

Reflection on FD

For FD, Juliet de Bairacli Levy made a lot of sense talking about rearing animals, "and, by inference, rearing children". However, this was the closest she came to any sort of enchanted human-nonhuman meetings in her entryways. Furthermore, the first part of FD's narrative was resolutely disenchanted in that her difficult engagements with professions were to the fore. In many ways she struggled with her professional life, identifying the problem of favouritism in her herbal training, as well as political difficulties arising out of being involved with the bureaucracy of organisations. Outside herbal medicine she encountered difficulties in her engagement with another therapy when her concern over the lack of non-herbalists' diagnostic skills eventually contributed to her decision to withdraw this therapy from her practice.

However, it is clear that in many ways FD was acting along the ethical guidelines that Wahlberg[42] has identified as being established for various CAM professions, irrespective of the therapy practised. Thus, for FD, the importance of conduct, competency, and responsibility in the activities of the profession as well as in practice can be seen in her manifest desire to see the influence of personalities removed from herbal training, to have bureaucratic processes in clinics that outlive the participation of individuals, to remove conflicts of interest in running clinics, to ensure that procedures are followed by organisations, and in raising the issue of poor diagnostic skills by non-herbalists. This combination of professionalisation and bureaucratisation may be seen as part of Weber's apparent disenchantment of the world. Furthermore, the near absence of therapy-specific details from ethical guidelines can be seen to be mirrored in FD's question about her own narrative— "Where's the herbal medicine in all this, because actually it's all politics, and that's been my career."

It is when FD starts to look outside the profession that we start to see meetings between humans and nonhumans, namely between FD and Jesus, and FD and plants. While FD has had a personal relationship with Jesus for most of her life, crossing the human with the divine in an enchanting relationship, it was only after her accident that she developed personal relationships with plants. After falling 200 feet down a mountain and having a "life review", Jesus told her that it was not her time to die, that she still had to "learn how to love". Following this event she found that she had lost interest in the "exotica" of herbal medicine, preferring to only use herbs that she knew as living plants, herbs where she has an "image in my head of the plant".

The enchantment of the voice of Jesus and of plants came together in FD's encounter with the branch of a tree, when she was told to put her arm on it, with the subsequent series of events, starting with a "healing crisis", leading to the improvement in her shoulder condition and the last-minute cancellation of replacement shoulder surgery. While FD's narrative started with various political disenchantments, her relationship with herbs later became pronounced in the necessity of knowing her herbal medicines as living plants. And paralleling this move towards knowing and using local plants there is also FD's move towards practising in a more informal way, as part of a community: an offering of love across the kitchen table rather than in the consultation room.

GA

Entryways

GA grew up in a family environment without any exposure to herbs, but remembers reading a book that got him thinking:

> I remember reading the Herman Hesse book, *Narcissus and Goldmund*, and Narcissus is a young monk at one point and he's asked to go out and pick some herbs. I think, in my head it's St John's

wort. I'll have to reread it and check whether I've got it scrambled over the years but the house I grew up in, herbs meant my mum's cardboard tube with little, like a squashed Smartie tube. A cardboard tube with a little plastic lid on it, "Pearce and Duff's mixed herbs" and it went down about three pinches in the eighteen years that I lived with my mum and dad and it was still in the cupboard another ten years later. So in my experience herbs were something you had this pinch of once every three years and in the book he's sent out to pick a, and he comes back with a sack of it and I remember reading the book and thinking, sack of herbs?

As a youth GA found refuge from council estate life by spending time in the countryside.

I grew up between, on the cusp of two housing estates, with the usual kind of working class shit that went on between boys at that time in the Sixties. So people from one estate say, you live on that estate, and they'd beat you up and the people on the other one, you'd just pick on people from the other estate because they were your enemies. Living in between both I got picked on by a kid from both ends and although I had friends I think it seemed quite attractive to me to just get away from the whole damned lot so I just spent a lot of time out in the countryside and as I grew older developed friends that liked to go for walks and bike rides and I used to just go out and at some point by about fifteen I just got interested in tasting plants as well as trying to identify them. So I was interested in birds, animals, I was very interested in frogs and toads, reptiles, gradually taught myself flowering plants and I think I got an early copy of *Food For Free* and started tasting things and didn't particularly pursue anything particularly herbal but it was just about getting to know my plants ...

His interest in Western herbs grew when a girlfriend was ill:

... a girlfriend of mine got ill and went to see an acupuncturist and the acupuncturist gave her some herbs and gave her some English herbs, well, a mix, amongst which I think was yarrow. I said, "Well don't buy it off her, I can go out and pick it for you," and it rekindled something about Western herbs.

GA then studied herbal medicine. He also spent time in the countryside:

> I lived on a little smallholding ... I lived about ten miles away ... and lived in a caravan and my rent for the caravan was a day's work a week on the smallholding, part of which involved growing herbs. So I felt I got an extra education by being in the countryside and growing stuff as much as being at the school really and was seen as a bit of a maverick in the school because I was somebody that just wandered around tasting things all the time and I assumed that everybody else would be the same.

GA was very good at plant recognition. He remembers one of his exams:

> ... they did a funny exam at the end of the herbal course in those days and ... would take you into a room and it was just to do with plant recognition, so it was a very minor thing. You'd be in there for fifteen minutes and you had about fifty plants laid out, just all around the room, it was in one of the labs, and he'd randomly pick out ten and he'd give you a score out of ten of how many you recognised and I went in and they said, "It's pointless doing this with you, you'll know all of them." He said, "I'm going to give you the one that nobody else has recognised, and it was gypsywort. I said, "It's gypsywort." He said, "Ten out of ten, get out."

Transformative energy

GA looked to bring other interests, from outside his training in herbal medicine, into his practice:

> From the early Eighties, when I began studying herbal study but formally, alongside that, I'd developed quite a strong interest in shamanic stuff and my reading of shamanic stuff was more anthropological than New Agey but it felt like there was something very important in there that I was trying to get hold of that I wanted to bring into my practice and I tried really hard with it the first couple of years and I thought, I don't know how to integrate these two and it was, there didn't seem to be any way of integrating the two interests to me, and I certainly don't want to bang a drum and sing

something to my patients. I just, I want some things, that kind of transformative energy in my consultation and I think I gave up, I couldn't find any way of doing it. I gave up.

In order to help patients change their habits he studied neuro-linguistic programming (NLP):

> I remember particularly having one patient who was a builder who had colitis, who between working every day and going home would drink several pints of beer … it would make a break between his work day and his home life, and I felt with him if I could make him change his habits I could probably get to grips with the other, his illness but I couldn't do it with herbs alone and I didn't have the skills to get him, to encourage him or to get him to change his habits and there must have been other people that had the, I had the same feeling about but I just remember him particularly and it gave me some incentive to do an NLP course because I thought it would give me those skills, and I did an intensive with Richard Bandler and, I've forgotten his name, McKenna, TV guy who's crap on telly but he's a brilliant lecturer, and it completely changed my practice and in a way it gave me some of that thing I was labelling shamanic. It gave me a way of working with a different kind of energy and it gave me a way of integrating with, finding a different way to converse with patients and it was interesting.

GA saw a theatre production based on the work of Arnold Mindell and his work with coma patients. This led to training in "process work" with Arnold Mindell, which enabled GA to help his patients to engage with their illnesses in a different way:

> A great little story, a mixture of storytelling, theatre, no props, the best, it had one examination couch and bits of tissue paper, that was it, and I was really interested. I'd listened to the show with a kind of NLP head on and I just thought, this is really interesting. If this is real representation of what this guy did I'm intrigued, and I decided there and then that next time Mindell was in the country I would do some training with him because I'd got in my head that he was old and I needed to catch him before he died. As it is, I've been doing stuff with him every year for about the last eight

or nine years and again, that resonated, it was just another way of working that's given me a basis for working with patients. So I think I've ended up with, I think the skills that I brought to being a herbalist were being quite good as a listener. Patients often say to me, "Oh, you're really good at being a listener. I tell you things that I've not told other people ..." I can't keep count of the number of times people have told me stuff and said, "This happened twenty years ago but I've never told anybody, I've kept it sealed up," and I felt like I needed an adequate response to that stuff rather than saying, "Oh, you should see a counsellor," especially because a lot of people in this country will engage with something that's seen to be about dealing with physical illness but they won't go and see a psychotherapist or a counsellor. So I had an aptitude to listen to people. I think the NLP gave me a few more skills about finding what resources people had inside them to make their own changes and break bad habits and the process stuff has learnt me to engage with people by talking about their metaphors for their illnesses as though they're reality ...

GA gives an example of a patient who was helped by his new understandings:

I had a policeman who used to come and see me, quite a heavy, high-flying armed response unit with ulcerative colitis and over a period of time we got him quite a lot better and then he had a flare-up. I changed the herbs, I tried to change my approach, couldn't quite work out what had caused the flare-up. So he was sat in front of me and I just said, "What's it feel like?" "I don't know, it just hurts." "Shut your eyes, focus in on what it feels like." He said, "Feels as if it's knotted up." "What's knotted up?" "I don't know, something inside." So try to, by finding language which coincided by him, his and getting him to focus in on it, just got him to follow the image and he said he'd got an image of guts being squeezed and it looks like something's been twisted and it, follow the end of it and I just followed him wherever it was leading and just kept prompting him to stick with it rather than open his eyes and come back to talking in a more normal way and it led to a succession of images and then suddenly he said, "It's about, he said, I'm at [X]." He was at the [X] disaster when it happened, tried to save some guy's life and this guy died in front of him. So then he talked about that and we talked in a more conventional way about that and what he remembered and he came back the next month and I thought, we'd had quite a weird, within generally day to day conversation, it was a very weird consultation that we've had. I was expecting for him, and he came back and it seemed like he had no memory of it. He just said to me, "Oh, I don't know what you've done but that last change of herbs seems to have sorted it out. It's all fine now. I've had no more bleeding from my bum, everything's gone and it's sorted, my pain's gone," and I think, sometimes because it's just off of somebody's normal map they, they've got no way of engaging with it, it just kinda vanishes.

GA describes how he helps a patient to engage with the metaphor of his illness as if it was real:

Another guy had really bad colitis pain and I just said to him, "If I had to be, I have to imagine your pain in me, what's it like?" And he said, "Oh, it's like three metal rods stuck into me ... it's like they're real metal rods." He said, "That's what it feels like." I said, "Well, this might sound a bit odd but just imagine getting hold of one." "Yeah." I said, "Well, pull it out." He went, I said, "What's that like?" "It feels better." I said, "Well, take the other two out then ..." So, and then people look at you in bafflement, so, oh, what's going on there? The, it's just finding those methods for, and little tricks that sometimes are a long-term cure for things, sometimes they only work for five minutes but some of those things for pain control work, teaching people effective pain control and stuff like that.

GA has his own particular focus when engaging with patients, in order to unravel illnesses, although he does not necessarily see this as being the "root" of their problem:

... I'm quite cautious about, I think we make a lot of wrong assumptions about the aetiology of an illness. So for my own approach, I tend to focus in on the psycho-spiritual end of stuff but that's just because it's my interest. I can think of osteopaths that maybe work with somebody with ME and saying, "This is tight here in this particular place. It's come from this." They think that because they can treat something by, because something is a successful treatment that the aspect of what they're treating is to do with the aetiology of the problem. My feeling is more that everything's connected and maybe what I'm tackling is not the root of the problem, it's just something that's interesting to me and if it works and if it works for them then that's OK but I'm not saying that because I'm tackling the psychological end that everything's psychologically ... psychological aetiology ...

A herbalist in a GP practice and in a CAM practice

GA works in a GP practice and also in a CAM practice. His patients in the GP practice tend to be unemployed working class, and in the CAM practice they tend to be employed working class. In the GP practice his patients are given a disclaimer stating that they will be given medicines that are not on the standard drugs lists. Also, a GP has to sign his prescriptions off. GA is unable to dispense his own herbal medicines—this is the responsibility of a pharmacist at a local pharmacy:

> The chemist or the gaffer there is an older guy who when I went round to negotiate with him I expected him to say no and he, he's known for moaning and cussing, "Oh, another bloody thing that ah ..." And he moaned for a bit and then he said, "Yeah, I'll do it." And it's proper medicine, none of this blister pack rubbish. It seems to be quite good to be involved in making something up and putting it into a bottle.

GA goes to weekly practice meetings:

> It is very much an old-style GP because when we have case history meetings somebody will say, "Where are they ... so and so, are they next door to the dealers and isn't so and so on the other side?" "It's his wife," and it's like, yes.

He feels able to speak freely:

> I think they respect that more than somebody who just sits in the corner and thinks, oh don't like these statins ... My work there initially was appraised and evaluated and seemed to having success but I think since then it's been mostly trusted that I'm going in a good direction

and I get, I talk to a lot to doctors in the corridor or somebody that's referred something. It's a lot of informal feedback. I'll just stick my nose in the room and say, "So and so that you sent my way ..."

Although GA is influenced by "transformative" NLP and process work, he also uses a purely medical approach if necessary:

> The more, the longer I've been there probably the more confident I am about describing things within my own terms. It'll depend sometimes on different patients. I had somebody referred to me with IBS stuff relatively recently and they just, they know I've got a good track record with that kind of thing. After I'd seen her the second time I just thought, this isn't IBS, this is gallstones, and I threw it straight back to the doctors and got them to refer through for ultrasound and yeah, it was gallstones. So sometimes it's very much a medical thing. It's like, actually, I've got this feeling, this person's presenting in this way but have they been, and I've often sent people out for blood tests or, so on that level I'm talking in very much pathology, anatomy, physiology terms.

GA is respected within the practice for his abilities with difficult patients. One of GA's patients had been to see a consultant:

> ... and basically the consultant was saying in the most tentative way [in a letter], this guy's an asshole. He was just really horrible, and one of the ... doctors showed it to me and I said, "Oh yeah, it sounds like him." I said, "Why are you showing me this?" And he said, "Just know that you're good at challenging him, maybe you can take it up with him?" I said, "OK, fine ..."

GA describes one of his GP practice patients:

> It's a bit of a nightmare at the doctors and I frequently ask people what they eat. One of those people that was late this morning, the fifteen-year-old boy, I just, who has got weird psychological things going on. Mum thinks he's got ADHD, doctor doesn't think he has. I just said, "So what do you eat? Just run through an average school day, yeah, a school day, what do you have on a school day?" "Well, I get up and go straight to school, maybe have a packet of crisps in the

break." He was there with his mum, fifteen and a bit. "What do you have lunch time?" "I have chips and a curry," which they go, he goes out and gets at the local shops. I know the shops, they're kind of horrible. "What do you have in the evening?" "Oh, it depends whether I come in at the, bit of pizza maybe." "Does he eat vegetables?" "Oh yes ... well, some days." So once a week, and that's quite frequent in that area and I just looked at him, I thought, he smokes. I said, "How many do you smoke?" "Twenty a day." I said, "You're at school, you're fifteen, how do you afford twenty cigarettes a day?" And his mum said, "Oh, he buys them out of the dinner money that I give him."

At his CAM clinic a patient is more willing to engage with dietary changes:

So it's just getting people to think about it and sometimes forcing them to. They come up with the answers. I had somebody in this room a couple of weeks ago, they said, and I, we came up, I said, "We need to discuss diet don't we?" And I kept throwing it back at her and in the end I didn't make a single suggestion. I said, "And then you know, if you did that what would be better?" "Oh, this would be better wouldn't it?" "But would you actually eat that?" "Well, that's a good idea but no, I wouldn't eat it." "But what would you eat? ... "Oh that, that, and that's crap. That one's good." So she just, she had built her own diet by then ... I thought, well this is good and I said to her, I said, "Have you noticed I haven't said any of this?"

St Cuthbert and the pleasure of small signs

GA uses mainly herbs local to him:

So I would say at least 80% of the herbs I use are either native to [the area where he lives] or grow in people's gardens around this area. So I may buy some in ... but unless I feel I've got a connection to the plant I don't really know what I'm doing with it.

When GA was starting out in herbal medicine he felt there was something missing:

I was desperate when we were training, I felt, really felt the lack of a unifying philosophy behind what we did.

However, he now is less concerned with having a philosophical or theoretical underpinning:

> The longer I've been in practice the more I don't give a damn really.

Instead, he feels that his practice is based on the firm foundations of his plant knowledge:

> I feel like I've always known my plants.

GA remembers a patient who had had insomnia for years. He made a suggestion to her:

> This might not have anything to do with [the patient], but felt I should offer it. Was there a need in her life to pray? "Pray?" she asked, "to whom? To what?" I made a guess as to what might be appropriate, "To the earth maybe?" Perhaps she should go to an ancient site? "No," she rejected that straight off. While she was not a Christian, if she was to pray, it should be in a church, a big church ... She thinks of the [local] cathedral as being nondescript, she decided to go to Durham ... Several weeks later she reported the results of her pilgrimage. Although it was far from natural for her, she had knelt and she had prayed, and in turn St Cuthbert had spoken to her. Her insomnia had gone, sleep was now easy. Now I resolved to visit myself. Maybe St Cuthbert would speak to me. Andrew came with me. We looked at what the cathedral had offered us. We climbed the tower but St Cuthbert was silent. Perhaps, foolishly, I was listening with my ears ... Sometimes I try too hard to hear the voices of the plants.

Despite not hearing the words of plants, GA reflects on the pleasure of being a herbalist, that he is "sustained by the plants all around". He remembers walking along a canal with another herbalist:

> ... looking for traces of the skullcap that grew there the year before. Jubilation at finding a dead twig and a couple of green leaves. The delight of a walk with other herbalists, taking half an hour to walk half a mile. "Oh look, a plant! ... Oh look!—there's another plant!"

Sometimes medical students sit in on his consultations. He remembers taking one on a walk:

> In a gap between patients, I take a medical student for a quick scout around the grounds outside the medical centre. It's a grim urban environment but there at hand is dandelion, mahonia, hawthorn. She tastes the astringency, the bitterness, and the gloopy mucilage in a leaf of plantain. We pick lemon balm with which she makes tea. Comparing the immediate generosity of this plant medicine with the sterile anonymity of pharmaceuticals, she wonders about retraining as a herbalist.

When he makes St John's wort tincture, he waits for a particular moment:

> Even if I made gallons, some of it has to be in a glass jar, for that magic moment when the green leaves and the yellow flowers turn the clear liquid instantly red.
>
> I rarely hear a voice, but in some way I have heard a little of what the plants have to tell … I let go of the need for some great epiphany. I revel in the offerings and omens of small signs—daisies by the wayside, liverworts by the steps. In the murmurings of the wind through the leaves the plants are speaking to me all the time.
>
> If I can listen to the voice of the owl and read the trace of the fox in its scent, and sense what the cow parsley says to me, perhaps today I may also hear the silent words of St Cuthbert.

Everything I do is herbal medicine

For GA, herbal medicine is difficult to define:

> … herbal medicine is the thing everything else feeds through. So if I read a novel, I only read novels that I'm interested, that I think I can learn something psychologically from. All the psychological learning, most of my CPD stuff the last ten years has been more psychological than herbal but it goes through this for everything, I think it just goes back through the herbal thing and so the books that I read or the music that I do give me more language and more metaphors and a wider possibility of communicating with people that I see as patients …

Herbalism is a bucket, or a compost heap or a treasure trove into which I put, or through which I process, all my learning and all my actions ... Anything that I do with the patient—*that* is herbal medicine.

And yet, somehow the focus on plants is a little narrow. Years ago, I had an interview for a job with the RSPB. "So, are you a bird-watcher?" the interviewer asked me. "No," I replied, "forgive me but I think birdwatching is stupid!" I explained that I would find the idea of going out to just look at birds, or just to look at plants, crazy. I want to look at everything. He offered me the job.

Reflection on GA

As a young man, GA spent much time in the countryside. He was interested in tasting and identifying plants. This concern for spending time in nature may be seen in his later narrative in that he mostly uses herbs that are native to his area or that are grown in local gardens, meaning herbs that he knows as living plants. He needs to have this "connection" with the plant. Without this, "I don't really know what I am doing with it," he says. Knowing plants this way, through spending time with them, is to be found as an entryway and in his later narrative.

However, in his youth, GA was also interested in wider nature, for example, in foraging, and in understanding birds and reptiles. This encompassing of something wider than simply herbs and plants may also be seen in his statement that "Herbalism is a bucket, or a compost heap ...," that includes, in his practice, knowledge of herbs but also his interest in the "transformative energy" of NLP and process work, as well as orthodox medical knowledge. As he recounts, when going for a job interview at the RSPB, he wants to look at everything. A second entryway, of realising that he could pick yarrow and use it as a medicinal plant for his girlfriend, is paralleled in his eventual career as a herbalist. Also, the early experience of living between two working class housing estates may also have been important for his awareness of the impact of social factors on patient health, which is seen in his narrative.

GA's entryways are not obviously enchanting, especially given his minimal exposure to herbs by his parents, who used three pinches of Pearce and Duff's culinary herbs in eighteen years, although his memory of thinking "sack of herbs?" when reading Herman Hesse may have subtly hinted at his future. However, GA's experience of spending time in nature and tasting herbs are sensual experiences. Also highly sensual is his engagement as a herbalist with helping patients to treat metaphors as if they are real. A visceral sensuality can be seen in the experience of two of GA's patients, one who pulled metal rods out of his abdomen, and another who followed his squeezed and twisted guts to a disaster scene.

Also enchanting are GA's description of sensual experiences—of the "pleasure of small signs" when he sees "daisies by the wayside and liverworts by the steps", when he anticipates the transformation of green leaves and yellow flowers into red tincture, when he is delighted at simply finding another plant on a herb walk and when a medical student tastes the "astringency, the bitterness and the gloopy mucilage in a leaf of plantain" and considers training as a herbalist. While he had no "epiphany" in his experiences with herbs, they "are speaking to me all the time" even if the words are voiceless.

These voiceless conversations with plants, which came after his entryways were completed, are meetings between GA and the nonhuman. GA's meetings with plants parallel his work as a herbalist, where he merges the two distinct spheres of orthodox medical knowledge and transformative practices. And furthermore, it seems likely that his sensual experience with plants and nature provides an affective energy that sustains his practice.

MN

Entryways

MN enrolled in medical school but left after one year:

> We disagreed on certain major philosophical points and it was their university so I left. But it was, it was a, it was a very surreal experience, it was a, it was a very strange experience … what I was offered was a medical training, learn this, do not think. Thou shalt not think. This is, this is the established stuff. There's just so much to learn, all the anatomy, all the biochemistry, all the physiology, here's Guyton … Learn this, and the human being is nowhere to be seen. So I'm afraid I didn't, I didn't really see eye to eye with it all,

which is a shame because that's what I wanted to be all my life, to be a doctor.

He decided to grow herbs:

> And people, 1980 people really hadn't heard of organic ... But I'd been fired up by what I'd discovered about the food industry, I became vegetarian at that point and so I earned some money, came over here and started growing herbs ...

The work of the French herbalist, Maurice Messegue, became important to him:

> ... he produced a beautiful herbal, *Health Secrets of Plants and Herbs*, which is a wonderful book, and I came here and started growing herbs. It just, that sang to me, well if I couldn't be a doctor then I was going to be a herbalist.

He heard about a herbal medicine course, but decided to delay enrolling, preferring to get practical experience growing herbs:

> But at that point I thought, well, I could go down there but they're probably going to talk about herbs that I can't grow here and they're probably going to talk a lot about the pharmacology of it all and how much are they going to be concerned about whether it's organic or not, and that whole bit. So at that point I decided not to go down there, and wait, and I lived here four years and grew herbs and read Messegue's book, that was a key thing. I had one herb book and it was, it's great, and that's enough.

When he had a firm enough foundation he decided to study herbal medicine formally:

> ... I decided I was going to go down to, now go down to the [herbal medicine school] and study and get, I was ready now, I felt I had my own philosophy and my own knowledge of, practical knowledge of herbs ... digging and hoeing and all the rest ... so I felt I was ready to go down.

Krebs cycle and Ayurveda

During his studies MN engaged with the science-based curriculum:

> It's not something we should be frightened of. The Krebs cycle is just beautiful, it's an absolute, you know, electron transport chain, it's awesome, awe inspiringly beautiful and yet it's taught in a way that, oh God, people groan about it, oh the Krebs cycle. Not fully appreciating that if it wasn't for their own Krebs cycle going on they'd be a pool of molten jelly.

In line with his herbal medicine training MN draws on orthodox medicine to model his consultation:

> And I see that, the first part of diagnosis is through a Western medical model, that's what we were trained in ... And so that's what you use. And I would, my argument is that it's not, there's nothing wrong with the Western medical model per se, it's just not done. Do you know? You take a detailed in-depth consultation, which you need an hour for, first visit, you do a detailed clinical examination on the basis of that. You work out a diagnosis on the basis of those two things combined, you come up with a differential diagnosis and then you come up with a treatment strategy.

He follows the medical clues that the patient reveals:

> I remember waking up in the middle of the night one night and going, Addison's disease! And this patient had been coming back, getting ill and couldn't quite work out what was wrong with her. And she had this amazing sun tan and yet it had been a crap summer ... But just being able to, it's like a detective story and my mind likes that, picking back, going back ...

While his training gave him lists of herbs for particular conditions, this didn't satisfy MN:

> And so I left with a lot of, with the idea that I would go into practice, and I had all my arthritis herbs and people would come in with arthritis, I would give them arthritis herbs, and they'd get better. And people came in with skin problems, I would give them,

I'd look at my best skin herbs, people talk about skin herbs, and I would give them that, and they, they would get better. But as Voltaire says, a third of your patients get better, a third of the patients stay the same, and a third of the patients get worse, which doesn't seem to me that, that good a batting average.

As well as valuing science, he also recognises another side to herbal medicine. He remembers meeting a herbalist:

So, and my first encounter with him was, he said, "So what do you think about raspberry leaf, mm.?" And I talked about the tannins, and all the rest of it, and all the stuff I knew about it, and he said, "Oh, that's interesting, because I've always thought of it as a warm furry blanket. And I was just like, ah ha … Stopped in my tracks, because here, here was somebody that obviously knew a lot and was brilliant in clinic, and wasn't entirely concerned … didn't share my concerns about the different acids … there was other stuff going on. And so that was a big turning point for me, that, that there was, the, the scientific side was interesting, but the artistic side of it was also equally interesting, and equally important.

After his training he decided to bring other influences into his practice in order to "break up your lists". He describes what he means by "energetics":

Well, I suppose it's a term we coined to encompass first of all the different traditions, TCM, Ayurveda, humoral medicine, as the three main strands of human, main human history in terms of that. And so you have an idea that when you're treating this complaint, I mean humoral medicine's interesting, for instance phlegm, if you're treating phlegm and you put too much heat in, in humoral medicine you can harden the phlegm at the beginning. So it gives you an energetic, I would say energetic's about treatment strategy as well, it's not just the herbs in terms of their energetic qualities, and that's quite simply hot or cold or moist or dry on one level. It's also about a treatment strategy so in humoral medicine you would loosen that phlegm before you put anything too hot in there, and that seems to make, still seems to make sense to me. It's arcane, archaic knowledge and language but it still, human physiology hasn't changed since Culpeper's day really, in that sense. You know, humans haven't changed physiologically that much, and going back to the whole thing about Hippocrates, and Hippocrates was very interested in climate and the effect of weather on people, and that makes a lot of sense to me. So it gives you, it breaks up your list. Is this a warming diuretic or a cooling diuretic, a warming expectorant or a cooling expectorant? ... I mean I think every system and every complaint has a potential to be examined in that light, because otherwise you might as well just open a shop and people come in with arthritis, you give them your arthritis mix.

Goethean science: knowing plants

As well as using orthodox and traditional energetic knowledge as resources for his practice, MN also seeks to include spiritual understandings:

> And I would say that you could look at giving herbal medicine on a physical basis, and treating a symptom and propping up a physiological pathway, but I think there's also, I would say there's also a spiritual element to herbal medicine. There's some indefinable thing that, what you would call the spirit of the plant, does something as well. Which is difficult to talk about, but I think it is important.

This meant seeing herbs differently:

> ... you should also encounter the herb as, give it the courtesy of looking at it as something, as an entity in its own right.
> ... I can certainly sense that, you know, when you're picking meadowsweet or something like that, there's a sense that meadowsweet's flowering all over the rivers of X ... And there's a sense of a wider entity than necessarily the individual plant you're picking ...

MN seeks to provide a method for bringing lost knowledge back to consciousness:

> We've lost that, as modern people we no longer have that innate capacity to, to read the book of nature, and I think we, traditional people would, certainly, maybe it's just heightened individuals

within that tradition too, but that's my experience. And so what we're trying to do is to bring that, what, the work we saw as doing, is bringing that into consciousness, that unconscious connection to somehow bring it into consciousness …

MN and his wife, also a herbalist, met a scientist who was investigating an "alternative approach to biology":

> … we encountered a woman called LT … and this was a woman who listened to plants. We thought that sounds like interesting stuff, and so we, we began to work with LT, and she'd been trained in Germany at the Goetheanum, in the Steiner tradition. She'd been a biologist, and then she wanted to, she'd, saw the way that that was going in terms of cloning and, and all of this, and, and reacted against that and did her training, studying an alternative approach to biology. An alternative approach to science, which is, and that's what we've done ever since, it's what, what we've based our, our life study on.

MN turned to the work of the German poet, naturalist, and statesman, Johann Wolfgang von Goethe (1749–1832), to engage scientifically with the subjective side of plant knowledge:

> … Goethe certainly sang to me, and, so a scientific method to embrace the subjective. Goethe saw science going very much down the, the, the microscope had just been invented, the telescope was getting better and better, this, these whole things were, were taking off, but he felt that the human being was the most perfect instrument. The human being if, if awake was the most perfect instrument to, to ascertain, to, to, to read this book of nature, and it's sticking a microscope on, onto somebody could perhaps just imbalance them, because you've increased the amount of input, but you haven't increased the amount of capacity to deal with that input. And so LT's point was that, that in Goethean science we're trying to improve the scientist, not just the machine …

For MN, Goethean science provides a way of understanding how the physicality of plants may be useful:

> And so it's immersing yourself, and it's spending time with it, learn its growing process, and what, what we do, what we talk about is

rebuilding that experience, and to give you an inner experience of that plant. So you know the physicality of it, you know its, its, its life cycle, and its, its growth patterns, and its history, and it, ultimately all, also it's pharmacology, and then you're trying to wrap around that Goethean scientist's saying, encompass all that, but put something else around that, that gives you a more holistic picture of what you're trying to study. And the physicality of the plant then has information, dandelion and horsetail are, are two diuretics, how would you use them differently? And if you look at the physicality of dandelions compared to horsetail, they're very, very different. Is there information there that's worthwhile? Does the physicality of how, how horsetail grows and reproduces, and, and its whole life cycle, is there information there alongside its pharmacology to guide you in its use? Seems a reasonable endeavour to me.

Goethean science is normally practised in groups. MN and his wife have developed a seven-stage process. The first of the seven stages is "first impressions", whose aim is to capture the "mood" of the plant through coming to the plant with an open heart. After meeting the plant each person tells the group one or two words which relate something of their experience of the plant.

So what we're, what we're attempting to do here is to then take to, to go to the plant, have a, have a, have a first impression, have a subjective impression of the plant, as if you, prepare yourself as if you're going to meet somebody, meet a person. And that is giving, for some people that's giving too much to a plant, saying that they have some kind of being ... I don't, I don't have too much of a problem in that consciousness if it's about, doesn't seem, for me it doesn't seem to stop. When I study physiology, that sodium ion seems to know what it's doing.

The remaining six stages are "exact sense perception", which involves the gathering of factual information from observing the physicality of the plant in minute detail; "exact sensorial imagination", where the facts are "put together" or moved between; "glimpsing the being", where group meditation "rebuilds" the plant from memory while participants simultaneously observe for their emotional and other responses to this process; "being the being", where participants join with the "essence" of the plant; "catching the essence", where the "intention" of the plant is sought; and "incarnating the idea", where the idea is "grown" into a remedy whose preparation and dosage is experimented with.

Throughout these stages the aim is to stay as close to the phenomenon of the herb as possible:

> The point being that as soon as you start to study an organic being, you've got a problem, because you, you're trying to stop it. Modern psychology stops the human body, and looks at the bits, but then it's very difficult to build that back up again from the bits. So how do you study it without stopping it, without killing it?
>
> And Goethe even says how quickly we kill something with a word. We're studying something, oh it's, it's a daisy, all the perceptions and the concepts come through, so how can you, how can you think without conceptualising, that's the, that's the challenge.

Goethean science: knowing patients

For MN, plants have more in common with people than others may suspect:

> Plants are inside out, upside down humans … because it's their, it's the amount of light, shade, water, climate, impinges entirely on their form, you can read, if you look round here, you can see the trees are windblown, you can see the wind in the trees, yeah? And whereas the human being, it's pretty much preformed, it doesn't, it doesn't keep growing after a certain stage, and it's the inner life of the human being that, that expresses whether people are succulent or dry …

It was MN's wife, RN who thought of using the same methodology to understand patients that they had developed to understand plants:

> So it was then, R who thought, well, could we apply this to, to the human being, and she's certainly embraced that, and probably done, we, initially we started off, the idea was to do it as a group, so we'd have the two of us in the, in the consulting room at one time …

They also identified the importance of patients making a decision to be well:

> And this is what R came to, she, she's saying, well, when people decide to get better, there's like, it can be like a snap decision, and they never look back from that. Sometimes it's the first, they, the first spoon of the medicine they take, I've heard that loads of time, it will be the first touch of that medicine, people hail me as a genius in taxis all over [the city], whether it's deserved or not, but that was their experience. They, this guy gave me this bottle, and I took it, the first spoon of it, I never looked back, OK, I went to see him for a few months after that, and we, we did this, we did that, and that was important, but it was that, that was initial, and R took that to say, did that person decide that that, did part of that person decide to become well at that point? It's difficult to say that, that physiologically the herbs had that effect.
>
> But here's an opportunity to, with, with our patients to really engage with them at a deep level, to really help them find out why they're ill. And if they can make a decision to be better, rather, if, if they can change their mind about being ill, it can change their, their blueprint in some way, if they can change something in there, then so much the better.

Herbs and intention are then brought together in the consultation:

> R talks about it in her Goethean consultations, that the herb is an indicator of your new intention, it's to remind you of your new intentions, taking the herb is a lot to do with that. And that's kind of the way I practise more that you're using the herbs less as something that's trying to replace somebody's physiology.

A Goethean consultation

MN meets his patient J for a first consultation. MN gives J some paper and pastels and asks him to do a drawing of how he is feeling at the moment, saying that he will do one as well:

> It can be as abstract as you like, the colour as important or even more important possibly than the form ... just let it flow.

MN says:

> You're coming to this with a question, is it fair to say? So focus on
> the question ... how do you feel about your general health, can you
> express that?

When they have finished MN asks J if he is ready to talk about his drawing. J describes how his picture reflects how he is isolated by pain and
lack of energy and that "things have got to change" and how he would
like to save his failing relationship and to continue being a good parent,
from which he gets most of his pleasure.

MN points out that there is a swastika shape in J's drawing, but that
it is in the Tibetan Bon direction rather than the Nazi direction. MN then
describes what he drew: that while he sees a bright happy side—"This
is your girls"—J also uses work to stop a dark, sad, melancholic side
from getting through.

They then discuss whether this makes sense to J. MN prompts J, who
talks about his relationship with his partner. MN then asks about J's
physical symptoms, pointing out how particular symptoms confirm J's
medical diagnosis, but J keeps returning to his relationship. MN points
out that if J had less pain and more energy he would have more time
for everything else, including his relationship. MN then asks questions
about J's medical history, family medical history and social life before
moving on to questions that cover each of the body systems.

MN then asks J to go into the herb garden:

> ... take your time walking, look at the plants and encounter and
> see what kind of plants really call you ... What we're trying to do,
> you've got a new intention ... get a fresh start ... it's making that
> agreement with yourself that things are possible. To take that back
> on board again. Together with the herbs and what you can do,
> hopefully we can get to the pain and break that cycle ...

MN asks J to keep his intentions focused. MN then leaves J alone in the
herb garden. J walks slowly and quietly in the garden, taking a route
around the herb beds, pausing to stand eye-to-eye with some fennel,
before moving to willows that border some of the herb beds and protect
the smaller plants from the wind. He stands there for several minutes,
before returning to the consultation room.

MN arrives and says:

> So what we are going to do next is ... what we call the rebuild-
> ing stage. Sit back, close your eyes ... we are going to rebuild you
> between us in our imagination, in our minds and there will be a
> natural progression from where you've been, where you are at
> onto, naturally progress onto where you want to be. So perhaps
> if I can, start, to give you a flavour of what we are talking about—
> sitting before us is J ...

MN then describes J, giving his age, occupation, and appearance before
saying:

> J gives off a sense of interest, excitement but underlying this is some
> deep sadness and pain in his life situation at the moment.

MN then says "Pass" and J understands that this means that it is his
turn to speak. J refers to himself as "J", talking about how he wants to
find a solution to his relationship as well as physical illness. "This is
what he wants. Pass." The conversation passes between J and MN like
this as they cover his medical history and how it has affected him. MN
describes how there may be an opportunity to:

> dispense with the need to be in pain, which you could look at as
> being the need to be punished, for, well, we all have long history of
> crimes in our head for what we have done, haven't done. So per-
> haps it is time to have a look at those things, and put them into
> perspective, to see if they actually are all relevant or if it's old stuff
> that we can let go of.

MN also suggests that J:

> has to make a conscious decision to open up his life—life has
> become a bit narrow for J, social life outside the family, there's not
> much he does, just for himself, sauna, swim, that side of things, has
> dried up ...

After this point J switches back and forth between referring to himself
as "J" and as "I" until he settles down into using "I". At this point,

MN refers to J as "you". They agree that J needs a courageous heart but that he also needs to be different so he can be attractive to his partner again. MN says that:

> ... possibly the best way to approach it is to be that different person, to come back as a breath of fresh air. Whatever happens to be that person ... to release outcomes, even though the outcomes seem to be crucial, in one sense take it out of your hands. So it's that flexibility that you talked about, to say I'm going to be me and enjoy the rest of my life, whatever happens around me, no other person has power over my happiness, I can be happy whatever happens, and that's kind of what makes us attractive ... So we see a new J with a new intention, flexible, spontaneous, fun-seeking J with a courageous heart, mainly to fight for something, able to relax about the outcome ...

MN brings J's attention back into the room, then says:

> Now we are looking towards a plant remedy that will remind us of that new intention and help the physicality and help our bodies to honour that.

The next part of the consultation involves both MN and RN and takes place in the herb garden. They each carry a garden chair with them. MN asks J to hold his intention and to go to wherever he feels drawn. J walks to the willows, as he did the last time he was here, and sits in his chair. A little while later MN and RN join J, all three sitting in their chairs in front of the willows. They sit quietly for about ten minutes. Then they discuss willow. J says that he had stated quietly, in his head, his intention to be strong, generous, flexible, energetic, pain-free, courageous, and Pan-like and that after being drawn to willow, had asked if willow could reveal something to him about itself. J reported getting a feeling of soft warmth in the middle of his chest when he did this and the feeling that this would be useful for helping his pain to go. MN and RN contribute to this conversation, saying that this willow is generous in its growth rate, growing up to nine feet in a year, and that it contains plant hormones that are often used to help other plants to grow. They suggest that this growth and generosity may be useful to J: it comes back well after being cut back, as J might be cut back if his relationship ends and he sees less of his children. They also point out its flexibility, that helps it bend to the winds without breaking, but which also provides support for others. It also transforms boggy stagnant areas into new life. They also suggest dock as a medicine, which is growing by the willow. They select it for its transformative abilities—it transforms minerals, particularly iron, into the plant. Vervain, a great herb of the druids is also suggested, to help transform J's intentions into reality and to connect the different parts of his body. The forms that the medicines should take are discussed, with it being decided that an amulet should be made out of the willow. J harvests the first young willow branch then gives the knife to MN who continues. Some vervain is then picked. They go inside and make the amulet by taking the leaves off the willow branch and then bending the young branch until it is formed of three layers in a roughly circular shape about three inches across. A chain is made out of the stripped outer bark of the other stems. Some willow bark strips are gently boiled in water, which turns a thin red colour. The decoction is strained and three cups are poured. They sit quietly as they smell and taste the medicine. Some strips of willow bark are given to J, along with the vervain, and a willow flower remedy in a brown dropper bottle that had been made on another occasion. MN suggests that J get some *Hyoscymus* to help with the pain, and reminds him to take some dock. The amulet is now finished. MN puts it over J's head so it rests over his chest, saying: "An amulet of osea willow to wear next to your heart." MN reminds J that the lion that was seeking courage in *The Wizard of Oz* was also given a medal.

Reflection on MN

MN's entryways relate to the rest of his narrative in a number of ways. First, he had always wanted to be a doctor and his continuing interest in orthodox medicine can be seen in his studying herbal medicine at an institution that was embracing science. It can also be seen in his engagement with orthodox case history taking and physical examination skills as being necessary, if not sufficient, for being a herbalist: the "detective" work of orthodox differential diagnosis is something that is required for his practice. MN's belief in the importance of spending time growing herbs as a way of developing a foundation in herbal medicine before studying it academically may also be seen in his later development of Goethean science as a formal empirical methodology that requires direct contact with living plants, often over their life cycles. Another of MN's concerns in his entryways was that the human being was "nowhere to be seen" in his experience of orthodox medical training. This concern can be found in his later attraction to Goethe, who saw the human being as the "most perfect instrument to, to ascertain, to, to read this book of nature". For MN, Goethean science seeks to "improve the scientist, not just the machine".

Given these two concerns present in his entryways, of the importance of the human being and of knowing living plants, it is maybe not surprising that MN, along with his wife, RN, later developed the methodology of Goethean science that eventually came to be applied to both humans and nonhumans, to patients, and to plants.

That such a methodology is possible suggests that for MN plants and patients have more in common than might be expected. Indeed, MN said that "Plants are inside-out upside-down humans." This implies some relationship between the human and the plant. Further similarities between the human and the nonhuman can be spotted in MN's understanding of herbs as "entities", both as "individual" plants that you can "meet", and also as entities that exist beyond individuals, "flowering all over the rivers of X". Goethean science seeks to bring lost relationships with plants to consciousness.

The various stages of Goethean science, particularly, "glimpsing the being", "being the being", and "catching the essence", suggest human-plant meetings. One way of looking at Goethean science is to see it as upholding the "epistemic virtue" of "truth to nature". Daston and Galison[188] define an epistemic virtue as "norms that are internalized and enforced by appeal to ethical values, as well as to pragmatic efficiency in securing knowledge". The epistemic virtue of "truth to nature" arose in the eighteenth century and sought to identify underlying types and regularities rather than the naturalism of individual objects. This quest for the "pure phenomenon" could be seen only in sequences of observations and not in time-frozen moments. Additionally, the "type" is "truer" to nature than any particular specimen. MN's Goethean science is epistemic in that it is certainly a pragmatic approach to securing knowledge, with its seven-step methodology requiring the human as the only instrument needed to read the book of nature. It is also epistemic in that it appeals to ethical values of interspecies connectivity. And it certainly is a "truth to nature" practice in that it is types, patterns, and essences that are sought rather than isolated instances. While Daston and

Galison identified truth to nature as arising in the eighteenth century, at the time of Goethe, it does not necessarily become extinct under new conditions, as long as it addresses a need for acquiring knowledge. And MN, a twenty-first-century practitioner, is not alone in Western herbal medicine, as we will continue to see, in identifying the importance of understanding plants outside the realm of orthodox "objective" science. Daston and Galison suggest that both the historical and contemporary focus on "objectivity" is in fact due to fear of the subjective. For MN, Goethean science seeks to find "a scientific method to embrace the subjective". MN's Goethean consultation with J is a structured method to embrace the subjectivity of the patient and guide him to listen out for a plant, in this case willow, which will help him to identify and maintain a new intention—"to be flexible, spontaneous, fun seeking, with a courageous heart, and relaxed about outcomes". Patients and living plants are brought together in the Goethean consultation. Given the above, MN's knowing of living plants, through spending time growing them and through Goethean science, may provide a sensual affective energy that helps to sustain his practice.

Visible entryway herbalists: the pull of enchantment

Although the power of clinical trials and techniques of science to enchant should not be discounted, they are based on the authority given by maintaining distance between subject and object, rather than their closeness. Hence, while TE walked the road of relative disenchantment, the following three cases revealed sites of enchantment that speak of proximity to a herbal medicine, to theory, and to woodland. CP related empirically, including via her own body, to particular herbal medicines which she subsequently uses in nearly all her patients, while EP was drawn to the sensuality of the theory of Chinese medicine that produces easier correspondences between diagnosis and treatment than she finds in Western herbal medicine, and JK talked of the "pure diversion" of spending time in her own wood, being nearly sure that this experience of nature does not cross over into her practice. None of these cases suggest that the enchantment of living plants impacts on the practices of these herbalists.

However, the cases of SB, FD, GA, and MN, while also describing visible entryways, do point to the importance of knowing living plants for their practices. Without spending time in gardens, knowing plants that grow nearby, and observing them through their life cycles, these herbalists would not be able to do what they do, they could not be the herbalists that they are. Indeed the "awe" that SB feels about living herbs may contribute to his "arborescent thinking" that helps him to follow clues to get beyond an orthodox diagnosis to the root of the matter. Following an accident, FD becomes aware of the need to know living plants so that she can prescribe them as herbal medicines, suggesting that meetings between FD and plants change which medicines she gives to patients. And herbs that are wordlessly speaking to GA suggest a meeting of realms that can also be seen in his method of nudging patients to treat metaphors as if they are real. MN, along with his wife, RN, developed a contemplative Goethean methodology for understanding plants using the human being as the best tool for understanding nature. They then applied the same methodological steps to their consultations with patients, suggesting correspondences between humans and plants.

We now turn to those herbalists who had hidden entryways, involving meetings with plants, often at a young age.

CHAPTER TEN

Hidden entryway herbalists

The next five herbalists, given the increasing professionalisation and engagement of Western herbal medicine with science, have somewhat surprising, hidden entryways to becoming herbalists. The first two herbalists, CT and VH, are arguably separated from the next three herbalists, AF, BC, and KA, by entryways that are different by degree rather than type.

CT

Entryways

CT grew up in a mining village and coins a term to describe himself as having, since childhood, a "naturphilic" predisposition, deliberately leaving out a letter to suggest a closeness, achieved simply through spending time in nature, particularly in broadleaved woodland.

> I wanted the woods and not the factory. That was really clear, I wanted to be above ground not under it.
>
> I had an orientation at the start that was naturphilic, I like nature, I felt comfortable in nature. That idea of the god Pan also being the

god of panic and being the god of the forests and the forests being a
forbidding place to be and nature being a dangerous place, I didn't
have that, nature was very much a refuge for me and a safe place.

He remembers being influenced by indigenous North American culture,
including the book *Touch the Earth*, by T. C. McLuhan:[189]

It said, the trees, the trees talk you know if you can listen in the right
way and they have things to say, some things, sometimes about
weather, sometimes about the animals, sometimes about events,
and I used to sit in the trees and listen to the wind go through the
trees and try and understand what they were saying to me. And
then one day I took a, there was a, at the animal sanctuary ... there
was a farmhouse and it had a library and I one day just took a book
off the shelf and I can't remember what the book was, but enclosed
in that book was a flyer for the School of Herbal Medicine, College
of Phytotherapy as it became, and I took this out, unfolded it, and
it was just a description of the course and the fact that you could do
a four-year full-time training in herbal medicine, and it was absolutely, straightaway I knew that was it, that's what I, that was it,
that's what I'd been looking for, that's what I needed to do.

Also important for CT in his arrival at herbal medicine as an occupation
was a "spiritual orientation", developed as a child, through his engagement with, and questioning of, Roman Catholicism.

So my thing of sitting at the top of the hill and listening to the trees and
hearing what they had to say to me, I was like, this is how God speaks,
he speaks from nature. And so there was always a sense of there is
something transcendent and something beyond but it's not this, it's
not Roman Catholicism so, but what is it? And finding that in nature.

CT regards having an "alternative mind-set" as also being important
for his genesis as a herbalist. In particular, it was Punk that influenced him:

That questioning thing resonated really and that thing, Britain was
rubbish at that point, it was boring and awful and grey and dreary in

the North at least and oppressive and that kick of, and also that kick of the Punk ethic of anybody can do it, you don't need to be able to play, you don't have to study guitar for twenty years before you can go on stage, you can get on and just make a noise. I still think of herbal medicine a bit in that way, just get some herbs and make a noise.

While having an affinity for nature is not unexpected in someone who ends up using natural products as medicines, his sense of "naturphilia", particularly seen in listening to trees, is a more surprising entryway to the realm of professionalised herbal medicine than has been described in visible entryway cases. He also spent time working as a sheep herder and living on the land in a tipi, and these were important for him in becoming a herbalist. CT sees his entryway to Western herbal medicine as being partly due to this "naturphilia", but also due to his religious orientation and an alternative mind-set. These routes are less visible entryways to professionalised herbal medicine.

Professionalisation and then de-professionalisation

CT has been actively involved in the political life of Western herbal medicine, for many years as a member of committees within the profession, and by vocally arguing for statutory regulation as being necessary for the survival of the profession. He is now drawn to an approach that sees practitioners as supporters of individual well-being rather than as treating conditions.

> I think because there's so much, the trajectory of professionalisation I think has been so fixed and to some degree I am associated with it because I have been involved with it, that there's a not hearing of some of the more radical things I've said lately at conferences and so on, and I think that marriage to the myth of what is I think a myth, or a delusion or illusion, professionalisation I think, has become so strong in the herbal community here that it's not very fertile ground in fact, it's very narrow. And I go [abroad] and they say, oh wow we wish we were in the UK where it's all developed and great and I'm like, no, you guys are the cutting edge, you're the cutting edge because you're the ones who are open to doing it in different ways and that's not how, happening elsewhere.

Influenced by Illich[37,190,191] and his understanding of professionalisation as manufacturing needs rather than promoting self-help, CT questions the professionalisation of herbal medicine.

> But in America there's, there is a sort of humility that's forced upon you by not being allowed to use some of the medical words and I think that's quite good. And so to think of you, yourself as a more, in a much more humble place rather than aspiring to be a doctor. A lot of herbalists in the UK, their leaflets say, I'm trained like a doctor but I use herbs, which is a rash and unfounded claim actually, but also a dodgy aspiration I think … rather than saying, no, I'm something different, I stand for empowering your well-being. And so the idea of a wellness advisor or a health facilitator or, rather than a practitioner, put yourself in a more humble role, more human role, drop that aspiration towards some kind of mystique or power, I think that would be good.

He sees this questioning of professionalisation as being in line with contemporary changes in health care:

> I think the best thing for the profession to do is to just look where the wider healthcare agenda is, so some people like Simon Mills, who's most notable in this I think, have looked at the self-care agenda in, that's coming up in conventional medicine in the NHS, and looked at ways in which herbalists might fit with the self-care agenda, so it does come into the areas of wellness advisors, wellness educators, healthcare decision maker, helpers, and trajectories like shared decision making and shared decision making tools and online decision making tools …

Pharmacology and psychotherapy

CT describes his approach of combining the prescription of pharmacologically active medicines with psychotherapy:

> I think my background really is conventional medicine, because ironically enough, because I like conventional physiology, I'm trained, that's what I'm trained in more than anything else,

conventional physiology, conventional biochemistry ... I think the way that the insights that science has brought, conventional science has brought to the functions of the body, that's where I base my thinking, I think of herbs as pharmacological entities mainly, that's my grounding. But then the psychoneuroimmunology is your thoughts, things you hear, experiences you have, they affect your physiology as well, so mine is very much a physiological pharmacological approach, but words are pharmacological agents and they produce physiological changes in the body.

I think we have something that's fairly unique in herbal medicine, we have one, on one hand through that process of the consultation we have the psychotherapeutic act and the psychotherapeutic potential, then we give medicines that genuinely do alter physiology, they do contain pharmacologically active compounds, unlike homeopathy, and so conventional medicine has the pharmacological compounds without the psychotherapy, homeopathy has the psychotherapy without the pharmacological compounds, everybody else is doing one or the other, and herbalists I think have this really unique position that we do tend to naturally be inclined to do both ...

He describes how the psychotherapeutic act in his practice can have a physiological effect:

... spending time gives us the opportunity to do more psychotherapy and to use placebo more effectively in a benign, loving, manipulative, but manipulative, way, and just being aware of what you're doing, just being aware of what you're doing and just being aware of how simple that is ... Kieron Sweeney talked about the power of bearing witness and he said, you're apparently doing nothing because a patient comes in with a condition you can't help them with and you just say, that must be really terrible, I'm so sorry that you're having to deal with this, and just sitting in silence for a minute and just letting that shared powerlessness but care sink in, and he said, the power of bearing witness we shouldn't underestimate ... including on physiology, of course on physiology, because nothing happens, nothing happens in the body that is experienced without a physiological mechanism underlying it, so the idea that somebody could feel something without a physiological change mediating that feeling, well of course neurotransmitters are changing levels, of course hormone levels are changing, of course immune cells are adapting. So, I think realising that, bearing witness is a physiological strategy, it's a psychophysiological strategy but it is a biochemical, it changes biochemistry …

Furthermore, he recognises that this approach of his is not a new one:

… it's long been appreciated … I think it's Thurston, a physiomedicalist, is saying that essentially it's a combination of the psychotherapy and the herbs and this is early 1900s.

CT gives an example of how he takes a psychotherapeutic approach in his practice:

My general thing is the idea of a transition zone or a deceleration zone. There's an architect called Christopher Day who, he designs anthroposophical buildings, Rudolf Steiner stuff, right? And he's in the UK, I'm not sure if he's still active, I read an interview with him years ago where he designed a school I think, I'm not sure if it was ever built but it was a school design with all the oval shaped windows they have and that kind of stuff. But what he talked about was that there would be a car park for the children to be dropped off or parents … and then rather than the car park be right next to the school there would be like a woodland walk or a meadow walk between the car park and the school. And he called it a deceleration zone, so that from the, yeah, I'm going to school, blah, blah, blah, arriving in the car park there'd be a little walk through the woods and then you'd get to the school and by the time you'd gone through the woods you were ready to be at school, so a deceleration zone or a transition zone. So when I see a new patient what I do is just go through the personal details, don't get my, the receptionist takes a few details and puts them on the computer, name and address … I like to check all those, go through those bits and pieces and treat that as a little deceleration zone or a little transition zone from arriving to the consultation starting proper, so rather than going straight into it. So I purposely have in mind that I'm just, the patient will be feeling me out and feeling the set-up and so it's that transition zone. And then usually I start with a similar kind of question along the lines about, along the lines of, so tell me what you'd like help with. And then my posture is usually to be, open my hands, sit back and it's about saying, I'm open and I'm ready to receive, I've got time, just tell me in your own words. And then if it works that way I'll generally just say to them, say to the patient, so tell me more about that, keep it as minimal as possible. And what I'm wanting is that the story will come out in their own way, their own priority. My assumption, I'll often say, what is it you would like help with? Because I want to reassure them that I am here to help, that's the whole point of it, and that they're open to tell me what they want to tell me ...

But my ideal is that I set the scene where I ask as few questions as possible and the patient somehow leaves feeling that they've been heard and they've told their story and so on ... And that would be my ideal thing that the patient's ability to articulate their story helps them to understand it better.

... but I do think about this, the extent to which I'm doing stealth psychotherapy under the pretext of herbal medicine. And, but I think any sensitive practitioner spending a lot of time with patients is doing stealth psychotherapy and it's just a question of being aware of that. And sometimes there's a great advantage to that because the patient is not labelling it in that way and you're not using that term and it is about herbal consultation but there's a freedom in which to explore things ...

For CT, doing psychotherapy means taking a broad approach rather than following a particular school:

I guess the thing that empowered me to think about herbal medicine in terms of psychotherapy is Carl Rogers ... he said, he said, you know look let's democratise psychotherapy, and his classic three characteristics to the psychotherapist that you have, you view your patient with empathy, unconditional positive regard and, the third one's not coming to me today. But if you do that then you've, he said, and he went on to write a book for teachers and for parents, so people in all walks of, friends, if you're having those characteristics you're doing psychotherapy, yeah. And at the end of his career he said, he said, all those things, what I really meant was "love", so, and I think too, in that liberated way.

In an observed consultation, CT describes to a patient, using techniques he has learnt from Chinese medicine, what he learns from taking her pulse. He then questions her on this and relates her answers to her childhood, before coming back to her pulse again:

CT: ... [your pulse is] not classed as fast but feels a bit stimulated, energy not massively deficient, if I press deep, yin level, but when I take the level off, yang, at both levels it is tight, stressed, if we relax that then the energy can come up. So you need a little relaxation. Have you learned meditation? ... or do you prefer intense physical activities? ...
(CT then takes her blood pressure.)
Patient: Sitting here feels like I could just fall asleep.
CT: Your pulse feels stimulated, tense, stressed. You find the energy but it would be nice to have a bit of rest. Maybe the relaxation phase just doesn't happen naturally. Maybe there is a need to curl up with a blanket.
Patient: I would feel guilty ...
CT: Feeling guilty tends to come from childhood, is that right? Tell me about your dad.
Patient: When I was thirteen he tried to commit suicide, he had a mental breakdown, he retired early, and hasn't worked since ...
CT: Childhood experiences go deep, is your mother someone who always keeps carrying on? ...
Patient: We were given chores at an early age. They were not big jobs but when you are a child, getting milk, unloading the dishwasher. Now I do everything for my son.
CT: Your father's early retirement, maybe that unsettled you?
Patient: He's lazy.
CT: Maybe you are saying, "I can do more, I will do more." Feeling guilty maybe. You *can* have a ten minutes lie-down during the day.
Patient: If I felt exhausted I would.
CT: Sow that seed to say that it is OK to have relaxing moments in the day, but also it will be very good for you, it will raise your energy. In the pulse the energy is there but it is pushed, it is stimulated.

A complex patient

CT finds that he uses fewer herbs than he used to in complex cases:

> And in really complex cases I'll often just use one herb now, what
> we used to call "simples", the way of working with complexity is
> often to begin with simplicity and not complexity, I've learned the
> hard way.

CT describes a patient with multiple sclerosis:

> I remember one particular MS patient, Lizzie, who was so chaotic
> I just couldn't get a grip on her ... I thought about her the next
> day, meditated on her for half an hour and thought the one thing I
> know about the patient is that there is so much heat, she is inflamed
> for a start, an inflammatory process, but she moves all the time,
> she doesn't sit still, she's flushed, she doesn't sleep, she doesn't
> settle, she never stops talking ... how can I cool her down? ... That
> is as basic energetics as you can get is a patient with excess heat.
> How to cool her down? I used certain herbs with her, like uncured
> *Rehmannia*, things to cool her down. And she phoned me in two
> weeks, she had this frizzy, friable hair that was all over the place it
> was so dry. Working with complex systems can lead to unpredict-
> able outcomes, OK? So she phoned me after two weeks and she
> said, "It's amazing." I said, "What's amazing?" She said, "My hair
> is glossy." The last thing on earth I would have expected her to say
> to me. But, in two weeks! She said, "It's hanging down, it's glossy"
> ... but, heat, cool her down!

CT reports that this patient was later told by her neurologist that he
didn't consider her as having MS any more:

> [Lizzie is] a fiery ... woman with really strong opinions and she's
> a memorable woman anyway. And she's somebody who doesn't
> suffer fools, so the fact that we've been able to work well together
> and get the result, she's the one, I haven't told you the rest of her
> story ... she's moved to Italy, so we do stuff by Skype now, but her
> neurologist in Italy discharged her two years ago and said, "You no
> longer have MS, I don't consider you as having MS." So she's one
> that we've been through a long journey with, I've been treating her

for seven or eight years, something like that, and after five or six years that happened. And she's completely convinced that herbs have saved her life and everything but then she is a drama queen, and I say that with great affection.

Complexity theory

CT looks to the cutting edge science of complexity theory to help him understand and develop his practice. Complexity theory seeks to explain complex systems such as weather patterns, insect colonies, the immune system and the brain.

> This is a quote from Francois Jacob, who is a writer in complexity, and he is talking about complexity and evolution and I love this quote because it sounds like us, see how it sounds to you. He says natural selection does not work as an engineer works, it works like a tinkerer, do you know what a tinkerer is, a tinker? OK. So this is what he says: "A tinker is somebody who uses everything at his disposal to make some kind of workable object, slowly modifying his work, unceasingly retouching it." So a tinker is like a gypsy in a positive sense of that, somebody who just has bits and pieces, and they say, "Hey, what can I do with this?" and they kind of try something. "No, that's not quite working, what if I put this on? Ah, that's good." Jacob says this is the complexity of life, this is what evolution is, evolution tries this on, what about if I do this, what about this colour …? To me that sounds like what I do with chronic patients … you work like a tinker, use everything at your disposal, dietary advice, meditation, referral to others, herbs, whatever to produce some kind of workable object, a treatment that helps, slowly modifying your work, unceasingly retouching it. Who gives the same prescription twice to the same patient? … you tweak things.

CT describes some of the characteristics of complex systems— "sensitivity to initial conditions", "attractors", "non-linearity", "self-organisation", and "emergent properties". He views both herbs and people as being complex systems "sharing many commonalities beginning at the cellular level", arguing that:

> Herbal medicine is a means of using plant systems to treat human systems—it is complex medicine … The traditional medicine practitioner typically stands in awe of the mystery of nature, content to modulate systems activity and modify emergent properties by, for example, "moving the blood" or "draining heat". As a greater knowledge of phytochemistry has been gained alongside more detailed information regarding the physiological effects of herbs, the potential for integrating traditional and contemporary insights into herbal practice has arisen. The potential has … been little realised but complexity theory offers a framework for this task.

Given this perspective he suggests new ways of thinking about herbs. These concepts include: simplicity, nudging, pushing, information, tuning, attractors/re-configuring initial conditions, working at the edge of chaos, self-organisation, and re-complexification.

CT argues that complexity theory has the potential to overcome the reductionism-holism dichotomy:

> Reductionism and holism are not incompatible … each approach can inform the other … when the two are separated from each other then the spectrum of understanding has been reduced at both poles. Reductionism set adrift from a holistic perspective tends to abstraction and irrelevance and even harm; whilst when holism eschews the insights of reductionism it gravitates toward flakiness and incoherence and inefficacy. The concept of "complexity" offers a means of renewing, integrating and transcending the reductionism-holism polarity … Above all the reductionist approach is a quest for certainty. The greatest gift of complexity to health care may be a means of living with uncertainty.

Reflection on CT

It has been argued above, via Weber, that professionalisation is closely linked to rationalisation, science, and bureaucracy and that the profession of Western herbal medicine has engaged with these trajectories. However, the case of CT suggests that, for this particular individual, while professionalisation has been necessary for political survival, it is unable to provide all the answers, and may even be problematic for practice with patients.

For CT, complexity theory has the potential to reconcile what are often seen as opposites—to unite holism and reductionism, and to bring traditional herbal knowledge together with science. This resolution of binaries is arguably more enchanting than Nissen's[103] assertion that the concept of holism is attractive to practitioners because it can accommodate many different meanings. CT's entryways also reveal something of the reconciling of opposites in the blurring of boundaries: a young man who listens to trees; transcendence found in nature yet not separate from an engagement with Roman Catholicism; and the influence of the DIY ethic of Punk yet also the finding of a profession. Looking beyond his entryways he was ultimately drawn back to his "alternative" roots in his favouring of the qualities of the "wellness advisor" over the "professional practitioner". And in his practice both words and herbs are pharmacological agents.

Through all these changes CT retains his "access" to "naturphilia":

> There's a default really, there's a default that I can access and I didn't realise it was, it, it's just, you just think, well this is how I am or you don't know, you don't think about it, but over time I've realised that I do have this basic feeling for nature, this basic confidence in nature.

CT's "naturphilia" is the enchantment that Weber said was disappearing from the world. Furthermore, on an experiential level, this "naturphilia", or enchantment by nature, including by herbs, is a sensual-affective energy, one that allows boundaries to be blurred and opposites to be negotiated and even reconciled. The pairs of holism and reductionism, science and tradition, nature and religion, punk and professionalism, advisor and practitioner, and words and drugs are easily brought together in one practitioner. Referring back to Bennett,[50] CT's engagement with the cutting edge science of complexity theory can be seen as an engagement with "interior reason"—the first wonder of the Kantian world, with his "naturphilia" referring to Kant's second wonder—nature itself. The complex worlds of the physiological bodies of humans and the phytochemical bodies of plants are both sites of enchantment.

VH

CT was drawn to the general principles of complexity science to help resolve opposites and to understand herbs and his practice. We now turn to a herbalist, VH, who was eventually drawn to a specific, if more peripheral, manifestation of complexity science.

Entryways

For VH, "My vocation was established at four years of age." He goes on to say that he, of course, "didn't realise it at the time". He remembers running and playing "Hc" on a farm, which had a gypsy caravan, on a warm sunny day. He fell over and smelt yarrow while lying on the ground face down.

> I didn't know its name then ... I kept my face in the grass ... I was involved with plants without being involved at all.

As a boy, he bought a botany book:

> You must remember that in those days, boys did chemistry, not biology.

He found at school that he knew things about the human body without having ever been taught them. When he was thirteen an older child of sixteen, who had found blood in his urine, approached VH:

> He said he was bleeding ... I found myself asking questions like "How long have you had it? Does it hurt?" Then I heard "kidney" in my head and I said to him, "If this happens again in the next 24 hours you should see Matron."

He also knew as a child that the herbs in his Letts diary were medicinal, he "just knew", no one had told him.

> How did I know that they were medicinal? *Viola odorata* was one of them.

He says he is not invoking some mystical capability, but rather:

> I have found words in childhood diaries whose presence there suggests that I knew the words, was not trying to be precocious and yet cannot explain how I came by the words or understood the concepts they expressed. A mystery in the sense of the unknown but not wilfully unknowable.

There was also his own illness, when as a young man in France, he was told by the matron that he had developed a *"crise de foie"* due to the mistral. She gave him a large bunch of thyme and told him how to infuse it. It was this that gave him the courage to look at his own illness history:

> The medical orderly came along with several neighbours to see how I was doing, made the infusion and explained that the trigger to the crisis was the notorious mistral, the wind that enters down upon the liver, heart and mind, depending upon the disposition of the person and the circumstances in which she or he had been so caught out ... The slow and sure healing process provided me with a meditation in which the medicinal plant served as an instructor in a way that the silence of previous mainstream interventions had never hoped to ....
>
> ... whatever illness it was that befell this twenty-two year old in the south of France, it was certainly calamitous and the strength of taste and smell of the herbal remedy appeared like a manifest ally and gave me the strength to contemplate the pathway that had led me to the crisis. The vigour of the thyme dispelled any sense of baffled victim that I might have entertained and gave me back not only courage and strength but also insight: the calamity that drove the illness had a richer history.
>
> The quality of that cure stayed with me and no doubt is why I eventually became a herbalist.

And finally, beyond knowing things without knowing how he knew them, his own experience of illness, the sensuality of the smell of yarrow and the taste of thyme, he remembers falling in love with a French aristocrat.

> It was dawn. I opened the kitchen door. She had little bunches of herbs.

So VH's beginning includes some visible entryways, such as his own experience of illness, but also some less visible beginnings including the importance of the smell and taste of herbs, and romantic love, and the arguably hidden entryway of knowing things without having been taught them.

Finding his theory of cure

VH went to a seminary, describing himself as a "religious child, not pious". His motivation was partly to please his great aunts, some of whom were nuns. At the age of fourteen he withdrew from that vocation, unable to commit to celibacy.

VH travelled to North and Central America, studying at various herb schools, trying to find a school that suited him. However, they all seemed to have an "implicit religiosity" about them, which he found unsatisfactory. And sometimes it was more explicit:

> The herb school I went to in Guatemala was run by Seventh Day Adventists—they didn't really want herbalists, they wanted missionaries and I didn't quite see myself in that role.

In the end he returned to the UK and studied with the NIMH. One of his teachers was Fred Fletcher Hyde, who we have already seen to be an influential political figure in Western herbal medicine in the UK:

> ... it was emphasised to me, especially by Fred Fletcher-Hyde, that we should treat the patient not the condition. "There is no such thing as eczema," we were taught, "but only a patient with eczema." If this were true, then the answer to the question, "Do you have anything for arthritis?" must be "No," because there is no such thing as arthritis, only someone with arthritis. Fred Fletcher Hyde gave quite a number of cold remedies and formulas for this and that condition ... so there was an inherent contradiction between a theory of cure and empiricism.

For VH the problem of empiricism can be seen in both orthodox medicine and in Western herbal medicine:

> I once had a patient with a big nasty intertrigo ... he went every week to a consultant dermatologist to sort it out ... but nothing worked ... at the last appointment the dermatologist said, "Oh, I dunno," and reached for the BNF [*British National Formulary*] as the patient clapped it from him and said, "No, *I'll* stick a pin in it and see what we come up with" ... that's when he came to me. In a fortnight he was better and had no relapse ... But "sticking a pin

in it"? We might as well at the same time have stuck a pin in the BHP [*British Herbal Pharmacopoeia*]—intertrigo—what is it?—a form of dermatitis—look up alteratives—what sort of alterative? So the patient in this anecdote is drawing attention to the arbitrary selection of remedies and it highlights the problems of empiricism ... empiricism is fine when it works ... but what do you do when the remedy fails?

The problem of empiricism is focusing on the phenomenon of the illness itself rather than the path that led up to it ...

The reason I am not an empiricist is partly because on leaving the School of Herbal Medicine I had these lists of things that did this but they didn't work, they just didn't. Hit and miss. Might get a bit better. So that's the reason I am not an empiricist—it's not very effective.

During his herbal education VH found that there was no "theory of cure", rather he just had lists of herbs with the same action (e.g., alterative herbs, diuretic herbs, carminative herbs, etc.), with little help on how to choose between herbs on any one list.

In 1987 VH went to Paris and came across Duraffourd's *Cahiers de Phytothérapie Clinique*[192] (originally published in five volumes between 1983 and 1996), which "spoke to me". The theory of cure that spoke to VH has a number of names including "endobiogenics", "endobiogeny", and "terrain theory". The other main text is Duraffourd and Lapraz's *Traité de Phytothérapie Clinique.*[193] VH felt at home in the French tradition. Initially he had difficulty understanding the endobiogenic writings but he kept reading. He describes himself as a "stoic wandering through treacle ... Suddenly, what you do not understand, you can." VH told an expert practitioner in endobiogenics about how he had had to admit when he was fourteen that he no longer wanted to be a priest. The practitioner recognised that that had "taken courage", and revealed how he had also been in a seminary but at the age of nineteen he heard some girls laughing and singing and could no longer commit to celibacy. Both had nearly been priests.

He eventually met Dr Lapraz in 1998. VH started to learn the "neuroendocrine theory of terrain" from the French texts and from Dr Lapraz and found that his practice improved. Endobiogenics is a theory of "terrain". Lapraz and Hedayat[194] describe terrain as being made up of structure and function, with the former based on genetic heritage and the latter being the expression of this constitution in maintaining structure and adaptive capabilities:

> In summary, endobiogeny is a theory of terrain. The terrain assures its own functioning through permanent movement: a constant and unceasing adjustment of its internal equilibrium in the face of inductive and reactive elements. The manager of this terrain must similarly be dynamic, ubiquitous, constant in its association with every aspect of the organism, and self-regulating. The endocrine system is the only system that meets these criteria, thus it is the manager of the terrain. In conclusion, endobiogeny is the study of how the endocrine system manages the terrain.[194]

Endobiogenics is a global systems approach to human biology. Hence it is part of systems biology.[195] However, it is regarded as differing from other approaches in three ways: it maintains a focus on the "global vision of the organism in toto"; it attends to the endocrine system rather than genes as the manager of the body; and it seeks to understand the reason for disease as well as simply the mechanisms.[195] Endobiogenics is concerned with understanding very detailed interactions *between* hormonal axes, something that orthodox medical practice is seen as ignoring in favour of the vertical relationships of hormones *within* axes. VH explains:

> Lapraz and Duraffourd ... realised that this was looking at an end-stage, when someone has Addison's or PCO or diabetes ... but that there was a horizontal relationship at the pituitary and a horizontal relationship at the hypothalamic level ...

Duraffourd explains why herbs are appropriate medicine: "The multiplicity, ubiquity, and polymorphous nature of the agents that disrupt normal physiological processes is perfectly matched by the plurality and polymorphous nature of the pharmacological activities of medicinal plants. This explains why we chose, very early on, whole plant extracts—or extracts that are as near as possible to this idea—in our attempt to grapple with the complex task of maintaining or restoring homeostasis."[196]

VH says that:

> Lapraz and Duraffourd found that herbs in very small quantities,
> very small doses, not homeopathic but physical material doses,
> influenced the relationships, influenced the relationships, every
> one of those relationships is modified by one plant or another …

During an observed consultation VH identified a patient's knee problem as being related to thyroid hormones and to gut health. The patient,
who had thrush, was complaining of a knee problem of several months
that wouldn't heal. VH examines the knee closely and says, "You have
a cyst—a baker's cyst … the knee problem is thyroid shock." VH has
a further look at the leg and notices hair loss on a specific area of the
lower leg. He says, "TSH resistance, low T4," and suggests that it is
necessary to "sort your bowel out to settle the cyst". The patient then
says that her bowels are not good, but are "eggy, on the verge of giar-
dia … I almost shat myself in the bath." VH gave her a tisane (a herbal
tea) of *Lavandula officinalis* (lavender), *Matricaria recutita* (chamomile),
Salvia officinalis (sage), *Thymus vulgaris* (thyme), *Lamium album* (white
dead-nettle), and *Menyanthes trifoliata* (bogbean). Also a tincture of *Foeniculum vulgare* (fennel), *Angelica archangelica* (angelica), *Salvia officinalis* (sage), and *Trigonella foenum-graecum* (fenugreek). VH's use of these
herbs is mostly based on the French clinical practice of endobiogenics
rather than English language textbooks and sources. He explained that
he gave *Foeniculum vulgare* (fennel) because it is an oestrogenic remedy
to help with the thrush that also stimulates the thyroid axis; the *Angelica
archangelica* (angelica) is alpha sympatholytic to help with the transition
from the vagus to the sympathetic; *Salvia officinalis* (sage) stimulates the
thyroid axis; *Thymus vulgaris* (thyme) stimulates cortisol and is used for
thrush; and *Trigonella foenum-graecum* (fenugreek) is vagomimetic and
anabolic. The patient's terrain is being treated via herbs that have endocrine actions. The symptoms are not being treated directly.

> This is a crucial point—if you get rid of a symptom, which the
> patient would quite like you to do, then you have to be careful that
> whether the symptom is the last gasp attempt to keep the boat afloat
> because if you remove that then you remove the very prop that the
> patient was relying on. This is where a very careful developmental
> history is so important. Something like migraine is an attempt to
> catch up because most migraineurs cannot operate so they lie down

in a darkened room, allowing the adaptive resources to rise so they can operate again. So if you are trying to treat a migraine ... identify which of the adaptive burdens the terrain is incapable of meeting and if you can assist in that way the patient will stop having migraines ... you simply switch them off at source. You certainly don't treat the migraine itself.

While endobiogenics necessitates a detailed understanding of complex hormonal pathways to treat the terrain, for VH this cannot be separated from knowing living plants by becoming habituated to them by simply spending time with them:

> Back to the theory of cure, if the therapist has a very clear procedure, a regulatory theory, it means that the quality of your attention improves and the patient appreciates and feels that. I am not saying that you can believe anything you like and it will help, but you have to have some regulatory theory of cure, and my experience of endobiogenics is that it satisfies me in that it is culturally attuned, one is able to validate certain aspects of it—it is not all subjective, and it is relational, it is about relativity, it is not about absolute states. In all the journeys that I have made in trying to find a theory of cure in North America and at the School of Herbal Medicine I waited for recognition of something that seems appropriate to the very thing that one is trying to use—medicinal plants, and I may be very naïve but if you're in the wild and you are surrounded by plants, we eat them and take them for medicine, and the primary notion is that you have to get to know them as creatures and if you learn a system of cure without that relationship then I think life becomes very difficult to practise herbal medicine. So I would make a case for always knowing the plants you use. I have never used a plant that I haven't grown or seen in the wild ... with the exception of culturally accepted plants like ginger. I am not into localism per se but to use a plant that you don't know directly I think limits your ability to find a theory of cure.

A priestly approach

VH's mother had said about him from an early age—"He'll sit and listen." VH had narrowly missed being a priest. And now he finds that quite a lot of his patients see him as something approaching a parish priest. VH says that he found his "path with heart" and that when a patient is diverted from his or her path with heart, they become ill.

> [Patients] need to find their path with heart and then they won't need the medicines.

While VH found his theory of cure in endobiogenics he also tries to create a space for patients to consider their problems "like spreading out a picnic whose contents are misremembered or were made by other hands". As well as having his theory of cure, which will reassure the patient that he is "more than a good and sympathetic listener", there is a parallel process of witnessing the patient and allowing a consideration of the problem at hand. For VH this parallel process is the main function of both the doctor and the priest. As VH says:

> In a way, one could summarise the sacerdotal agency as mediating the symbolic manifestation of a patient's problem, and contrast it with that of the "purely" medical as one that deals with technical manifestations. Of course, these problems, which seem "merely" mechanical, will almost certainly have symbolic origins. As an example, a lady came to see me last week. She arrived flustered and mumbling and continued to witter for some minutes. She became gradually more comfortable and relaxed from her journey and the stress of having to present herself as important. The problem of a fortnight ago surfaced and she broke into tears: as she herself said, and as everyone reassured her, it was a trivial problem—her home telephone broke. I treated her daughter for acne many years ago, then for her and her husband's infertility. Then Robert was born four years ago to the happy couple and this little boy gives this patient her reason for living. He arrived in time to be cradled by his maternal grandfather whom I treated in the final months of his life. All of this continuity means that she does not have to explain anything to me. This is the blessing brought by relationships, and is one of the benefits of the old system of family doctor. There needs to be some parallel processing going on: I have to listen out for her medical state as I provide her with the opportunity to interiorise in public, to display what is there for the benefit only of herself and her world.

These parallel processes—applying a theory of cure to select the right medicines, and the witnessing of the patient—in fact support each other:

> ... the quality of human attention is the usual conduit for medicine to be successfully introduced and for healing to take place.

Reflection on VH

VH's entryways suggest certain meetings, or blurring of the boundaries between the human and the nonhuman. This can be seen in his "being involved with plants without being involved at all", in the importance for VH of the smell and taste of herbs, and in his "knowing things" without a referenced source of information. The smell and taste of thyme was later important for him when he was struck down with a *crise de foie*. After VH had travelled a long road from England to France to North and Central America and back to England again he eventually found his theory of cure in Paris in the form of endobiogenics, a systems biology approach with a detailed understanding of the horizontal relationships of hormones at its centre. Like another practitioner, he gave up the enchantment of the priesthood and found endobiogenics. It was attractive to VH due to its language of science that meant it was "culturally attuned", and in its at least partial validation, as well as in its avoidance of viewing the body in terms of absolute states. VH's early experiences with herbs may be related to his selection of endobiogenics as his theory of cure, with both requiring meetings to occur. The first is between VH and plants, and the second is seen in endobiogenics' forensic examination of the relationship *between* hormonal axes where meetings occur, rather than simply following a single vertical axis, as is done in orthodox medicine.

Importantly, for VH, knowing plants, by simply "becoming habituated to them", was necessary for his arrival at his theory of cure, namely, endobiogenics. Without his childhood experiences, he may never have arrived at this need. This knowing of plants is an enchantment, or sensual-affective energy, that VH required to arrive at his destination. The other driving force was his desire to find a way to avoid having to choose from lists of apparently similar but ultimately different herbs that he was taught as a student. No more sticking pins in the *BHP*—the *British Herbal Pharmacopoeia*. Furthermore, VH's priestly approach to patients, seen in his attention to the "path with heart", is potentially enchanting.

Reflection on CT and VH

Both CT and VH, despite having hidden entryways, chose to engage with science. This coheres with the journey that the institutions of Western herbal medicine have been seen to be taking in the integration of scientific knowledge into teaching and practice and as a strategy of increasing the likelihood of its political survival.

CT, in his engagement with complexity theory, chose to work with the general principles of complex systems science. VH, in his attraction to endobiogenics, chose to engage with a specific manifestation within the field of systems biology, itself a sub-field of complex systems science. While both complexity theory and endobiogenics are "scientific", the former can be broadly seen as "cutting edge" and the latter can be viewed as more peripherally located within cutting edge science. Neither CT's nor VH's respective use of complexity theory and endobiogenics engages with elements of science that are taken for granted within the scientific community, and certainly not within orthodox medical practice. We now turn to the final three herbalists, whose entryways are arguably even more hidden, and whose narratives reveal rather different trajectories.

AF

Entryways

AF remembers the influence of spending time in nature on his eventually becoming a herbalist:

> I'd always been interested because my dad was very into natural history, when he retired, he was working, he did voluntary work on nature reserves and things. So we'd go for long walks on Sunday afternoons and look at the birds, and he'd say what they were, and the trees, and he'd say what they were. It never ceases to amaze me how little the students at university know about just the natural history around them. And things like going, we used to go to a favourite little meadow on the Downs, which was covered and

covered with butterflies. So many butterflies, you could run around and catch them, and let them go and catch them and let them go. You just don't see that any more.

AF sees a particular event as being important for his journey to being a herbalist:

> When I was five, that's when the plants called me, or the spirits of the plants called me. Because we had this typical suburban garden with a lawn and a vegetable patch and a bit at the end where you had the bonfire, and the bit at the end was always very exciting because it also had the air raid shelter, which hadn't been demolished then. And that was my favourite bit, and I seem to remember, around about the age of five, sitting there, and looking around at the plants, and suddenly becoming aware that plants were all different, they weren't all just general "plantosity". I think babies see the world as like a, everything sort of general and then they pick out their parents, they pick out another thing, they pick out another thing, they pick out things about their house and then they start to pick out things about the world. Anyway, the plant I became aware of was red dead-nettle, I didn't know what it was called or anything, but I became aware of it as a separate entity with a separate spirit, and that's my earliest memory and I think that's when the spirits of the plants called me.

While CT and VH had entryways such as "naturphilia", a critical religious sensibility, the importance of the smell and taste of herbs and "simply knowing things", that hinted at meetings between the human and the nonhuman, AF's early experience with red dead-nettle suggests a more active role on the part of the plant in relationship to the eventual herbalist that AF would become.

Three theories of cure

AF studied for a degree in physics and was a science teacher before he enrolled at the School of Herbal Medicine, graduating in 1983.

He also apprenticed himself with an older herbalist:

> I used to do that two days a week. And then she'd have, she'd call me in if they were interesting patients who didn't mind. And I'd

sit and chat to the patients, I learned a lot that way. It was a proper apprenticeship thing, in a way, because I had to prune her garden as well. I remember pruning a climbing rose, it took me a whole day to prune this massive climbing rose, got cut, really prickly things, climbing roses. I got covered in cuts. I remember cutting back the hawthorn, not the hawthorn, it was a rosemary, she had big rosemary bushes and she had … and a motherwort and all sorts of things growing there … So that was good, so then after I qualified I could always call on her.

When he qualified he set up practice from home:

And we came over here and set up this room, which is the front room, as a dispensary. And we built all those shelves out of skips, you used to find really jolly good stuff in the skips in those days, it's mostly rubbish these days …

AF knows VH, who found his theory of cure in endobiogenics.

What is my theory of cure? … I thought, well, you know, I don't actually have one. I have several. And I apply them according to the circumstances basically.

First theory of cure—working with physiology

When AF was training there was still a residual physiomedical influence on the curricula, with modules on physiomedical theory and dispensing, which retained an emphasis on physiology.

Pathology. I always try and ignore pathology, and work on physiology. And one of the best examples I had of that, was a patient … she had lupus, quite mild. And it mostly manifests on the skin but definitely also going inside, because her energy was very low, and I just, I started off, because I'd treated it before, just treating what it said in the books, that you use for lupus, didn't get anywhere at all, and then thought, well, let's use strong anti-inflammatories, and didn't get anywhere at all. And then I went back to the physiology book and it said lupus is basically a connective tissue disease, and connective tissue diseases affect, firstly and mostly, the circulatory system, so you need to strengthen the walls of the circulatory system, which is hawthorn and bilberry. I made her a tea, because she didn't take tinctures, hawthorn and bilberry in it and a few other things, and that was when we started to get results, that's by going back and looking at the physiology and what was really going wrong. So, part of my thing is physiology as orthodox Western physiology and the other herbs work with that. And I think there's still, I think quite a lot of herbalists work that way. It's a good way of working.

Second theory of cure—emotional causes of illness

While the first theory of cure is very much located at the physical level of tissues and organs, his second theory of cure looks to the role of emotions.

> And, when we first started ... we went and did the co-counselling network introduction course, that's all you need really, unless people are really bad, and basically just sit, shut up and listen. And listen, and then, listen to what people are really saying, and ... just feeds back a way of approaching people, which is incredibly important. It doesn't matter how clever you are, or how much you know what people need, they're not going to do it unless you get, unless you can speak to them on their level in some way.
>
> ... And then you give lots of space for people to talk, so people very often say, well, I don't know why I'm telling you this. Happens a lot that and some people say, "I've never told anybody this before," which is nice. Because, I mean, really people know the answer to their own problems, if you can just tease it, pull it out of them. Just tease it out of them. So I was treating someone the other day and she has depression and I used black cohosh because she used the word black and the word black just sprang out at me, bang, and then there's the old traditional thing about black moods and I very rarely use black cohosh for depression. Also there is, she had spinal issues. So I think, probably having used all the things that was normally tried and none, and nothing actually worked, I have great hope and great faith in, great hope in the black cohosh. Because then it's about fitting a herb to the person isn't it? So that means you need to get to know the person as well as you possibly

can, as well as you know the herbs. So you have to be thorough and you have to do the case history thing because people will forget or they'll de-emphasise things, which actually turn out to be quite important.

AF sees part of his role as helping patients to find the freedom to play with being something else.

> I need to be something else in order to be able to tell them to be something else. This is perfectly true.
>
> Then the other thing, the other way I look at it is you reach a place with somebody in the consultation and then quite often they'll go out feeling really happy and say, "I feel really happy and good and relaxed and content." You know it's not going to last because they're going back into the world, so in a way you give the bottle, it's like a distilled essence of the consultation to take with them.

As well as taking the consultation away with them in their medicine bottles, AF's patients also receive herbal medicines that may include restorative, relaxing or stimulating effects. Additionally, AF uses flower remedies to treat emotional issues. Flower remedies are mostly made by leaving freshly picked flowers in spring water in the sunshine for several hours before straining, adding a preservative, often brandy, and bottling. Many of AF's flower remedies have either been made by himself, other herbalists or friends, although some have been bought. AF uses a striped brown and amber pendulum, made from recycled Coca-Cola bottles, to douse for the flower remedy that is most helpful for the patient. The remedies are kept in home-made boxes that have collaged and varnished images of natural landscapes, including plants, a mouse, butterflies, a dousing stick, and horses that seem to be hiding.

> … it's a very useful way, I use it mostly integral with counselling, so you do the flower remedy, if a flower comes up, then you discuss what that flower remedy means to people, then they say, "Oh right." I have at the moment, I had a patient off and on, she's a psychotherapist … And she sends me her patients just to do flower remedies mostly … because then we can feed back to her, what

flower remedies come up, and it's ever so interesting. And another patient I've seen for years and years and years that way, and they would come in, you'd do the flower remedy, before they said anything, and they'd say, "That's the issue I've been discussing this week with my therapist," just like that, "that's what I need to work through." And then you do the remedy and it helps you to, facilitate that process. So that's really nice, I love working with her ...

Some of the flower remedies address understandings of human development:

> ... working through the stages of life. And that's a very interesting discussion, when they come out, and you can say things like, "What happened to you when you were fourteen?" and they say, "Horrible, nasty things happened when my dad left home," or whatever, and you say, "Well, your development is being stuck then. And you need to go back again and be fourteen again, you didn't do it the first time," and I see the effect quite a lot actually, you see it with people in their forties and fifties, whatever, being divorced and they're going out again and having a proper teenage thing and they start behaving outrageously. And, yeah good, that's what you're meant to do.

AF uses his pendulum to select a flower remedy in an observed consultation. His patient, John, previously had prostate cancer but has been told by his doctors that he is cancer-free. He also has a history of IBS. Mostly it is anxiety that John is seeking help for.

John says, "This health anxiety is terrible, it seems to have worsened the healthier I have got, these crashes, normally in the morning, it well kicks in, and velcroed to it is anxiety ... for example this [skin condition] can turn into kidney failure in a second ... Crashes and anxiety are more extreme but my system is stronger ... but it is such a battle with anxiety. I'd love to get on top of that a bit more. I'll get light headed."

It is a wide-ranging consultation that includes an abdominal examination and urinalysis, both of which reveal nothing abnormal. AF tells John that he's going to find a flower remedy for him. He gives the flower remedy boxes, one at a time, to John. AF holds the pendulum over the box in John's hands. The pendulum moves from side to side over each box. AF then stands up and says, "Better get the reserves out then," as he gets one more box off the shelf. This time the pendulum moves in a circle over this box. He then tests all the remedies in this box individually until he finds the only one that results in the circular movement of the pendulum.

AF picks up the remedy and says, "Bay flower—for bringing your dreams into reality. Does that make any sense to you?" John replies that in a way he already has lots of work. AF says that maybe it's about keeping that up, "like the Physicians of Myddfai say, 'proper diet, proper exercise and the esteem of your fellows' ... I think that'll do it. Can we do that for a month?" He also gives John a bottle of borage and skullcap tincture, and suggests chromium for blood sugar balance. John is concerned that "I drive myself, give myself a really hard time." AF finishes up by saying that "My thought is that you should be a bit more dreamy in life, do you know any dreamy people, that swan through life? See if you can pick up some tips from them? So probably this bay flower remedy is to help that." John confesses that he fantasises that everyone else's life is easier. AF replies that "That's usually from childhood, that's simple."

AF gives him the flower remedy, which he has put into a labelled bottle for John, saying, "It is a bit of a mystery, this remedy, so it'll be interesting to see what happens. Four drops four times daily." John gets up to leave and AF says, "Give me a ring if anything worries you and I'll tell you to stop worrying."

Third theory of cure—constitutional medicine and energetics

While the first and second theories of cure address the levels of physiology and emotions, the third theory of cure looks to more traditional understandings: namely, constitutional and energetic approaches. This learning was stimulated partly from conversations with Chinese medicine practitioners. However, he was particularly drawn to the work of seventeenth-century English herbalist Nicholas Culpeper, which nudged him on to further research:

> ... because Culpeper is very difficult to read ... Culpeper is famously choleric-melancholic—fire, earth and heat. He would write, he'd write so far and he says, if you can't work out the rest for yourself, then I can't be bothered with you. So you have to work it all out for yourself.

This search led AF to travel to the Wellcome Library in London. He read Anglo-Saxon medical writings, the Victorian herbalist John Skelton's work, also Parkinson, Gerard, and always Culpeper who he found intensely practical.

> They had, well, one interesting book they had was called, *Medieval Science Sourcebook*. It was basically just little snippets, but one of the snippets was on medicine and the, it was actual medieval stuff. So, that they just translate the documents for that and there was, the medicine one was a case study of someone who'd done a Galenic analysis of their patient, earth, air, fire, water, they were, earth three, air four, five, two, one and then they'd made out the prescription almost like, an algorithm, they'd done earth air fire water on the prescription, I thought, that's very, struck me as being reductionist, but that was quite inspiring.

AF was drawn to Galenic constitutional humoural medicine, which dominated European medicine from the second century to the seventeenth century AD. It divided people into various combinations of choleric, melancholic, sanguine, and phlegmatic "humours". Each of these humours is associated with an element—respectively, fire, earth, air, and water; and with qualities, respectively, of hot and dry, cold and dry, warm and moist, and cold and moist. People were categorised as certain types. If a certain humour is dominant in a particular person they tend to favour that humour which becomes excessive and needs rebalancing, which can partly be done by using herbs with qualities that oppose the dominant humour—treatment by "antipathy". In particular, he found that this approach helped him identify ways of relating to patients of different constitutions:

> … you know that sanguine people require a nice firm, authoritative hand, so you be as firm and authoritative. One of my problems is that, I suppose because I'm quite sanguine, is I tend to pick up from people, and I find if I get a completely scatty person coming in, I start to get scatty, so then I have to be quite strict about that. I've always found phlegmatic people the most difficult, which might be because phlegmatic people hide their emotion anyway, but it might just be because I have very little water, I don't know …

He now sees this categorisation into different constitutions as being too rigid:

> … you can't put people in boxes anyway, they don't fit in boxes, they've got arms and legs that stick out … in itself it's not that useful, it really isn't. It's much more useful to try and get a lower level, lower level, it's what we always try and do, get down to the real meaning of life …

AF prefers to use "energetics" now. He says:

> We all learn that plants have actions but that's just bollocks really … Herbs have interactions, they interact with a person, which is why different people respond to different herbs—that is the use of energetics—to find the herb to fit the person …
>
> When we study energetics we are not studying actions or constituents but we are studying the herb itself.

For AF, there are three main ways of studying the energetics of herbs, meaning the herbs themselves:

First, there are conversations with plants.

> I did an exercise a few years ago … we had a patch in clinic between patients and I took them [students] outside, and growing outside is a plant that I thought no one would recognise … That is Canadian fleabane … They didn't know it all. So we found the Canadian fleabane and I said, "Everyone go up to Canadian fleabane and introduce yourself, out loud, this is extremely important when talking to plants. You must talk out loud. Talking inside your head is how humans delude themselves consistently all the time. They think that because they think something inside their head that it has been done. It hasn't …" Anyway they did. They were quite brave. They talked out loud. You introduce yourself and you ask it a little bit of information on how it is in the world, its virtues. And there were half a dozen students there, and every single one, so we looked it up in the books to see what we could find. And every single thing in the books had been found by one or other of the students. And nobody had got anything wrong. On Canadian fleabane. And those were people on a BSc degree who were presumably quite logical and scientific. A lot of people say, "Oh, I dunno, I can't do this

intuitive stuff." You can, it's dead easy. All you do is go out and talk to the plants. You must talk. You must talk out loud.

Second, there is learning from texts over time.

> Pick a plant and read it up in all the old books you can possibly find. It's a thread … the plant has interactions with humanity throughout its history and if you can follow the thread all the way through from the old shamanic stuff all the way up to modern science including constituent pharmacology, after all even the constituents are made of the spirit, aren't they? And the modern uses, you can see the whole picture.

Third, there is learning from tasting herbs.

> Tasting will help you resolve tricky points on energetics. Too many people think that energetics is about reading lists of things, so many hot and cold … that is rubbish … it is about directly relating to the plant … you can't learn energetics from books, you can't learn about hot and cold and constitution from books … you can only learn about it by doing it and if you get involved in a dispute it is easily solved by tasting … We were doing a tasting … an Indian lady trained in Ayurvedic medicine said *Datura* was a warming herb … I thought that was strange … not a warming herb because it kills you basically … so we tasted it … it brings the heat in … it warms the centre … so in that sense it is a warming herb … but the periphery gets cold.

AF has developed a method of tea tasting that is usually done in groups. First of all a tea is made with a single herb, although not too strong, so as to avoid the taste being dominated by a particular constituent. No one is told the name of the herb.

> Try and approach it without any preconceptions, very hard as a herbalist, start by smelling it, do not drink it yet. I do think that, after sitting with herbs, tasting is the best way of approaching the energetics of herbs. … Herbs do not have actions, they have interactions … will interact with each of you differently so do not be embarrassed … If you want you can call it organoleptic testing, because you are using all your senses, toes and everything.

In AF's method, it is the smell that is assessed first—what does it smell like and how does it make you feel? General impressions are noted and medical language is avoided. Then the tea is tasted, sipped slowly, swished around the mouth; the texture is noted as well. What impressions does the taste give? A free approach to the language used is encouraged as well as whether it is, for example, bitter, sweet, sour, salty, pungent, dry, smooth or oily. Next, the "appropriations" are addressed, in other words those parts of the body—tissues, organs, and body areas where its activity is felt. What does it do there? Does it move outward, inwards, down or up? How does it move? Does it move slowly, expansively or lightly? Is it warming or cooling? Lastly, tasters are asked to finish the sentence "It is like …" and to be free with their language. During this process, AF draws a figure of a person and notes the answers down and highlights body areas as they are given out. In the end, there is an annotated image that describes what has been found. Then the name of the herb is revealed and its qualities and medicinal uses are discussed and compared with what the group had found in the tasting.

These three theories of cure are not used discretely. Rather AF draws on different elements as required. The ease of integration of these approaches can be seen when AF is talking about herbs. For example, when talking about lady's mantle he approaches it as a tissue herb for the womb. However, he also asked a patient every morning in May to gather the drops that it secretes as part of a wider emotional strategy for her. And when talking about sage he uses energetic terms:

> When you've tasted it I hope anyway you've felt the way it draws into the centre, it draws the vitality, the vital heat, the energy of life into the centre of the body, holds it there. Very good for scattered states, I use it a lot for after infections when everything has scattered and needs to be brought back to the centre again. Also of course for hot flushes, which is a scattered state, whether due to the menopause or fevers, low grade viral infections …

But just as easily he describes using it for prolactin secreting tumours of the pituitary gland:

> I've also used it, three times, in fact four times, for prolactin secreting tumours of the pituitary gland. Use tincture of equal parts thuja and sage, back that up with a couple of cups of sage tea just to really get the sage in there. Just to bring the prolactin levels down,

works very very well. I had three women there out of the four get pregnant, which of course is the main reason why women come to see me with prolactin secreting tumours. One woman actually had two babies each time with the sage, doing it, bringing the prolactin down again. It's a reasonable strategy, the orthodox strategy with prolactin secreting tumours is to give the drug for a couple of years and cross your fingers, because very often the whole thing will just go away and you don't have to do the operation, which is very tricky, so doing the same thing with sage and thuja is a reasonable strategy. Just measure the prolactin levels, see how you're going, and see if you're having success.

Spirit and a sense of place

For AF, it is only through his own spiritual development that he can help his patients:

> That is what it's all about. It's about plants and relating to the plants, and the way that plants help you relate to the spirit, and so the whole thing is about … the whole thing is not about patients, it's not about getting people better, it's not about being a healer, it's about you, and your spiritual development, that's what it's about. Because then, the more you can do that, then the more useful you are to people …

It is through knowing your local "patch" that spiritual development is possible:

> What is the first responsibility of the herbalist? … to my mind the first responsibility of the herbalist is to the earth … because that is where the plants grow … we look after our patch, it is looking after your patch that gets you in touch with the herbs and the earth and the energy of the earth in that place and no matter how many exotic herbs you may or may not use it is extremely important to understand the herbs growing in your area. Keep that conversation up so that you can keep up the conversation with the earth so you can know your sense of place. That is the spiritual dimension of herbal medicine. I regard herbal medicine as a spiritual path because the herbs relate directly to the spirit and help us to relate to the spirit …

AF knows his local area very well. He knows where to get which herbs at what time of year. He often leads herb walks for students and other herbalists. If you are late for a herb walk with AF there is no need to worry as they won't have gone far. The walk is less than a stroll, more of a shuffle, with lots of pauses. On one walk, inching slowly like a shadow on a sundial he shares his knowledge about cherry laurel, ginkgo, barberry, pignuts, creeping thistles, nettle, dock, pineapple weed, plantain, hawthorn, elder, hedge mustard, herb bennet, and enchanter's nightshade.

> I think the most important thing is about using local plants, you need to use as many local plants as you can, in order to build up your relationship, because you can only build up a strong relationship with the plants that are around you … I start building that up, and understanding it energetically, and its friends and relations, it's in that family that does, and it has that and so on. But I can't get as deep a relationship as I can with the stuff growing on my windowsill.
>
> And that's very important, and that, because in the end, even if it's just a handful of plants, my relationship with those plants is the key to me, and it's about building my own energy with the plants and my own relationship with the spirits through the plants which is about evolving me, so I think localism is incredibly important, for the herbalists themselves, maybe not quite so important for their patients, although the herbalists themselves, is important to the healing process.

This localism also extends to his patients. In one particular case AF treats a patient's "out of place-ness" with herbs and her condition improves:

> A woman, thirty-five years old, a student for her sins, very irregular cycle, no period for ten months, a bit on the chubby side, so you could think PCOS … prone to headaches especially migraines. She originally came because of tachycardia on exertion, nausea, heaviness to her digestion, very tired, all her life prone to depression, unsatisfactory relationship, not happy in London, father left home early, sluggish digestion, aches and pains. Migraine strategy of feverfew, betony, dandelion root and leaf … This strategy worked

well, in two months she was better, digestion improved, heart set-tled, energy increased.

But no change in her cycle. I tried, I am afraid to say, the stan-dard PCOS remedy—*Vitex*, liquorice, *Paeonia*, didn't work at all. Then we were talking about how she felt out of place [in a big city], she was brought up on the chalk Downs ... so I made up a medicine from my dispensary from all the medicines that grow on chalk ... a little bit of each ... vervain, St John's wort, pulsatilla, wild carrot, bryony, hemp agrimony, sanicle, cramp bark, clematis: 5ml a day. Her periods started in one month. I didn't want her to take 5ml three times a day—she might think it was a medicine. I wanted it to be a special thing—"Take a little hit of this" ... We used this medicine for her, over three to four months her periods became nicely established, but the flow was erratic so I added some lady's mantle tea ...

AF loves to harvest herbs. He sees it as helping to learn about herbs and connecting him with the ancestors.

And the hands speak directly to the heart. This is why doing things with your hands is so important ... Yes, I think your body learns doesn't it when you're picking because everything has to be picked slightly differently. Well, I don't know if I could put that into words, but the body learns about the plant when you're picking things.

It feels wonderful. Probably harvesting is the most important thing, that's why if I do a workshop I have as many people har-vest, it is just half an hour and to me that connects you with the ancestors ... I remember distinctly a few years ago picking, what was I picking, elderberries I think with a friend of mine ... and suddenly becoming aware of all the ancestors picking with you. So that's ancestral memory, tapping into that which is incredibly important, because we're distracted from that. So picking I think is invoking ancestral memory. I remember, another time it happened, not with picking, [at a summer school] they'd camp in the woods ... taking the camp down, I got this really strong ancestral memory, this is what people did, they took the camp down and they collect it all up and you could feel it, it was brilliant and in traditional society it's very important to keep that contact with the ancestors, otherwise you don't know who you are, you don't know.

Reflection on AF

AF's entryways of spending time in nature and being called by red dead-nettle are beginnings that resonate throughout his narrative. Spending time in local nature has been important for AF in his professional life, from pruning a climbing rose as an apprentice, to knowing his patch, harvesting his herbal medicines and in prescribing herbs local to where a patient used to live. And being called by red dead-nettle, as a human-nonhuman meeting, where boundaries between subject and object are blurred, is arguably an enchantment, providing a sensual affective energy that allows other lines to be crossed and other journeys to be made, including patients taking the consultation away with them in a bottle. For AF, talking to plants and the sensual tasting of plants became ways of knowing plants "energetically" as medicines.

Attention is given to the most "basic" level in order to help patients. AF has come to prefer energetics (knowing directly) rather than constitutional medicine (knowing by categorisation). Rather than treating disease he supports physiology, with physiology coming before pathology, enabling a patient's lupus to be addressed. And treating emotions, as causes of illness, with flower remedies is necessary when treating the body. And ultimately the only way to help patients is to acknowledge that "herbal medicine is about you", the herbalist.

A paring back to the most "basic" levels is always required, arguably in a similarly "arborescent" way that was described in the case of SB. This paring back and this closeness to plants reflect and reinforce each other. While having learnt his relatively traditional approach to herbal medicine over many years he still resources science, particularly physiology, and draws easily from his different sources as needed. The meeting of AF with plants allows his knowledge sources to sit comfortably together.

BC

Entryways

BC sees her route to becoming a herbalist as having started when she was very young, while "still in nappies":

> Every herbalist I've ever spoken to has a plant that called them. Their first experience of the plant world was something that was very emotive and significant. And, of course, as soon as someone's asked that question you want it to be the yew tree or the mandrake

or, and it's always something very humble. So at the time I wasn't aware of these things happening but with hindsight I can see a very clear trajectory so the very first thing that happened was that the plant that called me was grass. And I was, I was still in nappies. There's actually a photograph of me on that day and I crawled away from my parents in long grass and was surrounded on all sides by grass taller than I was so I couldn't see out. And the whole of the rest of the world fell away and I was in this still, beautiful complete world. And I remember really clearly feeling safe and a sense of wonder at this grass all around me and then was either come to be, was fetched or found my way out or called for help or whatever, but I remember so clearly the long summer grass and the short fresh green underneath it. And I remember looking around on all sides and being inside this wonderful space. And then when I was older, about five I guess, I was riding my bicycle up and down the street … and noticed grass growing through the paving stones. And again this sense of absolute wonder that these delicate small leaves had managed to push up. And I suddenly had this unfolding idea in my head of how nature is just behind the façade of the city and how easily it can push through. And I remember again this sense of enormity that came with it so that was my, if you like, the calling.

Her mother called her a "nature girl".

Why I chose herbs rather than any other form of medicine? My mum always used to say I was a nature girl. I've always felt very comfortable in nature, saw fairies for the first time when I was thirteen and in the woods. So and there's a picture of me. I'll show it to you. There's a photograph of me standing inside a tree. I think that she looks very comfortable there—that girl standing in the tree.
    … So I've always had a comfortable experience in nature, standing on the edges of cliffs, climbing up and down rocks, knowing my way up and down a tree, not being frightened to turn a rock over and find the creepy crawlies underneath and plants, always plants, so yeah …

As a young child, BC had extended stays in hospital where she was the object of investigations but where her subjectivity was denied.

I learnt to dissociate because as a child in those days they didn't believe that the nervous system or the emotional system of a child was fully developed so they wouldn't put you under completely and through an anaesthetic and so on and so forth. And also they never asked my permission to do these investigative, really invasive investigative diagnostic tests. And putting me in front of a classroom of students and saying this is the subject. I'm like, what? And actually having to say to them while they wheeled me down the corridor, am I having an operation? And then them saying, "Oh isn't she clever?" ...

So I, my, one of the results of that was I was like, oh my body doesn't belong to me. It belongs to these people here who remove parts of it and put you in a different bed than I was yesterday so my father can't find me when he comes into the ward. And my body doesn't belong to me. It belongs to these people to do with as they choose. So I learned to dissociate ... So it's possible that on some level I was taking care of my body. I don't know, anyway. But all of these things feed, the wounded healer and all of that, all of these things feed into it ...

BC's illness experience led her to choose to avoid orthodox medicine, preferring to learn to treat herself:

Our own illness is also a teacher. ... Although it's a very powerful gene in my family I always refused the tests. I always refused the medication. I always refused the hospital stuff ... But I was determined to find my own way through. So I started looking at diet, sugar ...

When she came to study at university she found that studying anatomy and physiology was "like remembering something". She realised that this was a continuation of formative experience all those years ago:

And within a few months I knew that I wanted to be on the herbal medicine degree course so I switched over. And as soon as I did it all fell into place and I realised that I had been on this road probably since the first time I was surrounded by grass.

Patients' stories

She sees herself as a "wound finder"—someone who patients feel comfortable confiding in.

And for one reason or another I've always been one of those people, as a journalist, as a person in this house with waifs and strays coming through, I've always been one of those people that people feel able to confide in. One of my pagan friends said, "God you're a wound poker!"... Really! And so I've tried to temper that down to wound finder rather than wound poker. But yes, I am. I can't help it. It's something that I have always been able to do. When I was younger people said, "Oh God, no you can, don't talk to her. How did you know that about me? Who have you been talking to?" I'm like, "Nobody."

She sees her role as facilitating patients' stories:

One of the things I now say is that my job as a herbalist is to help you, the wounded storyteller. So I'm the wounded healer. You're the wounded storyteller. There's a book called *The Wounded Story-teller*. So my, everyone, in fact I've spoken to several people about this and it's fairly well recognised. Everyone arrives at this ultimately on their own because it's so obvious. What happens is that you've got a, there's like a blanket that you're weaving. You're making a picture, a tapestry of your life with all the different threads. And sometimes those threads get tangled up. There's a knot. And sometimes people carry on but there's this knot left. Sometimes they can't carry on because the knot is too large or because they feel so defeated by it. And they bring this knot into me here and my job is to say, "Well where, this red thread, where does that end? Let's follow that back. Oh look, it's actually two red threads and it's actually helped unravel." And what I'm saying to the patient is, "What does this connect to? So I'm puzzled and learning, you're explaining and by explaining it you're understanding it." That's all my job is is to help you unravel that knot so that you can then continue to weave the pattern, to tell the story. And the herbs help to facilitate that process in many, many, many ways.

BC works from home. She begins observing her patients from when she opens the front door and follows them up the two flights of stairs. As well as covering the presenting complaint(s), the consultation covers the medical history, drug history, family history, lifestyle, and an enquiry into each of the body systems. After the patient has filled in an information sheet the consultation usually starts with BC asking, "So what brings you here to see me today?"

During the consultation she checks that she has understood the patient correctly:

> So I will stop them throughout the consultation to say, "This is what I'm receiving, is that accurate?" And sometimes when they hear it come back to them, there's this huge relief in them that someone's heard them, and is not trying to qualify it or change it or put their own reading on it. And that opens the floodgates.

For BC, the medical diagnosis and "what is the matter" with a patient are often different things:

> I want to know if the doctor gave them the diagnosis, or if it's something they've self-diagnosed. I'm happy to work with someone with a self-diagnosis. Sometimes, very often people are very well informed. But we need to explore the provenance of that. Sometimes they have a diagnosis from the doctor or the GP and actually it's not what the problem is. I had someone who came to me with a skin rash. And, when we came to talk about cardiovascular health it turned out that he and his brother both had, his brother had died of it, a congenital heart problem. And the rash cleared up after the first visit. And on his second visit he didn't even mention the rash, until I reminded him. He said, oh, he'd forgotten about it. What he was now speaking to me about was this physical coldness that would come upon him in the middle of the night when he couldn't sleep. And eventually we worked together towards a diagnosis of fear of the grave. So very often what brings them in to see you is not really what's going on. And it's, the storytelling part is about allowing them to come back to the central part of that story.

BC seeks to create the right environment for the patient to be able to identify the "truth of the matter":

> ... what I'm looking for is the point at which they start to ramble. They start to look more broadly. They'll start to look around the room, not look at me. They're starting to cast their eyes down into themselves, or up, into their own imagination. And I'll just be quiet and I let them go. Because this is where the interesting core comes, right? Now there's a book that I read called, oh, it was one of those

books about the consultation, the therapeutic relationship or some-thing. And I read one thing in one of those books that really went home to me. It was, if you have the patience and the courage to let, to be still, to be silent for, it said thirty seconds, actually it's longer than that, if you have the courage to hold the silence for thirty seconds, the patient will tell you what the problem is. And I don't interrupt that moment. So what happens is they become quiet, they become still … They're looking inward. And I'll sit and be very still and very quiet, very present, very focused, very alert, but quiet. And sometimes it can take up to a minute and a half. And I'm happy to wait, because I know that they're working in that time. And what they come back to me with after that silence, and sometimes it can be as little as ten or twenty seconds, is the truth of the matter, the heart of the matter. And, it may not be, it may be cryptic, it may be metaphorical, it may be symbolic, it may be a substitute, but it's the truth. It's the heart of the matter.

… So what comes back out of this silence is the heart of the mat-ter. And I have, I always say the diagnosis is in the history. I'm sure I'm not the first person to have said that. The diagnosis is always in the history, however mysterious, or complex or confusing it might be, the patient will tell you what the diagnosis is. Now, it might not be, I've got a skin rash because my detergent is wrong. The diagno-sis is going to be something else, be open. Be expanded in what that might be … I'm not talking about the clinical diagnosis, I'm talking about what's wrong with here [indicates her heart area]? What's wrong with, what's the matter? … For instance, this chap that I told you about who came to me with a skin rash and then he ended up telling me, he went into his drifty space, and I was waiting to hear what came of it, and he then told me that his brother had died in his sleep of a congenital heart problem. That was the crux of the matter for him.

However, for BC it is not her job to explain things to the patient, to put words in their mouths. Describing the patient above she notes that:

And I was, it would have been dangerous for me to say, so what you're saying is what's really wrong here is you're frightened of dying because your brother died in his sleep. It would have been dangerous, and unhelpful, and in fact, detrimental.

She explains this danger with reference to another patient:

> He came to me with bladder stuff, you know, ongoing repeating cystitis … And he was training as a counsellor, so I, as it turned out, foolishly assumed a certain degree of emotional intelligence and literacy, without checking my assumption was correct. So, when I started asking him about his childhood history, I asked him if he'd been a bed wetter. I asked if he'd had any bladder problems as a child. It turned out that he had been a bed wetter. He had wet his pants at school, it had been traumatic and awful. He was the youngest child in a family of five. It was all, five brothers, there'd been some dysfunction in the family home. And I said, "I wonder if some of the dysfunction in the family was becoming compressed in you, and spurting out in you." He said, "What do you mean?" I said, "Well what are you pissed off about? You're expressing this in your bladder, what is it that pisses you off?" And he looked at me, and he said, "You are." And I said, he said, "I didn't come for talking therapy, I came because I have cystitis." And he never came back to see me, and who could blame him, actually. I pushed him into a place where he wasn't willing to go. I assumed that he wanted, that he was comfortable and able to talk about … And I made the mistake of acting on my assumption, and he never came back to see me. And I don't blame him, and I learned a great deal from him, which is, don't act on your assumptions. Check your assumptions. Always check that your assumptions are true. It's not my story, it's your story. And, of course he was pissed off with me. If he's somebody that expresses his stuff by being pissed off, he's going to get pissed off. Right, I'm not helping by telling him that he's pissed off …

BC refers to Carl Jung to understand the importance for patients of the telling of their stories:

> Jung said, one of the most important lessons that he ever learned, Jung, you know the great shaman of the psyche. The modern shaman of the psyche, he talked about when he was at the Swiss clinic, doing his internship. He was just out of school. He said that the greatest mistake he made was assuming he knew his patient's story, even if he did know the story, it wasn't his story to tell. Never, ever, ever, tell the patient their own story. Ever. And that really went

home for me. I'm not there to tell a story, the patient is there to tell the story. I'm there to listen to the story. And that's how the unravelling happens.

BC's stories: a bowl of water, young maids, and nonhuman communication

As well as a desire to help patients to reveal to themselves the heart of their own stories there are BC's compellingly told stories about herbs and other things. In these stories, she makes observations about people, events, animals, and plants that pass by most people. These stories entail the blurring of boundaries.

A bowl of water: This first story refuses to separate metaphor from the patient. As a student, she saw something about how a patient moved that no one else did:

> ... there was this woman that came in and we were talking about her afterwards and I felt that I had a really clear understanding of what her great issue was that was manifesting this illness. And I realised that everyone else in the class was a bit puzzled by it ... the supervisor ... he was saying, "Well, what do you think the, what do we think's going on here?" And I, in the end I spoke up. And I said, "It's, when she came in here it was like she was carrying a very large glass bowl filled absolutely to the brim with water and she couldn't, she mustn't drop, spill a drop." And he said, "That's exactly what it is because that explains her gait, her caution, her sense of being distracted all the time." And I said, "What's in the water, what the water is is the question, whether it's something that we can help her with? Can we make the vessel larger? Can we remove some?"

Young maids: In this story BC took two "young maids" camping, one of whom had just injured her knee. BC listened to her intuition and found a medicine that she could not justify at the time.

> So August in my first year I was studying herbs, the beginning of August and I took a couple of young maids, about fifteen, sixteen years old, camping for their first time. And one of them, the younger of the two had a terrible injury. She still wanted to come

but she'd fallen and strained and twisted her knee. And she had, her knee had ballooned up. It was black and blue but, no, she definitely wanted to come. So there we were sitting in the woods with this girl that could barely stand. So I said, right, well, let's do some hedgerow medicine. Let's do some wild craft things. And I thought what have I got, what do I need? So, of course, I needed some comfrey and I wanted some white willow bark. And it kept coming up in my mind, meadowsweet, and I thought, pah, why would I need a digestive herb for this child? And I kept pushing it aside and it kept coming up. And I did a little invocation, a little prayer. I said, OK, well, I need to find if you don't mind, please, in this vast space I hope to find, intend to find comfrey and white willow bark. So off I went, off in a random direction and five minutes on the other side of the village I saw white willow growing by water and as I jumped over the fence I saw that there was swathes of comfrey underneath the white willow and all over the place meadowsweet. So I thought, OK, well I'm not stupid enough to turn down the meadowsweet. I'm going to, I don't know why, but since all three are here together …

… within hours [of using medicines made from these herbs] she was saying this feels much better and the next day she was walking and the inflammation and swelling had gone down and by the time I went home she was on the mend.

BC's attention to the circumstances and environment of where the knee injury occurred allows her to find wider meaning that she then reconnects with the herbs. The circumstances are more than incidental here:

She told me the story of the injury and what had happened was that she had, as she was coming out of school they were all talking, she and all her friends were talking about which college they were going to go to. And they were all so close and they all wanted to go to the same college. Yes, it was going to be wonderful but then she'd decided to do something different. So she had had to tell her friends in this dramatic way that children have, fifteen-year-old girls especially, I'm not coming with you. I'm doing something else. Shock, horror, despair. She felt that she'd betrayed them all, let them all down, rejected them and as she turned away from them she, to flee, she went to run up a set of concrete stairs, tripped and fell, landed on the front of her knee. And I thought, OK, well, in my Freudian, Jungian model that makes sense. She's done this terrible thing so she throws herself under a bus kind of thing … But also she's running upstairs so she's aspirational. There's all these kind of pictures coming up in my head. There I was in the woods and I was thinking, well comfrey and white willow bark makes absolute sense to me. Meadowsweet, meadowsweet. I understand her story as far as it's possible for one outsider to understand somebody's internal story, came home, looked up meadowsweet to find that it is, Elizabeth Brooke says that it's a wonderful ritual herb, especially useful for women, girls, females transiting from one life stage to another.

The injury is no longer a discrete event. It is not an accident any more. Biography is blurred with the knee joint. She also later found out that meadowsweet had other uses that were relevant to the "maid":

> … I didn't know at the time that meadowsweet was one of the places where aspirin was, I did not know that, I, at that point I did not know that. I subsequently learned it. So, of course, meadowsweet came up in that respect.

While BC pays attention to her intuition, and later relates it to scientific knowledge, she also questions it.

> And that for me was a really clear confirmation, that whole event, that whole experience was a confirmation for me that if a herb comes into my mind pay attention. Something's tugging at me. Pay attention. It's safer to look at it, learn about it and decide it's not appropriate for this case at this time than it is to ignore it and say I'm not going to bother because if nothing else it's an opportunity for learning.

Nonhuman communication: BC has dialogues with both animals and plants:

> I once walked across a field and noticed, at some great distance, a black dog standing with its people. Something in me immediately

loved the dog, and I thought, "Oh, dog!" and my heart opened to it. Even at a distance that would have necessitated loud calling to alert the humans there, too far to see the details of the dog's face, it "heard" me, or noticed me, and turned towards me and pricked up its ears and started wagging its tail. One paw up, it seemed to return my ... well, greeting, and I strove to continue the dialogue. It felt very much as if the dog was saying, "Oh! A human who speaks! Good! Hello there!" and then when I failed to follow up on my first greeting, the dog's whole physical demeanour slumped a little, and it turned away from me and back towards its own people. It seems to be saying, "Ooh ... what a pity, it only knows how to say hello, nothing else ... never mind ...."

Similarly with plants: those who have generously opted to stay connected to us, nettle, for instance, are open and eager for dialogue. Some others, daisy, for example, are so chatty that it doesn't seem to matter that we have been silent so long ... or perhaps, with daisy, its close association with us on lawns and in childhood has kept the channel open and active. Others, with whom perhaps in the past we had open relations but have since neglected, have given up waiting for us to respond and turned away, but are still willing to hear us readily. I'd include yew here, I think. Yet others, like, I suspect, *Datura*, always needed to be propitiated in some way before entering into dialogue with us.

BC learns directly from plants, who always tell her to pass on her knowledge of them.

> If I want to actively learn about a plant and its nature and to increase my understanding and thus my relationship with it, I would do a journey or a meditation with that intention. Like making a date, and then being on best behaviour and being my best and highest self for the meeting. And yes, if the plant has entered that with me, and accepts me and my ways, then of course we can have a great long conversation, with clear questions and answers and sharing of stuff. I always end with thanks, and the question "What can I offer? What would you like from me? Is there anything I can do in return for the favours I have received from you?" and the answer—always and every time—is, "Tell the people about us. Tell the people about us."

In a journey to find a particular plant, gallant soldier (*Galinsoga sp*), BC meets a moose in some woodland. He is "so relaxed, so chilled out. Like a confident stoned teenager." Seeing its huge antlers she asks it, "How do you move between the trees?" Moose replies, "I get by." On realising that moose *is* gallant soldier she later describes gallant soldier, as well as being relaxed and chilled out, as being strong, confident, friendly, and open. Moose's words, "I get by" have become a kind of mantra for BC.

> However tricky or challenging things seem to be, if I remain relaxed and gracious and unfazed, I'll find a way through: or more than that, the way through will become clear and open.

A local knowledge-holder

BC's stories reveal understandings of patients, events, plants and animals that others do not speak about. This world view is hidden within modernity. Its unacknowledged nature is highlighted by another story that BC tells about a visit to the anthropology department of a leading UK university by some indigenous shamanic healers from South America.

> And they were giving this seminar at [X] and it was filmed and afterwards somebody said, "Well, what would you like?" And they were like saying, "God somebody's finally asked us this. We know about Pachamama. We know what we know. What we really would like to learn is what you guys know? How do you people interact with your land? How, what is your understanding with, about Pachamama, the goddess, the mother? And this is [X], right, school of anthropology. Yes." And they were like, "Oh my goodness, we don't know anything about our indigenous local culture in terms of what you're talking about." Can you imagine?

Someone in the audience told them about some pagans who live at a stone circle. So fourteen tribal elders went to stay with them and they shared each other's rituals. This started a relationship between South American shamans and British pagans, who invited BC to talk to a ninety-six-year-old shaman.

So there've been seminars, meetings, all sorts of things and one of the things that happened was that I was starting to be invited as the herbalist to talk to these *vegetales* from South America, these people who have inherited their knowledge and wisdom through generations of teachers. And they're coming to ask me about British plants? It's quite extraordinary.

She told the shaman a story about a British plant. This was important to her because knowledge of British plants had not travelled in this direction before:

> … So there was one night when I was invited to tell the story of Persephone and the underworld and Achilles and the yarrow (*Achillea millefolium*). And as I started to tell the story it was being translated for a ninety-six-year-old healer of his tribe. And every so often he'd check a detail … "I noticed," I said afterwards, "I'd noticed that you were not ever saying the word Achilles." And he said, "Well, no, I was telling this story about one of our local warriors who's very similar to Achilles. It seemed pointless to introduce a whole new character when we have one that's very, very similar and would behave in these ways." And [the healer] would check every so often, "Have I got this right?" And at the end of the story I turned round to the room, almost everyone else had left the room so there was just me and the elder sitting there with the translator. And it had become quite an intense working between us. Anyway he said, could you show, could I show him the plants? "Gladly." We tried it together and he said did I think it would, did I think it might grow in the forest? And I said, "Well, it could. It's worth a try. I don't know how humid it is," but we talked about that. And he said, "We do have a plant that heals wounds in the way that you're talking about but this sounds like it could be really, really useful for our people." And the translator said he's going to tell this story when we go back. And I said, "Oh, that's great." And it wasn't until I was away from there and back here … I thought, bloody hell, I've facilitated the movement of Achilles to South America. I've told the story of Achilles and he's going to go home and tell his people about this, I have changed the myth cycle of his people by telling this story about a hero in my own myth cycle. That seemed really profound to me …. He in the end didn't take the plant back

to South America with him but he took the story back. And for me it was this massive validation because at no point did he say, "Do you really know what you're talking about or how can I trust what you're saying?" He treated me as the tribal herbalist. And here I was sharing information, talking the same language, I'm not talking about chemistry or anything but we were talking about plants in exactly the same way, exactly the same way.

Local medicine

While the anthropology department of a leading UK university stumbled over the possibility of UK indigenous knowledge, the shamans were at ease with BC. Similarly, BC's medicines may be particularly indigenous, very place-specific. After graduating BC didn't have the money to set up a dispensary of herbal tinctures. But she did have access to 300 dried herbs at a local health food shop. However, she knew that patient compliance with continually making herbal teas is often poor. Rather than prescribing teas or decoctions to be made up by the patients, as is the standard approach that is taught, she remembered a herbalist saying that a "well-made decoction" will keep for a long time. So she developed her own method of making a low dose concentrated decoction for her patients:

> How do I make a well-made decoction? So I thought, well, it's about concentration. So if I assume that someone's going to take three to five cups of tea a day how do I make that cup a teaspoon? So that was my thinking and I thought, well, I'll just start. Process is a good teacher. So the first thing that I, I started doing it with actual real patients. So I made the prescription and I was, I worked it out. I was like, OK, one teaspoon to a cup, three cups a day. I want a month's worth of medicine so I scaled it all up and I ended up with this enormous mound of herbs. And I thought, God how am I going to process this? And as somebody who is quite willing to trust my intuition and go with it and see what the outcome is it suddenly occurred to me that I didn't need to use three and a half ounces of, why not just use an ounce of? So I simplified all the recipes down to one ounce of whatever herb it was that I wanted, double it up if there was something mechanical that I wanted like

the mucilage or the astringent or whatever. Halve it if all I wanted was the energy, yeah but the material stuff wasn't necessary or it was a really pokey plant and see how I go. So I could at least fit it in the pot. And I thought, well, it doesn't, is there a better way than doing it on the top of the stove? Well, what's wrong with inside the stove? That way it gets heat from all sides. I can walk away. I don't have to watch it. The top won't rattle. I can leave it in overnight. So then I got a very large pot with a tight-fitting lid so its each step was dictating the next step kind of thing ... and I put it in the oven overnight. And I thought, well, if I'm going to decoct it for an hour or two is there any harm in leaving it overnight? Well, it was becoming really like a food, like a stock. But I also noticed because one of my concerns was that if it's just in water what's going to happen to the oils? But I noticed that cooking it for that long breaks down the structure to such an extent that the oils would come out. So I was ending up with really slicky stuff on top. And then I thought, oh what about the volatiles? It's all, it's well and good to have it inside a closed, but what happens because of course I've now got like, I've strained it and now got eight litres or ten litres of brown liquid. So I want to reduce that. So I put the heat under it very low just to let the top smoke. I'm not boiling it. So what about the volatiles? I'm obviously going to be losing the volatiles ... But of course it wouldn't be necessary in every case. If the volatiles are something that you want to retain then that would be theoretically one way of doing it. But you don't necessarily want the volatiles in every particular case. The other thing was I realised that once you get it down to 500 mils, a month's worth of medicine I could actually play around at that level. I can take it down to 200 mils and put cold spring water in if someone's hot because of course what I'm doing is I'm creating a lot of heat. So do I want to put that heat into the body? Possibly not. So reduce it down further, top it up with cool spring water so you're putting some coolness back in or I might want to put an aromatic water in or indeed a tincture. So you can take it down to below 500 and top it back up with some kind of medicine ... The other thing was that by reducing it that much to that kind of concentration I was removing so much water that it was making it quite difficult for any bacteria to really get a hold. The concentration of compounds in there to the water is not in a bacterial, a bacteria's favour. It is there. And also because it's heat treated, even if it's not at a boiling level, it is heat treated for a really long time. So that is also going to be preservative. I've got decoctions over there that are years and years old and I still use them for teaching. And they're still good. They're still efficacious. It's extraordinary.

We now come to what makes this medicine possibly a very local medicine:

> Somebody phoned me up and said it smells funny. And I said, well, pour it away. And then afterwards I thought, damn, I should have just asked them to bring it back to me. Well, what do you mean funny? And then not long after that somebody else said my medicine seems odd. And I said, "Well, can you describe it for me and can you bring it back to, for me?" And it had fermented. So I did some research because I thought, well, I don't, I'm not sure that this is necessarily a bad thing. And, of course, fermentation is a very healthy thing that we do to food. Sauerkraut, kimchi, yoghurt, beer, we rely on fermentation. And there's quite a lot of good evidence that shows that in order to keep the endogenous bacteria healthy and in balance with the environment it may, it's a good idea to have fermented food that has been fermented in the present, in the place, in the locale. Right. So there's an interaction where do we end and our, and the rest of the world begins? Well, it turns out it doesn't because our, if we're in a good state of health and living in a healthy environment our endogenous bacteria will, to some extent, reflect the exogenous bacteria and microorganisms, not just bacteria of course. So I thought, well, maybe it's not necessarily a bad thing that this stuff has fermented. And of course there's practical stuff like the bottle exploding and the flavour changes, the viscosity changes, the sweetness has gone, it becomes much more sour, becomes much more watery because the sugars have been eaten by the, you. But if the patient is agreeable to it I say go, I give them the option, "I'll make you a new one but these are the reasons why you might want to continue taking the medicine." And they all do actually. They all say, "Oh yeah, that sounds great. I'll continue taking it." And what I've found is that I've had some really profound deep healings following, I'm not saying because of, following on from using fermented medicines including somebody who's an HIV

positive man whose viral load went down to undetectable. And I
had a cancer patient who went into, apparently spontaneous remis-
sion after using the fermented medicines.

BC makes her medicines from scratch for all her patients and her house
is filled with the smell of the medicine being cooked. The earthy soup-
like smell is everywhere. The above suggests that her decoctions, particularly those that have fermented, may be very specific medicines,
specific to the microorganisms in the environment where the fermenta-
tion took place. This may have started in her kitchen, under which runs
a river. But it may also be specific to the patient's home, where they are
continually opening and closing the bottle. These medicines are potentially very "local", if not "indigenous".

Reflection on BC

BC describes being "surrounded" by grass when talking about her entryway of being called by grass and now she has developed a method of
medicine-making that means that she is surrounded by the smell of
the medicine being made overnight and during the day. The sensual
enchantment of her early experiences may have somehow motivated her
to engage with the process of making a new type of medicine that requires
her to be in such close and continuous contact with the herbs. Breathing
them in, even as she sleeps. While AF's narrative reveals the importance
of the sensuality of taste as a method of understanding herbal medicines,
BC's proximity to herbs via the aroma of her decoctions is another way of
knowing and being with herbs. Also, the sense of safety that she describes
in being surrounded by grass, and the sense of comfort in nature as "nature
girl", can be seen to be present in the way that she crafts the consultation such that patients feel able to open up and reveal the "heart of the
matter". And BC's own illness experience as a young girl, where neither
her story nor her permission were sought, and her subsequent questioning of orthodox medicine and the development of a self-help approach
to her own health, can be seen to be present in the importance that she
attaches to patients learning about themselves by telling their own stories.

The human-nonhuman meeting of being called by grass can, most
obviously, be seen in her later communications with a dog and with
plants such as gallant soldier. However, the blurring of boundaries can
also be seen in BC's refusal to separate metaphor from the patient. It is
also present in the case of the young maid, where BC uses intuition—an

immediate crossing between feeling and knowledge—to include mead-owsweet in the maid's medicine, and in her attention to the meaning of circumstances to understand the maid's "accident". What is more, in facilitating the journey of the story of Achilles and the story of the plant *Achillea millefolium*, if not the plant itself, to South America, BC challenges the boundary between "indigenous" and Western knowledge.

KA

Entryways

KA remembers her great aunt as having been an influence on her eventually becoming a herbalist:

> [She] sorted out the local community ... and she always had something for everything. Whether it was a crate of Guinness under the bed for iron, or whether it was some plants, or some concoction she'd made up. I thought that was interesting.

KA had an illness experience with bronchitis in her twenties that led her to taking herbs:

> ... and I got sicker and sicker ... kept going back to the doctor's, kept giving me antibiotics, as they do. And then someone said, "Oh, you should go and see a herbalist." And I thought, oh, what's a herbalist ... And this guy ran a health food store ... So I went to see him, and said, "Well, take all these herbs," and he, that's when the herbs were in jars on the shelves. So I got herbal teas, and some tinctures and things like that. Went home, took them and within about two to three weeks, it had gone. And I had been off work for the best part of two months with this chest, that had just got worse and worse, so I thought, hey, this, there's something in this, natural, it's really good, this natural stuff. So I wanted to find out more ...

While these two entryways are visible, there is a third, more hidden avenue that KA found in her journey to becoming a herbalist. Looking back at her childhood, KA remembers trees communicating with her:

> And sometimes, because when trees started talking to me when I was a kid, and I used to think, right, great. And then they stopped

for a while, and then they started again, a bit later on, and the ones that were the noisiest were the yew trees, and I'd be out, like we'd be out with a group of people looking round a stately home or one of these graveyard places, and you're sitting there eating your packed lunch, and all of a sudden this voice goes, hello, and you're like, you come to realise after a while that the tree is talking to you. And you're like, OK, I'm going to sit here quietly because people will think I'm mad, but this tree is talking to me, and you lean against it and then it went, you must take some of my leaves and little bits here and you must burn them, do a little ritual and burn them. I said why, well, we're all about death and rebirth, and some things you need to get rid of and offload and bury and you need to bring some new things in. I'm like, OK then, and then something lands on your head, and you think, ah it's a bit of the tree, that's the bit I'm supposed to have, then. Mmm, I think it's just listening and tuning in, I think anyone can do it, it's just that we've got this, we've had it bashed out of us as we've grown up that doing things like that is loony and weird, and we're not supposed to do it. We're not supposed to see anything beyond what is considered normal.

Talking with nature

When KA went to university to study herbal medicine she felt that she had to shut down her spiritual side:

It just seemed to be very apparent with the, within the framework of the course itself, and what we were studying, that there didn't seem to be any room for anything that was not scientific, not quantified, not evaluated in some way. That you couldn't say you felt this, it was always justify why you're doing that. You couldn't speak of any feelings, any sixth sense about anything, gut reactions, gut feelings. One lecturer you could possibly sit and talk to about that. Others it was almost, no.

As a student, a practitioner she knew saw what she was hiding:

Because he said to me, "Why do you hide what you do?" One day, peering over a book ... I went, "Sorry?" And then he peered over, and went, "What is it you can do?" And I said, "What do you mean?" He said, "You know what I mean." He said, "You seeing things and hearing things and stuff like that." And I hid behind a book and I went, "I don't know, stuff. I can do stuff. And he went, "Well, why do you hide it?" And I said, "Because I can't cope with it, I find this setting quite oppressive sometimes, and it's almost like, I didn't want to be perceived as a flake head of some kind, so it was just, be the model student that did this, did that, I just became that thing." And he said, "Now you're finished and you get out there," he said, "don't ever bury it," he said, "because, why do you think I'm so successful? Why do you think people come to see me? Why do you think people love what I do with the flair that I do it and stuff?" He said, "People love it, but I'm true to what I am and who I am, and you've got to be too." And I said, "Yeah, I know." So he said, "Well, off you go then."

After graduating and being in practice for a few years, one of KA's patients, Deborah, offered KA an acre of land on her smallholding that she thought might be suitable for growing herbs. Another of KA's patients was looking to make a financial investment and offered to back a herb farm. Together with KA's husband Tom they set up the herb farm to make fresh plant tinctures for herbalists. These herbs are tinctured within a few hours of harvesting. KA and Tom work full time on the farm, although KA still sees patients one day a week.

The land had been organic arable land but had been fallow for some years. It is surrounded by hawthorn hedges and trees, including oaks. The hundred-foot end beds had been cut out first—back-breaking work with a turf cutter. They then decided on a spiralling labyrinth design. They were influenced by the Findhorn community in Scotland and Perelandra gardens in America. KA and Tom drew on organic, bio-dynamic, and permaculture farming methods. They wanted to set up the farm in partnership with nature. It is from this partnership that the herbs were grown and the medicines made:

> Yeah, when I first met Tom, I read this book about Findhorn in Scotland … and reading this book about this guy and his wife who were just, they didn't really have a leaning towards anything, they had just heard things and saw things that you weren't supposed to see. And managed to contact, these devas [a Sanskrit term for supernatural beings] that looked after these plants, and did what they were told, and turned a derelict piece of land into this amazing

garden. And I thought, yeah, that's really working with nature isn't it. They say this is what you do, and you say, that's interesting, let's do it. Rather than, I'm the human being in charge, and I'm just going to do this. Because that's just us stamping our authority all over nature, and as you know nature can be a bitch and do what she wants to do. So, we thought, right, that was very important, and then that book really, well, yeah, it was a life-changing book to read. I thought this is amazing. So then I had little experiments. And it also explained why, when I was out in nature, that I thought things talked to me, and I thought I was going mad for a long time. Am I hearing voices? What's going on here? And then I realised no, that I could hear, and I could see, and I did have a connection with the land and the plants and the trees, some trees more than others. And I thought, there's got to be a way that you can bring this in. And then I started to read, we got into organics, and then we got into biodynamics. And when you start to read some of Steiner's stuff it's not that far removed, very much about working with nature as an entity in itself, and you think, yeah, there's something to this ...

Standing on the land that would become the herb farm, KA spoke directly to nature and a woman appeared to her:

And then I read a book by a lady who'd come over from America in the Seventies, late Seventies, she'd gone to Findhorn, and she had the same kind of experiences and she said, right I'm going to go back to America, and she had an amazing set of circumstances happen in her life, like I had in mine, that led you to a point where something like this is suddenly, comes your way, and you think, aaah!. And she worked exactly the same way, and her statement was just in the middle of the field one day, yelling out, "I want to work with nature, spirits, and devas, and the land, and we want to work as a co-operative partnership and this is what I want to do." And I thought, well, if it worked for her, it'll work for me, so I stood in the middle of a field and that's what I yelled out ... when I opened my eyes, there was this woman standing in front of me, and I thought, who are you? And I got an idea that it was probably either a personi-fication of the earth, or the mother earth, or goddess or something, and she just smiled and pointed, and I went, and it was said, you must plant a tree. And I'm like, OK, plant a tree, any particular tree? Just plant a tree. I was like, OK plant a tree, and then off she went.

And I was like, I was just standing in the field going, OK, fine, good, am I going mad? Very probably, so I thought, yeah. Plant a tree, and then the next day my mate went, I've got a pot-bound ginkgo, I'm going off to India, do you want it? Can you do anything with it? And I thought, put that in there, then. That will do nicely.

KA says that the woman who appeared to her was not human:

> An older woman, I suppose technically a definition of what you would think was a crone, sort of older, long white silver hair, quite a kind of otherworldly countenance about her, very shyly kind of a person, thing, spirit whatever you like to call it. And I thought, it wasn't like a, you've a ghost or something where they're not quite there. Or sometimes they are. I've seen ghosts of people that are quite real, and you go, oh blimey and then other times you see things that are not, that are almost transparent, but she was quite solid and quite there. And I thought, OK, and she, I couldn't work out what she was wearing, bits of different cloth and stuff. It didn't seem to belong to anything where you could say, oh there was some native tribal stuff going on there. She just seemed to be, and I thought, good enough for me ... Some people might interpret that as God, it might have been God in some way telling me something, or one of God's angels, but I like to think it was the Goddess, because that's what I believe and that's my. I always remember reading Micaelle's book, which we haven't got here that she said, when things appear to you, they often appear to you in the way your mind can understand and perceive them. So if you're going to see nature's spirits as little goblin fairy things, that's how your mind's eye will perceive them. If you're going to see them as people, that's how, your, but really they have no shape or form as such, it's only how we personify them. And we do, humans will personify everything so their minds can deal with it. There'll always be little people, little floaty things. Women, men, things that are not quite, you know they're not human, but you think, but they look human.

KA and Tom sought the advice of nature before making any decisions about the herb farm:

> And that was the first thing we did, and then the whole thing was very much, everything we did, we stopped and had a little chat

about it. What shape should it be in? What should we feed the soil with? What kind of mulch would you like? Should we put that there? And sometimes you'd get definites, no, no we want to be there. Or you'd get, well try it and see. There were no hard and fast things, and as with all things, some things work, some things don't.

Out of this working relationship with nature, they make herbal medicines that herbalists are impressed by:

> But the energy of the tinctures we produce, people keep saying they've never tasted anything like it. So we're obviously doing something, and people keep saying they've never seen plants that size, and plants with that much vitality, and so if herbalists, in particular, are noticing, they're noticing the vitality, so they're picking up on the energetics of the plant, whether they know it or not, that's what they're doing, because they're commenting on it. It's not like, isn't that plant big, they're like, oh I've never seen anything like it. You're like, no, neither have I, actually.

They grow about sixty herbs on the farm. They respond to the demands of herbalists, for example growing more wild lettuce, thyme, St John's wort, skullcap, and Sweet Annie as requested. They are also looking to bring back little-used indigenous herbs wherever possible. KA gives two examples—mouse-ear hawkweed and hemp agrimony.

> … we found out about mouse-ear hawkweed. Why use ephedra when we've got mouse-ear hawkweed? If you just want a good bronchodilator or something. It's interesting, yet no big scientific trials or studies have been done on it, but this is learnt from other herbalists who have brought this herb back again, and used it in a clinical setting and got results … Hemp agrimony, we're interested in looking at that, as we've heard it's supposed to be akin to a British echinacea, but saying that, echinacea grows well in our climate.

KA relates the story of meeting a deva of the hawthorn while working on the herb farm:

> I was working with a hawthorn once and then all of a sudden it was like this pair of eyes were just looking at me through the tree, like

this, and I thought, ah, it's a deva, it's a deva of the hawthorn. And
then it went back in and it was like a swirling kind of mist and then
it came and looked again, and then I'm like, oh hello, that's nice and
carry on picking. And they just watched. And I thought, well, have
you got anything to say to me? And it sort of, it just smiled and you
felt it in the heart, and you thought, oh, I'm with the hawthorn, and
it was almost like, well this is all about heart energy, you know. And
I thought, this is cool, pretty cool.

Understanding herbs as having personalities, KA describes how the
personality of *Hypericum* explains how it works as a herb for the nervous system:

> Some of them are quite grumpy and some of them, but yet again that's
> a personification thing, isn't it. Some of them, because that's how we
> are, so we can only relate in the ways we are. And that *Hypericum* has
> quite a dark side to it sometimes, it's all happy, happy, happy, but if
> you really get into, it's like it is, because its whole purpose in being
> here is to transform darkness into light. So it does have this dark-
> ness within it which is probably why it's so good as a mood uplifting
> thing that we give, because I said, it's not about being herbal Prozac
> at all, it's because that's what the plant does, you know. It just takes
> a load of dark rubbish and just *BLEURGH* and does that with it. And
> then, there are times, at certain times of the year, when you can feel
> it in the winter and it has that dark, it's all dark stuff, you know, and
> then it's almost now it's at its happiest, because it's done its transfor-
> mative work and here it is for you now, and now it's ready for you to
> harvest and give to people, so they can do their transformative work.
> And that's now, how I use St John's wort, I use it as a nervine as well,
> because, it's a good nervine. But that's why it's a good nervine.

Fieldwork

My first visit to the farm was on an open day on a muggy damp day in
June. Less than a week ago Deborah, KA's business partner, had died
from cancer but it was decided that the open day should still go ahead.
Herbalists and herbal students were present. There were several out-
buildings, including an open-sided barn where the tinctures were prepared, and a lorry-body for storing the finished medicines. There was

also a polytunnel, an old barge, the foundations for a community cen-tre, an old Greenpeace vehicle, a hay bale urinal for men, plus a solid waste eco toilet. A caravan marked the entrance to the herb field. We all started to walk around the plot, following the lines of the herb beds. We passed two small and nearly hidden *Vitex* plants, pungent and aromatic as we rubbed their leaves and took a nibble. Then passed the shim-mering motherwort, pokey mints, soft marshmallows, and giant mul-leins. During lunch in the open-sided barn I asked KA what was around the corner, pointing to a path leading into a wooded area. She replied, "Deborah, it's her grave ... would you like to see it?" It had started to rain. Deborah had died at home and had been buried two days ago, after permission had been granted by the local authority. Rounding the corner the freshly turned and beautifully prepared soil of the grave was bordered by cut flowers from the farm, and a slug moved across the grave. There was a little chair and a shrine with some Buddhist and Christian images. KA stood silent.

On another visit, as we rounded the corner into the herb field the heady over-sweet scent of valerian flowers was striking, very different from the "old socks" smell of the valerian root that is used in medicine. Tom told me that when digging the beds they had finally connected the two ends of the spiral pattern of the beds and he had felt a shock—"like I'd put my fingers in a socket". We carried on walking. The leaves of the mullein were as large as plates and as soft as rabbits' ears, with the yel-low flowers opening in their spikes. The sun was out now and had burnt away some clouds. I had forgotten to bring a hat so I put a burdock leaf on my head to keep the sun off. The orange of the marigold flowers was so bright that it hurt our eyes to look at them. A herbalist who was also visiting mentioned that *Macer's Herbal*, an Anglo-Saxon herbal, stated that just looking at these flowers would improve eyesight, saying that it had been discovered that marigold contains lutein, an antioxidant ben-eficial to eye health, which is used in macular degeneration.

I helped KA and Tom harvest some yarrow. We used some old but sharp cutting tools, which made a satisfying "snap" with each snip. When we had finished we took the herbs to the shredder where we fed them through till they were grabbed by the mechanism and pulled in, shredded, and passed out into another basket. The herb was then weighed and divided into batches in plastic tubs and a mixture of alco-hol and water added before being sealed. This would be left for several weeks before pressing out. We did the same with the lady's mantle: the plants were laden down with their flowers—the mass of green flowers was at least as great as the leaves.

On another occasion we harvested some St John's wort, the yellow-flowered herb reminiscent of the drawings in old herbals. Their unchanging form made them seem very old. Soon my hands were stained with small dark red spots from the plant oils in the herb. When we had harvested about half the stand we took it for tincturing. Within seconds of adding the ethanol and water when you pressed down on the herb the liquid became a deep burgundy colour. Tom said that they like showing this to kids because they can't believe how the red colour, hidden in the oil glands of the leaves and flowers, came out of the yellow and green plant.

On another visit it had snowed heavily the day before and a thick blanket of snow and silence had been laid down. I arrived early and visited Deborah's frozen grave. When KA and Tom arrived we pressed out eight buckets of hawthorn berries that had been macerating for six weeks. It was nearly frozen, as we were, and tasted something like brandy. We also tried some hawthorn tincture that had been pressed out several weeks before and noticed how it was darker and somewhat richer in flavour. KA speculated about the unknown processes that occur as a herbal tincture ages.

Reflection on KA

While KA did have two visible entryways—a great aunt who helped her community, and a personal illness experience resolved by herbal medicine—it is the third entryway, of communicating with trees as a child that is seen most in the rest of her narrative. Thus KA communicates with nature when establishing the herb farm, meeting a woman who is not a human—a nonhuman human. And KA continues to work with nature in making day-to-day decisions about the farm. She also sees other nonhumans in the herb farm, taking on the form of devas. There are many human/nonhuman meetings in KA's narrative which are made comprehensible to her in that she understands herbs as having personalities. This is how she sees humans as understanding the world. She relates to plants as persons.

However, she also spends nearly all her working days at the herb farm. It is constant physical work, in contact with the soil, the living herbs or medicines made from them. Amongst other things, KA digs, plants, sows seeds, washes off insects, enriches the soil, harvests, washes roots, shreds, macerates herbs in alcohol, and presses out the medicines.

Reflection on hidden entryway herbalists: from spirits to physical nature

While the hidden entryways of AF, BC, and KA bear some similarities to CT and VH, the human-nonhuman entryway meetings of AF, BC, and KA are somewhat different. CT spoke of the broad concept of "naturphilia" and VH was "involved with plants without being involved at all". However, red dead-nettle and grass "called" AF and BC respectively, and it was a yew tree, amongst others, that "spoke" to KA as a child. Such direct communication suggests enchanting human-nonhuman meetings.

A consideration of perspectives on shamanism resonates with the narratives of these three herbalists. We will briefly look at historical and contemporary scholarship on shamanism, which suggests that shamans believe in spirits. Narby and Huxley[197] look at how shamanism has been written about over 500 years. Their compilation of writings, as well as drawing from a long history (1535–2000), also visits a vast geography that includes Australia, Africa, South America, and the Far East. It shows how the construction of the definition of shamanism has changed, from being sorcerers working with the Devil, to the Enlightenment aspirations of a more measured and "objective" gaze, to the rise of social anthropology in the nineteenth century that initially retained a view of shamans as "primitives", to a self-reflexive questioning of the anthropologists' own biases in the twentieth century. By the mid twentieth century Narby and Huxley show that shamans had come to be seen as masters of religious ecstasy. And by the end of the last century they were moving towards being respected as complex producers of meaning on the same intellectual footing as the anthropologists living with and studying them.

Although there is an increasing academic respect for shamans, the understanding of shamanic practitioners as addressing spiritual matters puts them at odds with many of the perspectives that commentators have adopted to address this research area. Narby and Huxley note that "Many observers, especially those trained as scientists, are philosophical materialists. They believe that everything that exists is either made up of physical matter or dependent on matter for its existence. Shamans do not. They believe in spirits." DuBois[150] also looks to the centrality of spirits in shamanism, suggesting that the shamanic role is a calling, a personal relationship between a human and a spirit guide. DuBois refers to Backman and Hultkrantz[198] to argue that shamanism may be defined by the concept of spirits that are associated with the world's elements, and a cosmology of worlds inhabited by spirits, as well as the practice of spirit travel by shamans achieved through trance states. Looking at shamanic entryways, DuBois identifies several factors as being central to becoming a shaman. These include the importance for shamans of being called to their role by spirits; the variable volition of the future shamans in seeking out their roles; their sometimes acquiescence to spirits; the threat of terrible consequences if the call is refused; and transformative spiritual ordeals. The concept of spirits is central to most understandings of what shamanism and shamans may be.

The cases of CT and VH have elements of such shamanic considerations, even if they are relatively weak. Thus CT's "naturphilia" may be characterised as a gentle or "quiet" calling. Similarly, VH's quiet calling can be seen in his "being involved with plants without being involved at all" and in his "simply knowing things". Additionally, VH's own illness experience, where he found the courage to look at his own illness history, is a transformative illness experience.

However, it is AF, BC, and KA that resonate more obviously with some elements of shamanism. While BC and KA both had pivotal and possibly transformative illness experiences that helped them on their route to becoming herbalists, it is the centrality of spirits that requires our attention here. Spirits may be associated with plants in all three narratives. AF and BC were both called by plants, with the question of who or what is doing the calling suggesting the possibility of a spiritual explanation. Furthermore, AF refers to herbal medicine as a spiritual occupation, and BC journeys with plant spirits. Similarly, KA had conversations with plants as a child and sees them in her work on the herb farm. A spiritual explanation would put these herbalists within such a partial definition of shamans.

AF's descriptions of cases and his theories of cures are compellingly told, as are KA's meetings with nonhumans. Similarly, BC's stories of being called by grass and of meeting gallant soldier in the form of a moose are well told narratives. However, they do not add up to a cosmology, that is, a theory of the nature of the universe that could add weight to the argument of these herbalists as shamans. And there is no suggestion in the narratives that any communication they have with plants is achieved through the development of trance states. Instead, such communication is gained via direct and simple acts.

While the calling of some herbalists by plants, transformative illness experiences, human-plant communication and journeying with plants suggest that herbalists and shamans are not mutually exclusive, the lack of cosmology, trance states and threatening spirits indicates that seeking an alternative perspective may be required. For this reason, we look to a view of shamanism that prioritises the relationship with nonhuman nature, rather than with spirits. Abram[164], who we met above, argues that anthropology has been blind to the shaman's relationship to physical nature. Abram suggests that what defines the shaman is the ability to move out of her or his culture to contact "other powers in the land. Her or his magic is precisely this heightened receptivity to the meaningful solicitations—songs, cries, gestures, of the larger, more-than-human field." The shaman engages very closely with nature—arguably an enchanted meeting with elements from the more-than-human world. Abram draws on the phenomenology of Husserl and Merleau-Ponty in the primacy that he accords to direct experience. Importantly, this more-than-human world is not beyond the natural world: the shaman propels "his awareness laterally, outwards into the depths of a landscape at once both sensuous and psychological ..." And this allegiance to nonhuman nature is mastered by "long and sustained exposure to wild nature, to its patterns and vicissitudes". For Abram, the primary role of the shaman is to connect humans with the more-than-human by directly engaging with nonhuman intelligences. The shaman communicates with the more-than-human in the natural world rather than in a transcendent world. Everything is in the natural physical realm.

Using "communication with spirits" as the reference point, as discussed above, did indeed find some associations with the herbalists discussed. However, employing Abram's contention that shamanism is about contact with the natural physical realm, rather than spirits, opens up a possible explanation for how herbalists arrive at the knowledge that they do. Despite the enchantment of the narratives of AF, BC, and KA there seem to be few techniques involved, rather the way to gain knowledge is seen to be by being as direct as possible. AF asks living plants questions and also tastes herbal medicines; BC journeys with plants by simply going to meet them, and also has close and prolonged contact with the medicines by the aroma they produce as it fills her home; and KA is in close proximity to physical nature, working with the land and plants. Simply spending time with them in different ways. And the other two herbalists, CT and VH, also spend time with herbs, as medicines and as living plants. As VH says, it is necessary to become "habituated" to them as living creatures. Thus, knowing herbs through growing them, harvesting them, talking to them, tasting them, inhaling them and making them into medicines is argued to be central to Western herbal medicine. Herbalists are often in prolonged contact with plants and the medicines made from them. It is such contact that facilitates the awareness of spirits that we saw in AF, BC, and KA. However, rather than calling these herbalists "shamans" and seeing them as being somehow a lost link to far-flung cultures, which takes them away from their localities and fosters a discourse upon them, it is arguably more accurate to see these herbalists simply as practitioners of medicine, enchanted by plants.

The push of enchantment

The sensual affective energy of enchantment is visible in the entryways of CT and VH and is also present in their engagement with cutting edge science. The easy drawing together of influences that could be seen as divergent, and maybe even opposed to one other, such as holism and reductionism, nature and religion, punk and professionalism in the case of CT; and endobiogenics' forensic approach to working with the hormonal terrain and a priestly approach that recognises the importance of finding "the path with heart", in the case of VH, may be a consequence of herbalists' meetings with plants.

But enchantment is perhaps most obvious in the entryways of AF, BC, and KA and continues throughout their narratives. AF's easy drawing from his three theories of cure, namely physiology, the role of emotions and knowing plants directly, "applying them according to the circumstances", and BC's finding that studying anatomy and physiology was "like remembering something" while also being a maker of very local medicines and journeying to meet plants, may also follow on logically from the meetings of herbalists with plants, of species from one kingdom with species of another. And KA's working with nature allows her to meet a wide variety of nonhuman persons on her herb farm.

If we allow ourselves, for a moment, to fall into the trap of talking about science and tradition as if they are somehow inherently opposed, the presence of enchantment in the narratives of what we may clumsily call relatively more "scientific" herbalists (CT, VH) as well as in the narratives of relatively more "traditional" herbalists (AF, BC, KA) suggests that "enchantment" cannot simply be seen as meaning "traditional" and "disenchantment" simply seen as "modern" or "scientific". Rather, it suggests that enchantment is a process that spreads out, from herb-herbalist relationships, in the form of a sensual-affective energy, following the trajectory of interests of the herbalists. This may be called the push of enchantment, with this process having started before adulthood, and often much younger, in the lives of these herbalists.

PART IV

DISCUSSION AND CONCLUSIONS

CHAPTER ELEVEN

Beyond cases

C hapter 9 considered visible entryway herbalists and revealed the pull of enchantment by a herbal medicine, by theory and by woodland, albeit it with living plants having little apparent influence on practice. The possibility that orthodox clinical science is enchanting in its own way was also considered. Chapter 9 also revealed the enchantment of other herbalists whose experience of living plants supports their practices—to get to the root of the problem, to only prescribe medicines that are known as living plants, to treat metaphors as real and to understand patients using the same methods that are used to understand plants.

Chapter 10 looked at the push of enchantment in the lives of the hidden entryway herbalists—where "naturphilia" helps binaries to be resolved; where knowing plants is necessary to find a theory of cure; where a herbalist was called by red dead-nettle and knows plants and medicines directly through taste and talk; where a herbalist who was surrounded by and called by grass at a young age is now surrounded by the aroma of her own method of making medicine and who facili-tated the travelling of Western herbal knowledge to an indigenous com-munity in South America; and where a child who communicated with trees grew up to work with nature in growing medicinal plants.

Meetings and difference in Western herbal medicine

Resourcing these cases but looking beyond them, it is a contention of this book that the easy sitting together within these herbalists, and between these herbalists within Western herbal medicine of different influences, is at least partially due to the meetings of herbalists with plants and herbal medicines that we have seen in the hidden entryways and later narratives of the herbalists. This drawing together of such diversity would not have been possible without CT's "naturphilia"; or without VH's "being involved with plants without being involved at all"; or without AF being called by red dead-nettle and his energetic methods of working directly with plants that includes talking and listening to them as well as tasting them; or without BC being called by grass and surrounded by the aroma of the medicines that she makes; or without KA talking to the land where she grows herbs and makes medicines; or without the "awe" that SB experienced as a child in his gran's garden and the "magnificence" of the plants in his own garden; or without CP having herself experienced taking *Vitex agnus-castus* and *Chamaelirium luteum*; or without FD having had a serious accident and being offered help by Jesus and a tree branch; or without GA's experiences with plants that "are speaking to me all the time", even if the words are voiceless; or without MN's passion for spending time with plants, either growing them or observing them in detail throughout their life cycles and recording this information in a structured methodology.

It boils down to a simple proposition: if herbalists can somehow meet with herbs, if species from different kingdoms, namely humans and plants, have membranes that are more permeable to each other than is usually thought, then bringing diverse influences into the lives and practices of herbalists, as seen in the cases, is a simple reflection of this ability to accommodate, even welcome, difference. And if this is true for individual herbalists, it is true for at least part of Western herbal medicine.

Beyond the science/tradition dichotomy in Western herbal medicine

While cases are phenomena in their own right, they also have the potential to be relevant beyond themselves.[119] The cases discussed above will now be used as a resource to do theoretical work and to ask questions about Western herbal medicine. Hidden meetings between humans and nonhumans, between herbalists and plants, have been seen in the entry-ways of some herbalists. Such meetings have also been seen in the later parts of herbalists' narratives, both in those who had such hidden entry-ways and those who did not. This constitutes the "push" and "pull" of enchantment, a sensual affective energy that spreads throughout many of the narratives, sometimes starting before formal study begins and sometimes afterwards. Beyond the hidden entryways, later in the herb-alists' narratives, these meetings are sometimes between humans and nonhuman nature, for example where a near-death experience led to knowing living medicinal plants differently, or where a truth-to-nature methodology based on Goethe uses the human being as the "perfect instrument for reading the book of nature". However, such enchanted meetings can also be seen between humans and more simply material substances, such as a particular herbal preparation that had a physi-ological effect and then an affective effect on the herbalist. Enchanted meetings can also be seen in ways of thinking, such as when a herbalist who is in awe of plants also has an arborescent desire to get beyond the orthodox diagnosis to the "root" or "kernel" of his patients' illnesses, or when a herbalist identifies complexity theory as resolving incom-patibilities between holism and reductionism. Meetings between one realm and another can also be seen when a herbalist helps patients to treat their own illness metaphors as if they are real.

Importantly, these meetings have occurred in the lives of herbalists who draw on apparently more "traditional" influences as well as those who apparently draw on more "scientific" influences. "Apparently" is used twice here because it is notable that individual herbalists may draw easily and smoothly from both of these designations, suggesting compatibility and integration rather than tension in practice. Thus CT is influenced by both complexity theory *and* "naturphilia"; VH takes a priestly sacerdotal approach *and* focuses on the minutiae of the hori-zontal relationships between hormones; AF looks to physiology *and* to talking to plants; SB needs the awe of knowing living plants in order to practise *and* traces the cause of a patient's illness back, at least par-tially, to a gastrointestinal infection; EP practises orthodox first aid *and* differentiates between wind-heat and wind-cold; JK practises "proper diagnosis" derived from an orthodox approach to taking the case history and to conducting a physical examination *and* also draws on the "tissue states" of physiomedicalism; and MN, along with his wife,

RN, developed a Goethean science methodology *and* uses an orthodox medical approach to the case history and physical examinations.

Even if we choose to categorise some herbalists as either "more" traditional or "more" modern and scientific than others, the presence of enchantment within the narratives of both these groupings suggests that enchantment cannot be seen simply as some manifestation of residual tradition that will be eclipsed by the onward march of science and modernity. Rather the enchantment of meetings, often between herbalists and living plants, but also between herbalists and their many engagements with herbal medicine, is an energy that is present within the narratives and lives of herbalists and hence, at least to some degree, within Western herbal medicine.

Enchanted trees and rhizomes in Western herbal medicine

To understand how this energy spreads out we will return briefly to Deleuze and Guattari.[141] Arborescent thought, as introduced in the case of SB above, implies some sort of genealogy, where routes that bifurcate and spread out can be followed. In this book, the enchantment of herbs can be seen to be such an arborescent energy, found in the seed of the hidden entryways but also at places further along the narratives of some of the herbalists, in the stems and branches and leaves and flowers of their accounts. However, this is not the end of the story, because, in opposition to this linear, vertical and causal arborescent concept of enchantment, there are more "rhizomal" influences present within the cases. For Deleuze and Guattari, the concept of the rhizome, drawn from botany, is more about alliance than filiation. The rhizome is in the middle between things, it is multiple, non-hierarchical and made up of heterogeneous connections. The cases of the herbalists are rhizomes in that they draw on a wide number of diverse influences that they bring into their practices and that sit side by side without fear of contradiction. If herbalists and plants, and medicines made from them, can meet then herbalists can easily draw from a wide range of influences that others may see as being incommensurable. As GA said above, "I want to look at everything".

Cases versus paradigms, history, and the profession

We will now look beyond the herbalists' cases to consider how the cases relate to the initial sections of the book that considered social science work on Western herbal medicine, the history of Western herbal medicine and how the profession has engaged with politics and science.

The cases suggest that at the level of most of the individual herbalists, there has been less of a paradigm shift from tradition to science, from herbals to monographs, from expert practitioners to evidence-based herbal medicine, and more of an enchanting takeover by herbs, both as living plants and as medicines, that encompasses both the more traditional and more scientific approaches that herbalists bring into their practices.

While knowing living herbs is not important for the practices of the first four visible entryway herbalists (TE, CP, EP, and JK), it is important for the nine remaining herbalists, four of whom had visible entryways (SB, FD, GA, and MN), and five of whom had hidden entryways (CT, VH, AF, BC, and KA). And of these nine herbalists, three of them (SB, CT, and VH) draw heavily from mainstream and cutting edge science, while the remaining six herbalists (FD, GA, MN, AF, BC, and KA) draw relatively more from traditional knowledge, although as discussed above, differences sit easily together within herbalists.

The individual herbalists described here have more agency in their narratives than has been seen in previous social science work, which has tended to identify themes across data. Additionally, the herbs themselves, as living plants and as herbal medicines, are also seen to have more agency in their enchantment of herbalists than has previously been described.

So how might the narrative cases permit the early part of this book, which looked at the history of Western herbal medicine, its professionalisation and engagement with science, to be further understood? Even though orthodox medicine has separated itself from herbal medicine, herbal medicine is wedded to scientific knowledge, both in its training and in various manifestations of its practice. Of the cases represented here, TE is the herbalist who is most obviously aligned with orthodox medicine. Whether his approach reflects the majority of what goes on in Western herbal medicine in the UK is beyond the scope of this book, but it is an approach that the professional bodies and other institutions are likely to endorse in their engagement with science as a strategy for political survival.

The fragmented history of Western herbal medicine, as described previously, suggested that the separation of herbal medicine and orthodox medicine took place over a rather lengthy time period—ranging variously from the reign of Henry VIII in the sixteenth century to the demise of botany as the basis of medicine in Edinburgh in 1957. While there are undoubtedly many factors contributing to this being a rather long goodbye, the enchantment of plants may be one of them. After all, Henry VIII wrote and compounded his own prescriptions and was instrumental in the passing of what became known as the Herbalists' Charter. And Professor Bayley Balfour's physical contact with plants as a botanist may have impacted on his teaching of botany as the basis for medical education in Edinburgh. Furthermore, the historical attachment of herbalists to their "vegetable substances" in the seventy-five years leading up to the end of WWII could partly be accounted for by the enchantment of plants. Although we do not have these herbalists' narratives to be able to answer this question, the herbalists from then and from now both had and have a similar belief in the use of whole plant medicines or simple extracts as well as in what has come to be called the "synergy" of constituents within a plant. This does not mean that they related to or felt the same way about plants as the herbalists in the cases do, but it is a possibility that should remain open.

Let us look to the Thomsonian system of medicine, which influenced the development of Western herbal medicine in the UK as described previously. Thomson had borrowed heavily, although likely indirectly, from indigenous North American knowledge in the development of his herbal therapeutics and vapour baths.[19] He recalls, at the age of three or four, meeting "an old lady by the name of Benton" who made medicines from roots and herbs.[199] Thomson would go out with her to gather her medicines: "She would take me with her, and learn me their names, and what they were good for; and I used to be very curious in my inquiries, and in tasting everything that I found. The information I thus obtained at this early age, was afterwards of great use to me." Thomson knew these herbs as living medicines, tasting them straight from the plant. He could not read or write, but learnt from Benton and directly from the plant by tasting them. He remembers one particular plant, lobelia: "The taste and operation produced was so remarkable that I never forgot it. I afterwards used to induce other boys to chew it, merely by way of sport, to see them vomit." Thomson's engagement with herbs via tasting them has a sensual and experiential element to it, as well as an occasionally mischievous one, that speaks of a direct contact with his environment. This is not far removed from Abram's understanding of non-alphabetic cultures, and it is possible that these experiences could have provided a sensual knowing of plants, even an enchantment, although this word would not have been used, especially given Thomson's strict Christian upbringing. It is possible that this way of knowing plants supplied him with a sensual affective energy that contributed to the success of his system of medicine, which eventually spread over many states in America, and came to the UK. This is not to say that knowing plants in such a way is to be prioritised over historical, economic, political and other factors in explaining the success of a system of medicine, but it is not one that should be excluded either.

Let us now turn to the relationship between the trajectories of enchantment as seen in the cases on one hand, and the political history of the profession along with the profession's engagement with science, as seen on the other. This is a relationship of "purification", with herb-herbalist meetings being written in invisible ink. The story is a similar one as to why the enchanted entryways of herbalists are also necessarily "hidden" entryways, which was discussed above. As we have seen, with Latour's[47] "modern constitution" came the separation of science and objects and nature from politics and subjects and society— the nature/culture divide, for short. Any hybrids between nature and culture are swept under the carpet. Purification of nature from culture is valued and claimed, while hybrids are denied. Just as the enchanted entryways are, by definition, hidden in modernity, so are many other enchanted meetings between herbalists and plants within professional discourses. In seeking to engage with science they have no choice but to separate out subject from object, and culture from nature, and herbalists from herbs. It is a simple story and one that continues to be told. However, the narratives of herbalists suggest that while purification is present at the level of the profession, at the level of the individual, there are hybrids and meetings. And if this is true for some herbalists now, it is also possible for at least some herbalists, physicians and writers in the past. What would Fred Fletcher Hyde, Thomas Bartram, A. W. Priest, and L. R. Priest, Maud Grieve, Dr Coffin, Finlay Ellingwood, William Cook, Nicholas Culpeper, John Parkinson, John Gerard, William Turner, Leonhart Fuchs, Hildegard von Bingen, Galen of Pergamon, Pliny the Elder, Pedanius Dioscorides, and Aulus Cornelius Celsus reveal about their relationship to plants and herbal medicines and how this relates to the rest of their lives and to their writings or practice of medicine?

CHAPTER TWELVE

How plants enchant

We have discussed, thanks to Latour,[47] why modernity hides meetings between humans and nonhumans, including plants. However, this apparent blindness towards plants, viewing them solely as instrumental to human needs, has older origins. We will briefly discuss the marginal place of plants in Western thought before moving on to consider how it is that plants may be enchanting. To this end we will consider recent developments in plant science to understand plant enchantment through their similarities to humans, before considering developments in vegetal philosophy that help us to consider that plants may enchant by their very difference to humans, in the process of which they offer us hope of change. This will then be positioned within wider changes in the social sciences and humanities that are engaging with nonhuman agency. Just as herbalists experience both the pull and push of enchantment in their narratives, so plants can enchant through both similarity and difference.

Hall[200] argues that Theophrastus (371 – 287 BC), the "father of botany", deduced from observations that plants should be approached on their own terms as having their own purpose and not merely as being instrumental for humans. However, in the Western philosophical tradition, Theophrastus was overshadowed by Aristotle, Socrates, and Plato.

In this understanding the "vegetal" soul that represents botanical life was placed firmly at the bottom of the pyramid, with humans placed firmly above. Plants were ascribed only a "nutritive" level to the soul, denied access to the "sensitive" or "intellectual" levels. As already noted by Abram,[164] but worth repeating here, Plato writes that Socrates, in the play *Phaedrus*, says "I am devoted to learning; landscapes and trees have nothing to teach me—only the people in the city can do that." Marder[201] also looks back to antiquity and highlights the Platonic inversion of the plant where humans are rather upwardly "rooted" in the world of cognition and thought. Hall sees the non-perception of plants as continuing throughout history. He refers to Wandersee and Schussler's concept of "plant blindness". The symptoms of this condition remain largely present today and include the failure to see plants in one's life, the positioning of plants as a backdrop to animal life and the misunderstanding of the different timescales of plant and animal life. The disease of plant blindness, starting with the rejection of Theophrastus, has followed various trajectories up to this day. Hall[200] cites the impact of Francis Bacon, the Enlightenment philosophy of Descartes, the growth of rationalism as well as Christian doctrine that viewed plants as purely passive, lacking the "breath of life". Hall also discusses Eastern cultures, which are not simply portrayed as seeing what the blind West cannot. For example, in some major Buddhist schools and in some Hindu texts plants are relegated to a lowly status, although the Vedanta school of Hinduism is cited for its emphasis on the interconnections of all living things. Despite this, it is the Western conception of plant-hood that has viewed plants for the most part as purely instrumental to human requirements.

Enchantment through similarity—lessons from plant science

Within this trajectory of plant blindness there are signs that the perception of the marginal place of plants is changing. While Erasmus Darwin attributed to plants active sense-based engagements with their environments along with a modicum of mental processes,[202,203] it was his grandson, Charles Darwin, who is more widely remembered for his ideas that would contribute to the reconceptualisation of plants. In 1880, the publication of Charles Darwin's *The Power of Movement in Plants*, ended with the following assertion: "It is hardly an exaggeration to say that the tip of the radicle ... having the power of directing the movements of the adjoining parts, acts like the brain of one of the lower animals; the brain being seated within the anterior end of the body, receiving impressions from the sense organs and directing the several movements."[204] In a talk attended by the botanist Leonard Bastin, Darwin is reported as saying, "We must believe that in plants there exists a faint copy of what we know as consciousness in ourselves."[205] Bastin goes on to say that "In origin the animal and vegetable worlds appear to be indivisible, as though we may not dare to say that the plant is an intelligent being. There seems to be a field for a great deal of research, the opening up of which will form a new and fascinating branch of botanical study." However, it would be well over a century before Darwin's radical radicle idea and Bastin's hope were to produce visible, if contested, fruit.

An important influence on contemporary plant scientist Anthony Trewavas, and key to his thinking differently about plants, was Nobel Prize winner for physiology and medicine Barbara McClintock's 1984 statement, referring to plants, that "A goal for the future would be to determine the extent of knowledge the cell has of itself and how it utilizes this knowledge in a thoughtful manner when challenged."[206] Interestingly, Myers[207] notes that McClintock's research into the genetics of corn required intensive physical labour as she worked attentively with the plants throughout their life cycle in the hot summer sun. Her biographer quotes McClintock as saying, "I start with the seedling, and I don't want to leave it. I don't feel I really know the story if I don't watch the plant all the way along. So I know every plant in the field. I know them intimately, and I find it a great pleasure to know them."[208]

Monica Gagliano is a plant scientist at the forefront of recent developments in plant science. Gagliano and Grimonprez[209] note that plant science has begun to look beyond laboratory-based genetic engineering and molecular biology's explanation of plant growth, noting the re-emergence, this millennium, of an understanding of plants as active agents that demonstrate abilities to process information, communicate, and behave rationally within their ecology, including foraging for food, all of which are concepts that had previously been limited to the consideration of animals. Gagliano and Grimonprez call this new direction "a renaissance in plantness", and note that this has arisen out of the work of a relatively small number of research scientists "who have adopted ecologically driven approaches, where the 'cultural background' of plants is taken into account". Existing philosophical distinctions between plant and animal life as ontologically different are being eroded by studies that demonstrate plants as exhibiting intelligent behaviour, sensory perception, self-recognition, information processing, learning, memory, choice, decision making, foresight, behavioural control and resource sequestration with minimal outlay.[206,210-219]

Key figures, other than the already mentioned Monica Gagliano (University of Western Australia) and Anthony Trewavas (Edinburgh University), include Stefano Mancuso (University of Florence), Daniel Chamovitz (Tel Aviv University), Richard Karban (University of California, Davis), Frantisek Baluska (University of Bonn), and Susan Simard (University of British Columbia). While their endeavours haven't overtaken more conservative plant science activities, their contributions are significant, even if they have been controversially received. There now follows a necessarily incomplete, but hopefully indicative selection of some of this new plant science research and thinking that looks at plant senses, memory, learning, and intelligence, before considering their relevance to herbalists' enchantment with plants.

We will consider four scientists—Chamovitz, Mancuso, Gagliano, and Karban, who research plant senses and behaviour. Chamovitz[211] compares the human experiences of sight, smell, touch, hearing, awareness of location, and memory, with that of analogous physiological and chemical reactions in plants. For example, plants can distinguish between lights of different colours. They know if you come near them or stand over them and can tell if you are wearing a red or blue shirt and they know when the sun is about to set. They can sense gravity via specialised cells that function similarly to human inner ears such that the roots can sense which way is up and which way is down. They are aware of aromas: if a willow is damaged by tent caterpillars the tree releases a cloud of chemical volatiles that nearby willows sense or "smell" and respond to by building up chemicals in their leaves that are toxic to the caterpillars. Many plants that are attacked by insects release volatile chemical signals that attract the predators of the insects that are attacking it. If you touch the branches of a beech tree "the tree will remember it was touched. But it won't remember you." Mancuso and Viola[214] note that some of these volatile chemicals, including methyl jasmonate, send a clear message of "I'm not well" to warn other plants as well as other parts of the same plant. Plants can be seen to have "palates", for example, roots are able to identify mineral salt in minute concentrations. Mancuso and Viola tell the story of the famous scientist Lamarck (1744–1829) who asked his collaborator to push some small *Mimosa pudica* specimens, plants that are known to retract their leaves when touched, on a cart through the streets of Paris, reporting back that at first all the plants closed their leaves in response to the bumping vibrations of the cart but soon reopened them when the experience proved not to be dangerous. Continuing to think about touch, Mancuso and Viola note that root tips find their way past obstacles and that climbing plants also demonstrate touch in their aerial parts with, for example, the pea vine producing sensitive tendrils which curl up within a few seconds when they find something to grip onto. Another example of touch, or rather the awareness of the lack of it, is "crown shyness", where some trees avoid touching each other's crown even when growing very close to each other, implying an agreement to not disturb each other, to keep their crowns to themselves. Plants sense vibrations conducted through the earth via mechanosensitive channels found throughout the plant, with sound exposure being able to activate genes. In a study in Montalcino, Italy, grape vines exposed to music for five years demonstrated better growth, earlier ripening, richer flavour and colour, and higher polyphenol content with less insecticides needed. Mancuso and Viola note that it is the sound frequencies, not the type of music that affects the growth, with bass sounds promoting seed germination, growth, and root lengthening. Roots also produce "clicking" sounds, possibly due to the breaking of cell walls during growth. As roots can both perceive and emit sounds an underground communication system may exist, with one possibility being that plants use a form of growth-derived echolocation with clicking sounds acting as the source transmission.[215]

Gagliano[220,221] is at the forefront of this emergent field of plant bioacoustics, revealing that plants produce sound waves in the lower end of the audio range as well as ultrasonic sounds, and is exploring their ecological significance, both among plants and with other organisms. There is now evidence that sounds are produced independently of cell elongation or peristaltic water transport, with speculation that sounds produced by plants may facilitate plant competitive ability. Furthermore, sound emissions may influence the behaviour of insects such as wood borers and even warn close neighbours of impending herbivory. And if bacteria can communicate using ultrasonic waves, Gagliano[220] asks if it is far-fetched that plants could do the same. In an experiment, Gagliano et al.[221] found that plants, in the absence of moisture in the soil, were able to use the vibrations caused by water moving inside pipes to locate a water supply and grow towards it, demonstrating the ability to sense moisture without need of access to moisture gradients. However, when both moisture and acoustic cues were present, roots used soil moisture rather than sound vibrations to find the water source, selecting the most advantageous cue. They also found that noise affected the abilities of roots to respond appropriately to the soundscape, suggesting that acoustic pollution can negatively affect plants. Karban[222] notes that plants can differentiate between shade that is caused by light-competing plants and that caused by inanimate objects and will choose to grow away from their competitors. Karban[203] also notes that some climbers' tendrils have been found to have a greater sensitivity to touch than humans have and that touch can delay flowering and produce reduced inflorescences. Even more interesting is the possibility that plants may have additional, as yet undescribed, senses: in one study, closeness to a neighbouring plant induced seed germination even when cues associated with light, chemicals or touch were blocked. Some plants have inflorescences that can produce more heat as the external temperature drops, with this being achieved by changes in mitochondrial respiration with respiration rates as high as those of a hummingbird in flight having been recorded for some plants, suggesting that plants are able to sense temperature and regulate respiratory rates.

Another aspect of plant behaviour is discerned in the possibility of kin recognition. Dudley and File[212] show that a beach weed called sea rocket (*Cakile edentula*) can sense whether it was growing with siblings or unrelated plants of the same species. Allocation of resources to roots increased when placed in pots with stranger plants, but not when groups of siblings shared a pot. It was suggested that root interactions provide the cue for kin recognition. The possibility is that the related plants are less competitive and more cooperative with each other than unrelated plants, preferring to use resources for aerial growth, and hence kin reproduction, rather than battling for resources. Gagliano and Grimonprez[209] suggest that volatile emissions of plants are more effectively received among kin than strangers and that related plants may be recognised through leaf "gestures", with this pointing to a process analogous to "cultural transmission" in humans.

Suzanne Simard,[216-218] has found that the forest shares its resources. Using radioactive isotopes injected into Douglas firs she found that these trees provide carbon-based food to young fir seedlings and to fungi via underground mycorrhizal fungal networks that connect the trees' roots. In return these networks provide the trees with nutrients. Simard[215] describes the oldest trees functioning as the most active "hubs", branching their connections out to more trees than just the younger trees. These "mother trees" were able to deliver nutrients to shaded seedlings that included their offspring, until they grew enough to access light. However, not only did the evergreen firs communicate with their own species but they exchanged nutrients with deciduous birch trees, lending them sugars when they had a surplus and receiving sugars back at a later date. These arrangements led to more robust and resilient health of the forest as well as a larger total volume of photosynthesis. Needless to say, this has been named the "wood wide web".

The possibility of plant learning and memory has also been investigated. We will consider two studies co-authored by Gagliano. In the first study,[223] a similar experiment to the one described above by Lamarck was conducted, except that the *Mimosa pudica* plants were repeatedly dropped and responded initially by retracting their leaves. After repeated dropping they stopped further retractions, remaining open, demonstrating a behaviour in response to learning the non-dangerous effect of the droppings. However, Gagliano et al. also found that after a month with no further droppings they still did not retract their leaves after being dropped. Gagliano suggests that a cellular calcium signalling network may be responsible for the apparent memory accessed by the plant. In a second study, Gagliano et al.[224] sought to show that plants are able to learn by conditioning, similar to the well-known Pavlov's dogs experiment. In their experiment, Gagliano et al. used pea plants (*Pisum sativum*), air flow via a fan as the cue and light as the reward— instead of dogs, the sound of a bell and food, as in Pavlov's original experiment. The plants conditioned by the air flow grew towards the fan even without the presence of light, appearing to demonstrate associative learning in plants, seen in their choice of direction of growth based on their prediction of where the air flow, and hence, light source, would come from. The study suggested epigenetic reprogramming at a molecular level as an explanation for learning across taxa, including in plants.

Looking beyond senses, behaviour, and learning, in an interview, Chamovitz,[225] expands on plant memory:

Plants definitely have several different forms of memory, just like people do. They have short-term memory, immune memory and even transgenerational memory! I know this is a hard concept to grasp for some people, but if memory entails forming the memory (encoding information), retaining the memory (storing information), and recalling the memory (retrieving information), then plants definitely remember. For example a Venus Flytrap needs to have two of the hairs on its leaves touched by a bug in order to shut, so it remembers that the first one has been touched. But this only lasts about 20 seconds, and then it forgets. Wheat seedlings remember that they've gone through winter before they start to flower and make seeds. And some stressed plants give rise to progeny that are more resistant to the same stress, a type of transgenerational memory that's also been recently shown also in animals. While the short-term memory in the Venus Flytrap is electricity-based, much like neural activity, the longer term memories are based in epigenetics—changes in gene activity that don't require alterations in the DNA code, as mutations do, which are still passed down from parent to offspring.

We will now turn our attention to two key points made by Pollan[215] in his 2013 assessment of developments in plant science and its willingness to engage with concepts of behaviour, communication, and intelligence. First, the controversy within plant sciences is more about the interpretation and naming of discoveries, rather than the validity of the data itself. The questions that stir up the most heated debates include whether plants can "learn", "remember", and "make decisions", or whether these words should be "reserved for creatures with brains". The second point that Pollan makes is that intelligence can be defined in two ways. It can be seen as requiring a brain, from which reason, judgment, and abstract thought arise. However, intelligence can also be seen as "less brain-bound and metaphysical", and instead a behavioural definition can be emphasised, with intelligence being the "ability to respond in optimal ways to the challenges presented by one's environment and circumstances". Unsurprisingly, the plant scientists discussed above are drawn to this second definition. Mancuso and Viola[214] argue that "intelligence is the ability to solve problems", and indeed that it is "a property of life" with the difference between human intelligence and the intelligence of others being quantitative rather than qualitative, with intelligence being distributed throughout the modular structure of plants rather than localised in particular organs.

Trewavas[206] similarly concludes that "intelligence is quite simply the capacity for problem solving" and suggests that the different timescale of plants, along with activity hidden at the molecular level, have been barriers to seeing what is in front of us. He chooses the concept of physical intelligence, which opposes the common view of intelligence as supposedly always an intellectual activity. Chamovitz[211] argues that the important question is not whether or not plants are intelligent but, rather, whether they are aware. His answer is emphatically "Yes". Certainly plants, without having hands, noses, ears or eyes, have a wide range of senses analogous to human senses and maybe additional ones. Like humans, they can learn, make decisions, forage, share resources and remember. Chamovitz asks whether, given these similarities, we see ourselves when looking at a plant?

It is interesting that it is science that has arguably, through the chosen experimental designs and descriptions of behaviour, anthropomorphised plants. However, Bennett[171] has suggested that anthropomorphism may well be a price worth paying in order to oppose anthropocentrism. Seeing human-ness everywhere may be a partial solution to the problem of human exceptionalism. The possibility that is to be raised here is whether photosynthesising life that is (mostly) rooted to the spot and exists at an apparently slower pace, yet which, in its own way, can see, smell, hear, taste, touch, evaluate, remember, decide, and act, enchants herbalists precisely because of similarities to humans. Enchantment may partly be a recognition of similarity in something that is also very different. And it is this similarity that allows herbalists and plants to meet in the first place. While there is no suggestion that herbalists are tenured plant scientists, the relations that herbalists have with plants, based on time spent together, and medicines made from them, could generate an enchanting realisation of the similarity between humans and plants.

Consider the following propositions: TE's prioritisation of empirical scientific herbal knowledge is paralleled in Gagliano's study of associative learning by the pea plant that demonstrated a rational decision to move towards the cue for light. CP's use of *Vitex agnus-castus, Chamaelirium,* and other herbs to treat female infertility, developed through taking them to promote her own fertility and which resulted in the birth of her son, is reflected in the Douglas firs' sharing of resources with those that they identify as kin and in the exchange of resources with other species. The sensual qualities found in EP's engagement with Chinese medicine, for example, in the diagnosis of phlegm or wind-heat, or in JK's attention to her patients' physical tissue states that variously require protection, astringency or stimulation, are also seen in the ability of *Mimosa pudica* to differentiate between the touch of wind or of rain or of a human. SB's desire to get to the root of the matter is present in the ability of roots to seek out the source of the sound of running water. FD's change to only using herbal medicines that she knows as living plants, where she has "an image in [her] head of the plant", is also found in the ability of plants to grow in a new direction after differentiating between shade caused by other plants and that caused by inanimate objects. GA's voiceless conversations with plants are seen in the possible use of echolocation by plants that we are unable to hear. In GA's practice, the therapeutic treatment of his patients' metaphors as if they are real are also found in the language that is used in the recent developments of plant science whereby plants can see, smell, taste, touch, and hear. MN and RN's use of the same methodology to understand patients as they use to understand plants is present in Gagliano's selection of the same experimental design to understand associative learning in plants that has been used for studying animals. CT's reconciliation of opposites, including holism and reductionism, nature and religion, and punk and professionalism, is played out in the way that the "wood wide web" both cares for kin and develops beneficial relationships with stranger plants. Something of the complexity of VH's endobiogenic approach to understanding the horizontal relationships between hormones is also manifest in the complexity of the underground mycorrhizal network that facilitates communication and response. AF's desire to understand plants "energetically", through knowing them directly, including by taste, is found in the ability of roots to detect trace mineral concentrations, the grip of a vine's tendril and the detection of warning signals in clouds of volatile chemicals produced by neighbouring plants. BC's facilitation of the space where patients' stories can be told is also present in the occurrence of "crown shyness", where trees agree not to touch each other's crowns, allowing each other access to light and hence growth. And KA's relating to plants as persons is visible in the ability of plants to tell if you are wearing a blue shirt or a red shirt.

The above suggests that similarities exist between plants and herbalists. This is enchantment through similarities where meetings with creatures from another kingdom, namely plants, provide a sensual affective energy in the practices of herbalists and in Western herbal medicine. We next turn to vegetal philosophy, to see how enchantment may arise through difference.

Enchantment through difference — lessons from vegetal philosophy

Recent developments in plant science show us that humans and plants have common ground, giving us the enchanting warmth of recognition when we consider plants. Yet plants are also different from us, and it is this very difference that offers up enchanting possibilities of change, something that is particularly relevant to health care. To this end we now turn to philosophy, mostly to the work of Michael Marder, to identify enchanting ways of thinking about plant difference. One of Marder's[201] assertions of the meaning of "plant thinking" is that human thinking is "to some extent, de-humanized and rendered plant-like, altered by its encounter with the vegetal world". Meeting plants and knowing them by simply spending time with them and adjusting our rhythms to theirs is an enchanting possibility. Marder[226] points out that while at times we grow and decay, the pattern of constant change is the domain of plants rather than of humans. Marder suggests that knowing plants "face-to-face" is not possible: they change before we can meet them, and then we do not stay with them, whether that is due to lack of patience or ability. This book suggests that enchantment by both similarity and difference is a form of knowing and does happen, largely by spending time with plants, side-by-side, rather than face-to-face.

We will now briefly consider eight entwined philosophical plant enchantments. First, Marder[227] points out that plants, unlike humans and other animals, may not have the power of locomotion but they do demonstrate Aristotle's other three types of movement, namely growth, decay, and change of state. Humans move and so relocate to another environment, or excavate and build boundaries around themselves, while plants change themselves through phenotypic plasticity and modular growth and so change the environment, from which they are inseparable. Plants change their state all the time, with their internal busy-ness and their growth reminding us to consider our own potential for change. Second, Marder[228] suggests, putting modular growth to one side, that it is the world that comes to meet the plant, rather than the plant venturing outside its locality, with sessile life demanding the ability to adapt to local changes. Marder argues that "[A] rooted mode of being and thinking is characterized by extreme attention to the place and context of growth and, hence, sensitivity that at times exceeds that of animals." Furthermore, as plants grow they change the places where they are found, with their own sense of place depending on their intentional positioning of new leaves, shoots, and roots.[227] Being with plants can help us to develop or fine-tune a sense of place and an awareness of ourselves within it. Third, looking back on the history of Western thought, Marder[229] notes that plants, unlike animals, are regarded as "non-oppositional being(s)" to the point of "merging with the milieu", with plants not being "other" to their environment.

Referring to Hegel, Marder suggests that "The plant is all about a visible extension without interiority." Pouteau[230] notes that the plant "body center(s) is (are) already 'around', whatever this 'around' may represent in a non-Euclidian space". Furthermore, they have no "psychic interiority" and have no metaphysical distinction between "inside" and "outside".[231] Seeds give a visible understanding of this plant non-separation: they germinate "in and as the middle", growing shoots up and roots down, with no separation or traumatic break, as occurs in humans and other animals,[232] with flowers and roots turned into "variegated extensions of the middle".[233] As it is arguably the human sense of separation that has fuelled much conflict, both internal and external, the consideration of plants is an offering of hope. Fourth, Marder[227] quotes Canguilhem's definition of organismic life, where "To live is to radiate; it is to organise a milieu from and around a center of reference." However, Marder argues that plants do not fall within this definition, stating that "the plant does not organise its milieu", instead arguing that plants are made up of internal biochemical, hormonal, and synaptic communication networks as well as external communication routes that connect the plant to its environment. "It is, thus, an open system, coupled with its environment ..." This openness is also considered by Houle,[234] who notes that scientific speculation includes the possibility that the external plant cell wall is a descendent of the original external wall of the zygote, meaning that plant cells inherit an outside identify.

Houle describes how, in animal and human embryogenesis, the process of "gastrulation" occurs, that is, invagination of the embryo resulting in the creation of an inner space, which is an internalisation of what was facing outwards. The human mouth, oesophagus, stomach, small intestine, colon, and anus were all originally outward facing. Biologically this is an early dualism in human development. But plants do not do this. Houle quotes Pouteau, who says that plants live as "unsplit beings (having neither an inside nor outside) … in an undivided, unlimited, non-centered state of being … Plantness faces only outwards."[234] Houle asks whether we can "learn to face only outwards and in all directions at once, like plants?" Continuing to think about direction, Pouteau[230] notes that biophysical research shows that plants and animals develop along distinct "fields of hydrodynamic forces", with the spiral arrangements of plant parts along a stem being ruled by axial forces, such that the plant body remains open, perpetually coming into being and declining. The "twisting, curling, folding and bending" of leaf attachments to stems never leads to invagination. On the other hand, she describes how tetrapods, including humans, are ruled by concentric forces that start in embryogenesis and reach a closed, self-referential state that is bound to limits. She argues that this results in plants and humans as "incommensurable beings".

Pouteau[230] notes that to understand plants we must understand what it is to be a decentralised entity with no front or back, no left or right, but with a top and bottom. For humans, who have all these binaries, such an understanding of non-binary open orientations may prove difficult, but would move us to more fully appreciate vegetal life. The open orientation of plants has much to offer in moderating human tendencies to contraction and expansion, defence and attack. Fifth, Marder[228] notes the modular development of plants, where the same plant structures, such as leaves, flowers, branches, and roots, are replicated. This means that plants have no vital organs. They can lose much of themselves and still be alive and vital. Plants also have an indeterminate number of parts, that is constantly changing, with severed plant parts having the potential to become other plants.[235] Marder[233] notes that the head "loses its transcendental privilege", in that flowers can be lost but the plant can remain vital. Marder[233] suggests that, metaphysically speaking, plant life is superficial as it does not have a "deep essence", seen again precisely in that it can lose virtually any part without losing its life. Valuing superficiality is inherently difficult for humans, but seeing the benefits to plants could help us to move beyond our interiors.

Marder,[233] referencing Deleuze and Guattari, suggests that a plant can be seen as "a body without organs". While a human body without organs takes us to images of death, the modular structure of plants offers up the enchanting possibility of a vital life without vital organs. Sixth, a corollary of modular life is that intelligence is not contained in a specific organ but is found in the entire living being. Marder[236] further explores "plant-thinking" and refers to "the non-cognitive, non-ideational, and non-imagistic mode of thinking proper to plants (hence, what I call 'thinking without the head')". For humans, while we jealously guard and protect our cerebral cortexes, being with headless thinkers could open new ways of being in the world. Seventh, Marder[235] quotes Theophrastus on the diversity of plants—"We cannot here seize any universal character which is common to all," noting that this became a guide rather than a hindrance to Theophrastus, who sought to become "attuned to the singularity of each plant species". The term "plant" may be metaphorically violent, destroying the differences between a mayflower and a palm tree, or between a moss and a raspberry bush.[233] Focusing on individual plants avoids the human obsession with unity and can be seen as demystifying, arguably assisting us in knowing ourselves and other humans.

And finally, Kalhoff[237] argues that the concept of "flourishing" has two useful meanings for understanding plants. It is empirical, in that plants can be observed to complete life cycles, manage challenges as well as having capacities that are expressed in shapes. However, it is also "evaluative" in that flourishing indicates the "good life" of a plant. Applying the plant yardstick of flourishing to our own lives could help us move to more satisfied ways of being.

We have briefly looked at how plants, through their very difference, draw our attention to change, a sense of place, non-separation, openness, a modular life, distributed thinking, diversity and flourishing. The cases reveal parallels with these concepts. Change is obviously a key motivation in health care and the herbalists discussed use a wide variety of knowledges, including clinical trial data, complexity science, endobiogenics, Chinese medicine theory, Goethean science, and the emotional affinities of flower remedies to bring about a wide variety of changes in the internal states of their patients, including in receptor site activation, levels of complexification, dampness, decision making, and emotions. The apparent ease with which plants change could be one reason that they have persistently been used for health and well-being by humans. The cases also reveal the importance of a sense of place, seen in, for example, the value to SB of knowing his grandmother's garden; FD's preference, over "the exotics", of using plants that she knows as living plants in her garden and elsewhere; MN's patients, who go to meet plants in his garden; AF's attention to looking after his "patch" and knowing herbs that grow on his windowsill the best; and BC's highlighting of the indigenous knowledge in Western herbal medicine, seen in the travelling of the story of yarrow to South America, and her production of place-specific fermented medicine.

Non-separation is also found in the cases. VH, in his use of endobiogenics, resists orthodox medicine's separation of vertical hormonal axes, instead identifying relationships between hormonal axes as being key for human health; CT sees both herbs and words as pharmacological agents in the consultation; AF sees the spiritual development of the herbalist as necessary for being helpful to patients; EP's use of Chinese medicine theory means that diagnosis necessarily leads to clear treatment principles; and GA, in his attention to patients' stories, does not separate metaphors of illness from reality. A sense of openness is found particularly in consultations: in CT's sitting back and being "ready to receive"; in VH's "priestly approach" that witnesses the patient; in MN's instruction to his patient to go out and meet the plants; and in BC's listening to patients' stories in such a way that they get to the "heart of the matter" themselves. Looking to modular life, this is present if we look at the cases *in toto*, with all contributing to the life of Western herbal medicine but none being essential, precisely because knowing plants allows diversity to be brought into practice. One or two or more could be lost but Western herbal medicine continues, despite being changed, just as a plant will regrow differently after being cut back, but it is still the same plant. Similarly, distributed thinking and distributed intelligence are present in that the cases demonstrate some common ground between practices, for example, between TE and CT, who both see conventional physiology as the basis of their practices, even if there are also differences between these practices such as CT's engagement with complexity science. And if CT was to retire, VH's practice of endobiogenics would continue a specific manifestation of complexity science.

The diversity of herbalists is self-evident. Whether it be the differences between or within the visible or hidden entryways, or the desire to get to the root cause of an illness versus helping patients to make decisions to be well, or an enchantment with empiricism or with theory, differences abound in the cases. And finally, flourishing patients, one way or another, are the goal of these herbalists, both in the empirical sense of the content of patients' lives, and in the evaluative sense of patients finding their "path with heart". Maybe some of all of this is down to plant difference.

CHAPTER THIRTEEN

Plants, nonhumans, agency, and Western herbal medicine

W e have considered how it is possible, for herbalists and other humans, to be enchanted both through their similarities and differences with plants, almost as if there is no escape. We now broaden out from the specifics of plant science and of vegetal philosophy to look at the growing social science and humanities interest in plants and, more generally, in nonhumans, to further develop an understanding of Western herbal medicine.

Critical plant studies

Marder is a central figure in the small but expanding field of what has come to be known as critical plant studies, plant studies, or human-plant studies[202] that has been developing recently in the social sciences and humanities. For the arguments of this book other key figures include Matthew Hall,[200] John Ryan,[238–240] Patricia Vieria,[241–243] Randy Laist,[244] Prudence Gibson,[245,246] Lesley Head,[247] Natasha Myers,[207,248–251] Michael Pollan,[215,252] and Luci Attala.[253]

A central motivation of critical plant studies is to overcome plant blindness and, to this end, it draws widely from philosophy, ethics, communication, linguistics, poetics, art, literary studies, feminism, and aesthetics and explores concepts such as agency, cognition, language, and intentionality.[202] As Head et al.[247] note, the case is being made in plant science, philosophy, and other humanities, particularly literary studies, for plants to be engaged with respectfully as subjects rather than as objects, and is tied to environmental concerns. Gagliano, who we met above, is a plant scientist who brings philosophy into her plant science and plant science into her philosophy. Gagliano's recent book[254] *Thus Spoke the Plant: a Remarkable Journey of Groundbreaking Scientific Discoveries and Personal Encounters with Plants*, is a "phytobiography" of stories, each written "in partnership with a plant", that reveal the dynamic agency of the plants that have "helped along the way" in her research into plant cognition and communication.

Critical plant studies engage with developments in art. Gibson's book *The Plant Contract*[245] is an explicit plant specific endorsement and development of Serres's *The Natural Contract*. While Serres promised that the natural world would no longer be human property, but rather a symbiont with humanity, Gibson refocuses from nature in general to new plant thinking in art in particular, in "an effort to un-mute nature". She notes that much of the artwork around developments in plant science is performance art, addressing the temporality of plants. Gibson suggests that art can help us to reconceive the vegetal world and oppose plant blindness. Aloi's recent book *Why Look at Plants?*[255] examines plant-presence in contemporary art in the Anthropocene through the eyes of artists, curators, and academics. Also, Gibson and Brits'[246] '*Covert Plants: Vegetal Consciousness and Agency in an Anthropocentric World*' is an interdisciplinary approach to "thinking with and through vegetal life", which explores the impact of this re-evaluation of plants on the arts and culture, arguing that it is important to seek to express vegetal life rather than simply to represent it.

Plants are also being reconceived within literary studies. Randy Laist[244] explores how literary and cultural products express human relationships with plants, and seeks to promote a sensitivity to our "photosynthetic brethren". Ryan[238] is at the forefront of "botanical criticism", a disciplinary approach forged out of ecocriticism. He looks at how Australian, American, and English poets relate to plants in their work. This book can be fruitfully read alongside Marder's directly philosophical work. Ryan and Giblett[240] look at the cultural and natural history of old-growth forests in south-western Australia, held together by the narrative of the Giblett family.

Head et al.[247] note that within cultural geography the agency of trees, gardens, crops, and seeds is being taken seriously. Their development of plant studies challenges political thinking that confines itself to humans, and documents, through ethnographic methods, both collaborative and antagonistic relations between plants, humans, and others. They show that human-plant relations can help us to rethink the political. Jeffrey Nealon[256] suggests that animal studies have reinforced the idea of the human as a noble independent animal and investigates how discourses on biopower, that is, the power that is exercised over bodies, as well as discourses within animal studies, change if plants are introduced to the discussion.

Feminist plant studies are an important thread within critical plant studies. Luce Irigaray, in her personal, philosophical, and political written conversation with Michael Marder in *Through Vegetal Being*,[257] applies her work on the sexual differences in being human to a vegetal world. Irigaray[258] argues the case for learning from plants and their focus on *becoming* rather than the human fixed sense of *being* as well as from how they work with rather than against their environment. And Elaine Miller, in *The Vegetative* Soul,[259] through her reading of nineteenth-century German thought, compares animal-derived understandings of the individual subject with plant-derived understandings where interconnection and change are highlighted. She also explores how the "vegetative" subject can help to reconfigure the association of the feminine with nature in politically useful ways for women.

Matthew Hall[200] could be described as a plant animist philosopher and has been central to the recent "turn" to plants in the social sciences and humanities. In an attempt to urge a reconsideration of the moral and ethical standing of plants, Hall adopts the concept of "plant personhood", derived from the work of animist scholars such as Graham Harvey and Irving Hallowell. In this approach, plants, as "other-than-humans", are related to as persons. Human interactions with plants are seen in terms of kinship links and relationships between persons. Hall suggests that viewing plants as persons allows the "voices" of nonhumans to be heard. Plant personhood is not concerned with anthropomorphising, with projecting human-like qualities onto plants, rather plants are seen as living beings with their own perspectives and modes of communication. For Hall, "Personhood thus emerges from a focus on relating and the recognition of shared volition and intentionality in natural beings." Furthermore, this understanding of plants as persons must be learned and even the transmission of ancestral knowledge and wisdom can only play a supportive role to the active learning that is required. Drawing on the philosophical ecology of Kohak, Hall urges us to develop "manners of speaking" that are "modes of interacting with reality which render our world meaningful and guide our actions therein". Plant personhood is part of this wider project.

Gagliano et al.[202] point out that discussions within plant science on plant behaviour often use "correspondences to the animal world" so that they may be taken seriously as sensitive and intelligent. Hence plants remain somehow secondary to humans and are not addressed in their own terms. Gagliano et al., drawing on the biosemiotics assertion that language is present in all life, prefer to conceive of language as "an ecology produced by organisms in interdependent and multispecies interrelation". This approach to language includes both humans and plants, does not require an emitting "individuated living subject" and opposes plant language as being simply metaphorical, allegorical, symbolic or a figure of speech. Gagliano et al. suggest that "phytosemiotics" sees plant language as expressing physiology in semiotic terms and suggests that it is necessary for humans to be open to speaking without words. They look at linguistic processes from an ecological and biological perspective, suggesting that language is a "meaning-making activity" at the core of all life, including plants, with the nonhuman world being rich in language. They seek a more universal understanding of language and propose an embodied view of language where language is viewed in terms of what it enables organisms to do. Gagliano et al. propose that perceiving the language of an ant, sunflower or bacteria, for example, could be a matter of "attuning" to their vocabulary of gestures, postures, displays, brief chemical, and electromagnetic signals. They show how plant chemical language, for example, can attach new meanings to old chemical words, and suggests that plant language, like human language, emerges from the interplay of biological evolution, individual learning, and cultural transmission and can be seen, for example, in the recognition of kin by specific leaf gestures. Language is a consequence of the meanings made in an environment, and "engraves the very identity of that organism and its physical embodiment in its world". Marder[260] argues that "To hear plants speak we must listen to the lacunae and silences of language, leaving plenty of room for the untranslatable and hence unspeakable, in these practices of translation." He suggests that the language of plants is "an articulation without saying", with articulation referring both to expression and the joining of two or more things: plants articulate themselves as they proliferate. "They form a world, by which they, themselves are shaped." Ryan[239] develops the idea of the non-verbal, ecological, and corporeal voice of plants, with humans being able to recognise this through the sense of taste, touch, smell, and proprioception.

Michael Pollan[252] addresses issues of plant enchantment when he argues that food plants and flowers have been considered simply as passive participants in evolutionary history while, in fact, the converse is true, plants have actively domesticated humans, using us as "human bumblebees". He looks at four plants, the apple, tulip, marijuana, and potato that meet human desire for, respectively, sweetness, beauty, intoxication, and control, with their successful domestication of us resulting in their cultivation, proliferation, and care by humans. Interestingly, he argues that the success of cannabis is due to its skill in turning off, rather than on, the human mind, giving it a rest from memory so that it can be more attentive to direct experience. And, of course, since the publication of Pollan's book the medicinal uses of cannabis, from pain management to cancer treatment, are being debated as they never have been before. Chamovitz[211] makes a similar suggestion, arguing that for some species we make excellent allies in their propagation, in return for which we receive flowers, colours, fruits, fragrances, and flavours.

Which brings us to Luci Attala,[253] who further explores plant abilities through the benefits of being eaten by humans. Attala suggests that "Being edible can be repositioned as a phytochemical communication strategy that some plants use to initiate affective relationships with the human animals that consume them." Attala points out that while ethnographic accounts highlight plants as chemical communicators with humans via ingestion, plant science, although increasingly addressing plant agency, keeps humans excluded from plant awareness and behaviour. She asks, given evidence that plants utilise their phytochemical resources to persuade other species to provide them with assistance, "Is it likely that humans are exempt from their charms and are not beneficiaries of their instructions?" Attala suggests that "Ingestion of another can be usefully repositioned as part of a long-term chemical dialogue rather than a destructive event." From this perspective, being edible is a mechanism that plants utilise to develop relationships with humans. Attala gives the example of the Amerindian hallucinogenic plant preparation ayahuasca that is used in ritual healing, the ingestion of which enables long-term relationships between human beings and plant beings. For Attala, being edible is more than simply promoting seed dispersal. After being picked, plants endeavour to retain human attention through taste, chemical breakdown, and assimilation. Attala gives the example of how physiological addiction to plants, such as coffee, tea, cocoa, sugar cane, opium, cannabis, and tobacco means that "Addicted individuals work extremely hard to retain access to their substance of choice." Attala suggests that both plant-induced hallucinations and cravings for plant foods demonstrate plant "proficiencies" in provoking "caring responses from humans, who protect, seek out and proliferate plants they are attached to because of these capabilities". Regarding Western herbal medicine this raises a particular question: do herbs cultivate relationships with humans, including herbalists, through being medicinal? This is one way of looking at the agency of herbs. It is interesting to note here that many of the phytochemicals that have been shown to be medicinal, including alkaloids, glucosinolates, terpenoids, phenolics, and glycosides, are classified as "secondary metabolites" that are not involved directly in growth, metabolism, or reproduction and are not essential to the life of plants. After all, a plant that is medicinal is likely to be looked after. And many of the herbalists in this book either grow or wild harvest or care for herbs in one way or another. From this perspective, the professionalisation of herbal medicine along with its engagement with science and its historical battle to maintain the right to practise and the right to access herbal medicines can be seen in part as a response by the profession to the enchantment of herbs such that herbs are cared for and allowed to flourish.

Other engagements with plants

Anthropology's ethnographic study of human societies' relationships with plants has included agricultural settings, cooking and plant processing, human health, ethnomedicine, and poisonous and psychoactive plants. While it is argued in medical anthropology that plant knowledge arises locally in social relationships and that medicinal plants have to be coaxed if not seduced by healers,[261] it is multispecies ethnography,[262] emerging out of the intersection of science studies, environmental studies, animal studies, and anthropology, that has recognised plants as key actors. While Ogden, Hall, and Tanita[263] point out that plants (along with animals) have been conceived of as holding totemic power, structural order, sexual suggestion, symbolic ecology in the age of globalism, and indigenous ecological knowledge, it is multi-species ethnography that aims to be "attuned to life's emergence with a shifting assemblage of agentive beings. By 'beings' we are suggesting both biophysical entities as well as the magical ways objects animate life itself." Ogden et al. argue that multispecies ethnography seeks to attend to the nonhuman, with stones, birds, bees, animals, and plants having the power to bring about change.

Kohn's *How Forests Think*,[264] a multispecies ethnography of the montane forests of eastern Ecuadorian Amazonia, identifies life as being the only prerequisite for a self and challenges human symbolic systems, including language, instead revealing non-verbal signs articulated among many species in the "semiosis of life". Language is not required for agency and becomes just one way of communicating. Kohn's anthropology "beyond-the-human" develops an approach to semiology where iconic signs, which have much in common with what they represent, and indexical signs, which have a geographical or temporal association with what they represent, are central because they are the signs that nonhumans also resource. Despite this inclusiveness plants are not considered substantively, which is odd given the title of Kohn's book, instead preferring to consider dogs, jaguars, giant anteaters, and monkeys, although a non-stinging nettle, ephiphytic cactae, and vulture's pacai are marginally present.

One exception to this marginality is Tsing's *The Mushroom at the End of the World*.[265] If we can overlook the human placement of mushrooms in a kingdom separate from plants, Tsing's following of the highly prized gourmet matsutake mushroom through its commodity chains highlights the relationship between the wrecking effects of capitalism and cooperative multispecies survival. Along the way, she reveals that to be human is to be in interspecies relationships. Similarly, Ogden et al.[263] argue that the human emerges out of relations with multiple organisms and that multispecies ethnography must be a "mode of wonder" that, paraphrasing Stengers, makes us "think, feel and hesitate".

Someone within multispecies ethnography who addresses plants in her fieldwork is Diana Gibson[266] who draws on changes since 2000 within anthropological research relating to ideas and practices around medicinal plants, as well as ethnographic research in Namibia and the

Western Cape, to argue that in relationships with humans, plants can instigate political and other changes and that they can be regarded as nonhuman subjects with non-intentional agency. Gibson[267] also developed, in her ethnographic research in the Western Cape, methodologies that sought to be more attentive to plants while avoiding anthropomorphising them, a task which is understood to be tricky for any human. Techniques included slowing down and seeking to "stretch our perceptual skills: visual, olfactory, auditory, gustatory, and tactile as part of a sensorial toolkit" by ingesting, drawing, and photographing plants in order to know plant life, in the process of which the author entered into relationships with environments, weather, and creatures including insects and larger animals. This approach is a step towards answering questions that Abram[268] poses: despite lacking central nervous systems what does it feel like, to a decentralised, distributed, and democratic being, to be rooted in a place, sipping minerals, drinking sunlight? What does it feel like to transmute sunlight into material?

Natasha Myers addresses the "more-than-human" and documents the "affective ecologies" between plants and people and other relations. For example, Myers[250] looks at how human-plant relations are produced in botanical gardens. Myers[248] tries to figure out what matters to a black oak savannah, whose existence depends on the force of fire to keep the grasslands well and promote oak regeneration. The savannah needs humans with particular knowledge, thus forming a savannah-human relationship that can be called a "naturalcultural" formation. Myers,[249] in response to the arrival of the Anthropocene, calls for humans to make allies with plants and for a "planthropology" to document the affective ecologies between plants and people. Myers[251] also calls for "photosynthesis" to be a keyword for "these dire times" to remind us that we are not alone, that we have powerful allies.

The rise of the nonhuman

Critical plant studies reflect broader changes in the social sciences and humanities where the nonhuman is being attended to more centrally in an attempt to mitigate the destructive effects of human exceptionalism. In fact, Hall,[200] discussed above, quotes Harvey's key statement that "Animists are people who recognize that the world is full of persons, only some of whom are human, and that life is always lived in relationship with others."[269] Persons are simply those with whom other persons "interact with varying degrees of reciprocity". Importantly, Harvey points out that the term animism has two main usages, the older of which has its origins in colonialism and which regarded indigenous people as un-empirical, believing in spirits and lacking the ability to distinguish things from humans, while the newer usage refers to a moral, political, and environmental concern with knowing how to relate to and behave with both human and nonhuman persons in multispecies naturalist, rather than metaphysical, communities. Harvey[269,270] refers to animism as "the attribution of enchantment to these other-than-human loci".

Grusin[271] notes that the nonhuman has a long history in human cultural outputs, from Lucretius's first-century BC didactic poem "De Rerum Natura" that was taken up in the early modern period, to the literature of Emerson, Thoreau, Whitman, and Dickinson. He suggests that this thread was strengthened by Darwin's deliberate non-separation of human and nonhuman species when it came to the laws that governed them, and by William James's argument that human non-material emotion, thoughts, will, and habit are inseparable from and reliant upon nonhuman physical processes. Despite this, attention to the nonhuman has recently escalated in many spheres of life, including academia, in response to awareness of the impact of human life on nonhuman others. While animism is arguably as direct a way to establish new relationships with nonhuman others as can be imagined, a number of more tangential academic "turns", or shifts in academic focus, have been important for re-engaging with the nonhuman. Grusin points to several of these, including the ecological, evolutionary, ontological, and affective varieties. While the relevance of the first two to the nonhuman are self-explanatory, particularly in the Anthropocene, the remaining two require some attention. The ontological turn, articulated particularly in anthropology, was itself a response to the "writing culture" turn of the 1980s, initiated by Clifford and Marcus,[272] which sought to describe multiple cultural representations of a single reality. However, the ontological turn opposes the view that while people may understand the world differently the world is still *the* world, instead suggesting that there are multiple worlds.[273] This position forces us to more actively consider nonhuman worlds. Looking to the affective turn, affect, as discussed previously, is not simply feeling or emotion but is rather a bodily experience of intensity. The affective turn suggests that material bodily forces require consideration when seeking to understand our capacity to engage with others.[274] This, along with the argument that affect is resistant to language, and can only be experienced,[275] is useful in considering how we may know others who are not like us, including plants, and with whom we do not have a common language.

Notable influences on the nonhuman within these academic turns, traced by Grusin,[271] include actor-network theory, especially the work of Latour; affect theory as made manifest in psychology, philosophy, and queer theory; animal studies, with Haraway being central; the work of Deleuze, particularly his assemblage theory; the new materialisms found in philosophy, feminism, and Marxism; the ascendancy of object oriented ontology; and systems theory, including its ecological varieties. Grusin suggests, nodding to Latour, that the nonhuman turn demonstrates that we have never really been human, that we have always been indistinct from the nonhuman, having evolved with, existed with, and collaborated with the nonhuman. Stark and Roffe[276] suggest that it is now impossible to consider the human without the nonhuman, with the nonhuman turn challenging human privilege and placing the human within the "more than human world". They suggest that the nonhuman turn asks us to question the dualisms of the organic and inorganic and the subject and object. We are also asked to question the place of the human within nonhuman timescales, with the identification of the human as a "momentary blip" in deep or geological time leading to a re-evaluation of human-nonhuman relations. Crucially, this refocusing on geological time humbles conceptions of human agency while highlighting evolutionary and nonhuman agency.

We will now briefly turn to posthumanism, where the nonhuman has also been highlighted. While Grosin points out that the very idea of the posthuman runs the risk of an assumption of human progressive development there is also a nonhuman focus within posthumanism. Anthropologist Descola[277] refers to posthumanism as "the project of repopulating the social sciences with nonhuman beings and thus of shifting the focus away from the internal analysis of social conventions and institutions and toward the interactions of humans with (and between) animals, plants, physical processes, artefacts, images, and other forms of beings ..." Descola traces the posthuman concern with the nonhuman back to science and technology studies in general and actor-network theory in particular, and also to Levi-Strauss and the ambition to avoid "some of the great anthropological dualisms—nature and society, individual and collective, body and mind", while also maintaining that differences are not flattened in the process, but are meaningfully retained and understood. Braidotti[278] explores some of the trajectories that have led to posthumanism, including humanism, anti-humanism, and post-secularism. For Braidotti it all started with "He: the classical ideal of 'Man', formulated first by Protagoras as 'the measure of all things' ... and represented in Leonardo da Vinci's Vitruvian Man." Braidotti argues that, in this particular model of human perfectionism, humanism has limited what counts as human. For Braidotti, posthumanism functions to explore alternative ways of thinking about the human subject. One such way is through "the nonhuman, vital force of Life, which I have coded as zoe". Braidotti goes on say that "Zoe as the dynamic, self-organizing structure of life itself ... stands for generative vitality. It is the transversal force that cuts across and reconnects previously segregated species, categories and domains." For Braidotti, such an approach looks to identify and create enhancing connections between all that lives, whether it breathes or not, which necessarily challenges the primacy of the human in general, and the male subject in particular.

Actor-network theory and the writing culture movement both originated in the mid 1980s and were part of the academic debates and lineage that led either directly or indirectly to considerations of the other-than-human in the social sciences. However, there is another major influence of the same time period that is important for the academic evolution to the posthuman and nonhuman. Donna Haraway's[179] 1985 paper *"A Cyborg Manifesto: Science, Technology, and Socialist-Feminism in the Late Twentieth Century"*, later published in a collection of essays, introduced the metaphor of "the cyborg" to argue against assumptions of essentialism in feminism and to prompt feminists to engage with technology. Addressing "the cyborg" drew attention to the blurring of boundaries between the human and the machine in order to enable radical politics. *"A Cyborg Manifesto"* ends with the statement, "I would rather be a cyborg than a goddess." For Haraway, technology breaks down long-standing Western dualisms such as mind/body, male/female, and self/other. Instead, we are cyborgs. Her prolific writings have influenced much of social science including cultural studies, women's studies, political theory, philosophy, science, and technology studies and anthropology. However, attention to the non-technological nonhuman is also seen in a more recent work, where Haraway[279] turns from technology to look at "companion species", a term which does not refer simply to "pets" but which suggests that humans and other species are networked into economies, societies, biologies, and concepts. She explores our entanglements with "critters"—"a motley crowd of lively beings including microbes, fungi, humans, plants, animals, cyborgs and aliens". While Haraway's concern is more about dogs than other species, and less about plants than other "critters", it leaves the window open for a vine to find a way in. In an interview, Haraway[280] gives her most direct reference to the place of plants in her intellectual history and vision, describing the impact on her thinking of "my sense of the intricacy, interest and pleasure—as well as intensity—of how I have imagined how like a leaf I am. For instance, I am fascinated with the molecular architecture that plants and animals share, as well as with the kinds of instrumentation, interdisciplinarity, and knowledge practices that have gone into the historical possibilities of understanding how I am like a leaf."

Agency, assemblage, and grafting in Western herbal medicine

There are correspondences between, on one hand, Western herbal medicine and, on the other, developments within plant science, vegetal philosophy, critical plant studies, anthropology including multispecies ethnography, and the nonhuman and related academic turns. The pull and push of enchantment; the enabling of multiple differences in herbal practice through herbalists' relationships with plants and herbal medicines; and going beyond the science/tradition dichotomy in practice all sit easily with the enchantment of similarity as revealed by plant science; the enchantment of difference as revealed by vegetal philosophy; the consideration of plant language in critical plant studies; the possibility that we are human bumblebees for plants, including medicinal species; the attention to nonhumans in multispecies ethnography; the search for ways of overcoming dualisms in anthropology; and the decentring of the human in the nonhuman turn.

These correspondences are importance for two reasons. First, as Western herbal medicine is a politically marginal profession, it is arguable that it could benefit from forging links with the ideas, institutions, practices, and persons (human and otherwise) that have been discussed in these last three chapters, rather than deny their relevance and power in the hope that it is possible to somehow catch up with the idea of modernity, when everything will somehow be alright. Second, these correspondences all point to an increased sense of the agency of plants. The herbalists' cases that describe the push and pull of enchantment, as well as the recent turn to the nonhuman, including plants, inevitably raises questions of agency and challenges assumptions of human exceptionalism. Agency, however, is a contested term, with rich intellectual trajectories, including within practice theory, which explores how the world is transformed by social beings (Williams,[281] Gramsci,[282] Giddens,[283] Bourdieu[284]), as well as language studies (Butler,[285] Ahearn,[286]), gender studies (Gardiner,[287] Davies[288]), and actor-network theory (Latour,[289] Law & Hassard,[290] Callon[291]) and made particularly manifest in ethnographies such as Ahearn,[292] Mahmood,[293] and Kohn.[264]

However, it is to Jane Bennett[171] that we return to situate the agency of plants and herbal medicines within Western herbal medicine. Her book, *Vibrant Matter*, is a key text for vital materialists, and was influenced by thinkers including Latour,[289,294] Thoreau,[295] Spinoza,[296] Bergson,[297] and Deleuze and Guattari.[141] Bennett's arguments seek to dissolve many boundaries, including those between life and matter, organic and inorganic material, subject and object, nature and culture, and human and nonhuman, in a strategy to produce openness to the vitality of materials. Bennett uses the concept of "thing-power" for the distributed agency that emerges in groupings of all sizes, to start to think beyond these binaries and to demonstrate remnants of aliveness in materials, both man-made and not. Bennett illuminates the meaning of agency through other terms that gravitate around it, including "efficacy", where something new happens or occurs, but without a singular subject being at the root of an effect; "trajectory", where movement is made away from somewhere; and "causality" where snooker-ball mechanical models of effect are "impossibly rare". For Bennett, agency is a form of creativity, "a capacity to make something new appear or occur". Agency becomes "distributed" among a confederation of various elements, both human and nonhuman. Rather than agency describing the intentionality of a subject whose will causes things to change, there is no subject as the cause of an effect, instead there are a "swarm of vitalities at play". Bennett argues, "There was never a time when human agency was anything other than an interfolding network of humanity and nonhumanity; today this mingling has become harder to ignore." She asks us to recognise "the force of things", both natural and constructed, that enables things "to exceed their status as objects and manifest traces of independence and aliveness". Bennett borrows the term "assemblage" from Deleuze and Guattari,[141] the Dolce and Gabbana of continental thinkers, which also owes much to the relational thinking of Haraway and Latour, with Bennett's assemblage referring to ad hoc groupings of heterogenous human and nonhuman elements, "vibrant materials of all sorts", "conglomerates", "confederations that are able to function". The agency of assemblage is chosen over human will and intentionality in vital materialism's attention to decentre the human. This agency is produced when things in an assemblage form alliances, with agency being the ability to make a difference in the world. While this approach to agency highlights relationships rather than object-bound individualism, this democracy does not mean that the various actors are somehow all equally endowed with agency, rather they have different capacities. Bennett is able to highlight relationships and alliances while recognising what Graham Harman[298] calls the "echoing, resounding, vibrating, unexpressed metaphysical reality of objects" that make up assemblages.

The argument has been made that plants enchant. However, the medicines made from plants have also been seen to be enchanting in herbalists' narratives, for example, in CP's personal experience of using plants for her own fertility and now for her patients, in AF's knowing plants through tasting them as medicines, in MN's Goethean science process that involves "incarnating the idea" into a medicine, and in the aroma of BC's medicine that fills her home as she decocts her herbs. This enchantment is achieved partly through what Bennett refers to as the "remnants of aliveness" that these medicines are, as well as through their specific places in individual narratives. Following Bennett, these medicines "exceed their status as objects and manifest traces of independence and aliveness". They have a certain force to them.

Bennett's use of the term "efficacy" as a way of attending to agency is useful in that it suggests that in Western herbal medicine it is the "swarm of vitalities" found in the combination of the herbalist, the medicine, and the plant that produces something new. We have seen many different "assemblages", or "ad hoc groupings of heterogenous human and nonhuman elements" in the herbalists' visible and hidden entryway cases, whether that be, for example, in FD's accident, a helpful tree, knowledge of herbal medicines that she knows as plants, offerings of love, and her kitchen table; in JK's "proper diagnosis", orthodox clinical examination, use of physiomedicalism, and the love of her wood; in SB's grandmother's garden, search for root causes, going beyond orthodox medicine, and his feelings for plants; or in GA's pleasure of small signs, treating metaphors as if they are real, and everything he does being herbal medicine. In this application of the term "assemblage" the elements from which they are made are found along narratives rather than located at a particular time-point or zone, with these narratives bringing us powerfully to the present and no doubt impacting on possible futures.

Given the agency of plants as described in this book and the increasing attention being paid to the nonhuman in a more-than-human world, the concept of "graft" is borrowed from Marder[299] to make it possible to think specifically about the herbalist-plant-herbal medicine assemblage in Western herbal medicine. Grafting is a technique where tissues of plants are joined in such a way that they continue to grow together. Marder, in his vegetal philosophical engagement with the notion of the graft, points out that, in agronomy, grafts are the twigs or shoots that are pushed into slits made in a tree, changing the tree, which either produces flowers and fruit with features of the graft, or with the features of the graft and host existing alongside one another. Both host and graft are changed in the process of grafting and in the process unusual meetings, mixtures, and surfaces are formed. As Marder says, "Membranes, tissues, liquids, and surfaces must be exposed to one another in all their nudity for a graft to work, to exercise its transformative influence."

This is also true for the herbalists' cases discussed in this book, with enchantment resulting in unusual meetings, where assemblages are formed out of herbalists and their narratives, plants, and herbal medicines, and where the surfaces of the elements of assemblages meet each other and ultimately meet patients. In horticulture, the different plant materials retain agency in the grafting process. In the herbalist-plant-herbal medicine assemblage, or graft, agency is distributed among the different elements: in the herbalists and their narratives that bring in diverse influences, facilitated by meetings with plants and herbal medicines; in the plants, that have enchanted herbalists through similarity and difference, and in the herbal medicines which, as vital materials derived from once-living beings, hold power. Grafting also implies work on the part of each element, in the process of which each is changed. Notably, in the process of grafting in Western herbal medicine, the herbalists, the plants, and the herbal medicines may each be the host and/or the graft, with agency variably and unpredictably distributed between them.

The positioning of plants and herbal medicines in assemblages with their herbalists begs a particular question that is relevant to medicinal plant practice and is where this book has brought us: what is the relationship between living, ecologically situated plants and plants human-made into medicines? To move beyond approaches that consider simply the materiality, constituents, and qualities of dead plant matter we turn to herbalist Christopher Hedley, to whom this book is dedicated, who noted that "How the plant is in the world is how it will be in you." Recent developments in plant sciences and in vegetal philosophy, as briefly introduced in this book, could help to explore the insight that this comment suggests. How does recognition of the enchanting power of plants, partly achieved through their similarity to us, including through their sensing, kin recognition, learning, memory, and intelligence, help us to rethink what it means for plants to be medicinal? And how does recognition of the enchanting power of plants, partly achieved through their very difference from us, including their affinity for change, a sense of place, non-separation, openness, a modular life, distributed thinking, diversity, and flourishing, help us to rethink what it means for plants to be medicinal? Furthermore, looking beyond what goes into the patient, the love that herbalists have for the plants that enchanted them should not be ignored therapeutically. While "biophilia", a term introduced by E. O. Wilson[300] in 1984, can be seen as the urge to know and even love other life forms, "phytophilia", the urge to know and even love plants, born of enchanting relationships with plants as described in this book, and which provides a sustaining energy for herbal practices, can also, given the rise of practices such as forest bathing[301-303] and horticulture therapy,[304,305] be seen as a therapeutic strategy which herbalists are particularly well suited to develop with their patients.

REFERENCES

1. Stewart, C. (2010). Hermeneutical phenomenology: experiences of girls with Asperger's syndrome and anxiety, and Western herbal medicine. PhD thesis. Edinburgh, UK: Edinburgh Napier University.
2. Nissen, N., & Evans, S. (2012). Exploring the practice and use of Western herbal medicine: perspectives from the social science literature. *Journal of Herbal Medicine*, 2: 6–15.
3. Jackson-Main, P. (2005). Western herbal medicine—gender, culture and orthodoxy. In: C. O'Sullivan (Ed.), *Reshaping Herbal Medicine* (pp. 87–98). London: Elsevier.
4. Scheid, V. (2002). *Chinese Medicine in Contemporary China: Plurality and Synthesis*. Durham, NC: Duke University Press.
5. Tobyn, G., Denham, A., & Whitelegg, M. (2010). *The Western Herbal Tradition: 2000 Years of Medicinal Plant Knowledge*. London: Churchill Livingstone.
6. Barker, J. (2007). *History, Philosophy and Medicine: Phytotherapy in Context*. West Wickham, UK: Winter Press.
7. Stobart, A., & Francia, S. (2014). The fragmentation of herbal history. In: A. Stobart & S. Francia (Eds.), *Critical Approaches to the History of Western Herbal Medicine. From Classical Antiquity to the Early Modern Period* (pp. 1–22). London: Bloomsbury.
8. Griggs, B. (1982). *Green Pharmacy*. London: Viking.

9. Griggs, B. (1997). *New Green Pharmacy*. London: Vermilion.

10. MacLennan, E., & Pendry, B. (2011). The evolution of herbal medicine as an unorthodox branch of British medicine: the role of English legislation from antiquity to 1914. *Journal of Herbal Medicine, 1*: 2–14.

11. Pitman, V. (2005). The relationship of classical Greek medicine to contemporary Western herbalism: an exploration of the idea of "holism". In: C. O'Sullivan (Ed.), *Reshaping Herbal Medicine. Knowledge, Education and Professional Culture* (pp. 99–114). London: Elsevier.

12. Pitman, V. (2013). Early Greek medicine: evidence of models, methods and *materia medica*. In: A. Stobart & S. Francia (Eds.), *Critical Approaches to the History of Western Herbal Medicine. From Classical Antiquity to the Early Modern Period*. London: Bloomsbury.

13. Grieve, M. (1996 [1931]). *A Modern Herbal*. Canterbury, UK: Tiger Books.

14. Williamson, E. (2014). Foreword. In: S. Francia & A. Stobart (Eds.), *Critical Approaches to the History of Western Herbal Medicine: from Classical Antiquity to the Early Modern Period*. London: Bloomsbury.

15. Withering, W. (2014 [1785]). *An Account of the Foxglove, and Some of Its Medical Uses: Practical Remarks on Drops and Other Diseases*. Cambridge: Cambridge University Press.

16. Guthrie, D. (1961). Plants as remedies: the debt of medicine to botany. *Transactions and Proceedings—Botanical Society of Edinburgh, 39*(2): 184–195.

17. Brown, P. S. (1985). The vicissitudes of herbalism in the late nineteenth- and early twentieth-century Britain. *Medical History*, January, *29*(1): 71–92.

18. Webb, W. H. (1916). *The Standard Guide to Non-Poisonous Herbal Medicine*. Southport, UK: W. H. Webb.

19. Winston, D., & Dattner, A. (1999). The American system of medicine. *Clinics in Dermatology, 17*(1): 53–56.

20. Caldecott, T. (2008). *The History of Physiomedicalism*. [http://www.toddcaldecott.com]

21. Cook, W. (1998 [1869]). *The Physio-Medical Dispensatory*. Sandy, OR: Eclectic Medical Publications.

22. Thurston, J. M. (1900). *The Philosophy of Physiomedicalism: Its Theorem, Corollary and Laws of Application for the Cure of Disease*. Richmond, IN: Nicholson Printing.

23. Wood, M. (2002). The six tissue states: the energetics of Physiomedicalism. *Journal of the American Herbalists' Guild, 3*(1): 28–33.

24. Menzies-Trull, C. (2003). *Herbal Medicine—Keys to Physiomedicalism including Pharmacopoeia*. Newcastle, Staffs, UK: Faculty of Physiomedical Herbal Medicine.

25. Priest, A., & Priest, L. (1983). *Herbal Medication: a Clinical and Dispensary Handbook*. Saffron Walden, UK: C. W. Daniel.
26. Shelley, D. (2014). NIMH—celebrating 150 Years. Avena. Spring 2014. *Journal of the New Zealand Association of Medical Herbalists*. [http://www.nzamh.org.nz]
27. Denham, A. (2014). Herbal practice: just how complex an intervention? In: H. Brice-Ytsma & F. Watkins (Eds.), *Herbal Exchanges: in Celebration of the National Institute of Medical Herbalists 1864–2014* (pp. 57–66). London: Strathmore Publishing.
28. Moffatt, D. (1986). *A Review of the Extent and Influence of Thomson's American Medico Botanic System in Industrial England, 1880–1930*. Unpublished MA thesis. Centre for the Study of Social History. Coventry, UK: University of Warwick.
29. Brown, P. S. (1982). Herbalists and medical botanists in mid-nineteenth-century Britain with special reference to Bristol. *Medical History, 26*: 405–420.
30. Shelley, D. (2014). A brief history of the National Institute of Medical Herbalists. In: H. Brice-Ytsma & F. Watkins (Eds.), *Herbal Exchanges* (pp. 3–10). Exeter, UK: NIMH.
31. McIntyre, M. (2005). Herbs and herbalists: professional identity and the protection of practice. In: C. O'Sullivan (Ed.), *Reshaping Herbal Medicine: Knowledge, Education and Professional Culture* (pp. 115–130). London: Elsevier.
32. Footler, P. (2009). *Henry VIII and the Art of Herbal Healing. The Pharmaceutical Journal*. [http://www.pharmaceutical-journal.com]
33. Saks, M. (2002). Professionalization, regulation and alternative medicine. In: J. Allsop & M. Saks (Eds.), *Regulating the Health Professions* (pp. 148–161). London: Sage.
34. Robbins, C. (1994). Fred Fletcher Hyde. *European Journal of Herbal Medicine, 1*(1): 29–33.
35. McIntyre, M. (2011). Statutory regulation—a legislative basis for herbal practice. *Journal of Herbal Medicine, 1*: 30–32.
36. Saks, M. (2002). *Orthodox and Alternative Medicine. Politics, Professionalization and Health Care*. London: Sage.
37. Illich, I. (1974). *Medical Nemesis: the Expropriation of Health*. London: Marion Boyars Publishing.
38. Cant, S., & Sharma, U. (1999). *A New Medical Pluralism? Alternative Medicine, Doctors, Patients and the State*. London: UCL Press.
39. Wahlberg, A. (2010). Rescuing folk remedies: ethnoknowledge and the reinvention of indigenous herbal medicine in Britain. In: R. Moore & S. McClean (Eds.), *Folk Healing and Health Care Practices in Britain and Ireland* (pp. 130–155). Oxford: Berghahn.

40. McIntyre, M. (2013). Herbal regulation in the United Kingdom—the stop start process. *Herbal EGram, 10*(12), December.

41. Walker, D. (2015). Report on the regulation of herbal medicines and herbal practitioners. 26 March. UK Government. [https://www.gov.uk/government/publications/advice-on-regulating-herbal-medicines-and-practitioners]

42. Wahlberg, A. (2007). A quackery with a difference—new medical pluralism and the problems of "dangerous practitioners" in the United Kingdom. *Social Science and Medicine, 65*: 2307–2316.

43. National Institute of Medical Herbalists (2015). *National Institute of Medical Herbalists Code of Ethics and Practice.* The National Institute of Medical Herbalists. [http://www.nimh.org.uk]

44. National Institute of Medical Herbalists (2015). *National Institute of Medical Herbalists Continuing Professional Development: Guidelines for Medical Herbalists.* The National Institute of Medical Herbalists. [http://www.nimh.org.uk]

45. Health and Care Professions Council (2015). *Standards for Prescribing.* Available from: Health and Care Professions Council. [http://www.hcpc-uk.org]

46. Professional Standards Authority (2015). *Standards for Accredited Registers* [online]. Available from: *The Professional Standards Authority.* [http://www.professionalstandards.org.uk]

47. Latour, B. (1993). *We Have Never Been Modern.* Cambridge, MA: Harvard University Press.

48. Shapin, S., & Shaffer, S. (1985). *Leviathan and the Air-pump.* Princeton, NJ: Princeton University Press.

49. Pickering, A. (1994). Book review—*We Have Never Been Modern. Modernism/Modernity, 1*(3): 257–258.

50. Bennett, J. (2001). *The Enchantment of Modern Life: Attachments, Crossings and Ethics.* Princeton, NJ: Princeton University Press.

51. Wahlberg, A. (2008). Pathways to plausibility: when herbs become pills. *Biosocieties, 3*(1): 37–56.

52. Colquhoun, D. (2011a). Herbal medicines fail test [online]. Available from: [http://www.dcscience.net/2007/10/04/herbal-medicines-fail-test/]

53. Colquhoun, D. (2011b). Why does the MHRA refuse to label herbal products honestly? Kent Woods and Richard Woodfield tell me. 1 April. Available from: DC's improbable science. [http://www.dcscience.net]

54. Weiss, R. (1988). *Herbal Medicine.* Gothenburg, Sweden: Arcanum.

55. *The British Journal of Phytotherapy, 1*(1). Bucksteep Manor, UK: The School of Phytotherapy.

56. Editorial. (1994). *European Journal of Herbal Medicine, 1*(1). Exeter, UK: National Institute of Medical Herbalists.

57. St. George, D. (1994). Biomedical research or new paradigm? *European Journal of Herbal Medicine*, 1(1): 38–39.

58. Pendry, B. (2011). Editorial. *Journal of Herbal Medicine*, 1(1): 1.

59. Evans, S. (2008). *Changing the Knowledge Base in Western Herbal Medicine*. Social Science and Medicine, 68: 2098–2106.

60. Treasure, J. (2014). Back to the future—Herbalism 3.0 Part 1: Foundations. *Journal of the American Herbalists Guild*, 12(1): 18–26.

61. British Herbal Medicine Association (1983). *British Herbal Pharmacopoeia 1983*. Bournemouth, UK: British Herbal Medicine Association.

62. Tassell, M. (2007). Posology in herbal medicine: do we have a sound basis? Unpublished MSc thesis. Isle of Arran, UK: Scottish School of Herbal Medicine.

63. British Herbal Medicine Association. (1996). *British Herbal Pharmacopoeia 1996*. Bournemouth, UK: British Herbal Medicine Association.

64. British Herbal Medicine Association (1992). *British Herbal Compendium. Volume 1. A Handbook of Scientific Information on Widely Used Plant Drugs*. Bournemouth, UK: British Herbal Medicine Association.

65. Swale, M. (1994). British Herbal Compendium—review. *European Journal of Herbal Medicine*, 1(1): 49–50.

66. Graham-Little, E. (1935). Medical herbalists. *British Medical Journal*, 13 July: 86–87.

67. Burns Lingard, W. (1958). *Herbal Prescriptions from a Consultants' Case Book*. Exeter, UK: National Institute of Medical Herbalists.

68. Priest, A. (1959). *Studies in Physiomedicalism. Paper 2. Principles of Diagnosis*. Exeter, UK: National Institute of Medical Herbalists.

69. Priest, A. (1961). *Studies in Physiomedicalism. Paper 3. Principles of Medication*. Exeter, UK: National Institute of Medical Herbalists.

70. Priest, A. (1962). *Studies in Physiomedicalism. Paper 4. Materia Medica*. Exeter, UK: National Institute of Medical Herbalists.

71. Colquhoun, D. (no date). *DC's Improbable Science: Truth, Falsehood and Evidence: Investigations of Dubious and Dishonest Science*. [http://www.dcscience.net]

72. Sense About Science (2015). Proposed registration of herbal medicine practitioners. [http://www.senseaboutscience.org]

73. Nightingale Collaboration. (2015). Herbalism on the NHS: complaint upheld. [http://www.nightingale-collaboration.org]

74. Goldacre, B. (2015). UCL, Colquhoun, and Dr Ann Walker—a victory for common sense. [http://www.badscience.net]

75. European and Traditional Herbal Medicine Practitioners Association (2014). *Core Curriculum for Herbal and Traditional Medicine*. [http://www.ehtpa.eu]

76. European and Traditional Herbal Medicine Practitioners Association (2007). *Core Curriculum for Herbal and Traditional Medicine.* [http://www.ehtpa.eu]

77. Mills, S., & Bone, K. (2000). *Principles and Practice of Phytotherapy: Modern Herbal Medicine.* London: Churchill Livingstone.

78. Bone, K., & Mills, S. (2013). *Principles and Practice of Phytotherapy: Modern Herbal Medicine. Second Edition.* London: Churchill Livingstone.

79. Conway, P. (2010). *The Consultation in Phytotherapy.* London: Churchill Livingstone.

80. Hoffmann, D. (1983). *The Holistic Herbal.* Shaftesbury, UK: Element.

81. Hoffmann, D. (2003). *Medical Herbalism.* Rochester, UK: Healing Arts Press.

82. Holmes, P. (2007). *The Energetics of Western Herbs. 4th edition.* Cotati, CA: Snow Lotus Press.

83. Barnes, J., Anderson, L., & Phillipson, J. (2007). *Herbal Medicines, 3rd edition.* London: Pharmaceutical Press.

84. Braun, L., & Cohen, M. (2010). *Herbs and Natural Supplements: an Evidence-based Guide.* London: Churchill Livingstone.

85. Owen, N. (2013). *Principles and Practice of Phytotherapy—Modern Herbal Medicine. Bone, K. & Mills, S. 2nd edition.* Book review. *Journal of Herbal Medicine,* 3(3): 120–122.

86. Barker, J. (2001). *Principles and Practice of Phytotherapy: Modern Herbal Medicine.* Book review. *British Journal of Phytotherapy,* 5(3): 155–157.

87. Bone, K. (2013). An evening with Mills and Bone. Recording of talk given by Simon Mills and Kerry Bone. Tuesday 16 April. The Pullman, Brisbane, Queensland, Australia. Available from: Integria Healthcare. [http://www.integria.com]

88. Snow, J. (2016). Context effects in Western herbal medicine: fundamental to effectiveness? *Explore,* 12(1): 55–62.

89. Niemeyer, K., Bell, I., & Koithan, M. (2013). Traditional knowledge of Western herbal medicine and complex systems science. *Journal of Herbal Medicine,* 3: 112–119.

90. Niemeyer, K. (2013). Personalizing Western herbal medicine: weaving a tapestry of right relationships, a grounded theory study. Unpublished PhD thesis. Tucson, AZ: University of Arizona.

91. Fisher, C., Adams, J., Frawley, J., Hickman, L., & Sibbritt, D. (2018). Western herbal medicine consultations for common menstrual problems; practitioner experiences and perceptions of treatment. *Phytotherapy Research,* March, 32(3): 531–541.

92. Hiller, S. (2013). Vitalist strategies in contemporary Western herbal medicine. *Focus on Alternative and Complementary Therapies,* 18(4): 190–194.

93. Bitcon, C., Evans, S., & Avila, C. (2016). The re-emergence of grass-roots herbalism: an analysis through the blogosphere. *Health Sociology Review*, 25(1): 108–121.

94. West, V., & Denham, A. (2017). The clinical reasoning of Western herbal practitioners: a qualitative feasibility study. *Journal of Herbal Medicine*, 8: 52–61.

95. Braun, L. A., Spitzer, O., Tiralongo, E., Wilkinson, J. M., Bailey, M., Poole, S. G., & Dooley, M. (2013). Naturopaths and Western herbalists' attitudes to evidence, regulation, information sources and knowledge about popular complementary medicines. *Complementary Therapies in Medicine*, 21: 58–64.

96. Nissen, N. (2015). Naturalness as an ethical stance: idea(l)s and practices of care in western herbal medicine in the UK. *Anthropology and Medicine*, 22(2): 162–176.

97. Yates, A. J. (2016). "Considering there's supposedly nothing wrong with me, it's not a life": women's narratives of distress, visiting herbalists, and being well in the 21st century. Unpublished PhD thesis. London: University of Westminster.

98. Waddell, G. (2015). The Enchantment of Western Herbal Medicine. Unpublished PhD thesis. London: University of Westminster.

99. Nissen, N. (2010). Practitioners of Western herbal medicine and their practice in the UK: beginning to sketch the profession. *Complementary Therapies in Clinical Practice*, 16: 181–186.

100. National Institute of Medical Herbalists (2015). Snapshot survey of herbal practice, March 2012. Personal communication.

101. Whitehouse, J. (2014). Research informing herbal medicine practice. In: H. Brice-Ytsma & F. Watkins (Eds.), *Herbal Exchanges: in Celebration of the National Institute of Medical Herbalists 1864–2014* (pp. 77–86). London: Strathmore Publishing.

102. Nissen, N. (2008). Herbal healthcare and processes of change: an ethnographic study of women's contemporary practice and use of Western herbal medicine in the UK. Unpublished PhD thesis. Milton Keynes, UK: The Open University.

103. Nissen, N. (2011). Perspectives on holism in the contemporary practice of Western herbal medicine in the UK. *Journal of Herbal Medicine*, 1: 76–83.

104. Casey, M. (2009). The practice of Western herbal medicine in Australia. PhD thesis. Newcastle, UK: University of Newcastle. [http://www.ogma.newcastle.edu.au]

105. VanMarie, E. (2002). Re-presenting herbal medicine as phytotherapy: a strategy of professionalisation through the formation of a "scientific"

medicine. Unpublished PhD thesis. Yorkshire, UK: White Rose University Consortium.

106. Little, C. (2011). Patient expectations of "effectiveness" in health care: an example from medical herbalism. *Journal of Clinical Nursing*, 21: 718–727.

107. Snow, J. (n.d.). A physiology relevant to herbal medicine. Asheville, NC: American Herbalists Guild. [http://www.americanherbalistsguild.com]

108. Nissen, N. (2013). Women's bodies and women's lives in Western herbal medicine in the UK. *Medical Anthropology*, 32: 75–91.

109. Nissen, N. (2010b). The storied patient-practitioner relationship in the practice of Western herbal medicine in the UK. *European Journal of Integrative Medicine*, 2: 200.

110. Scheid, V. (2016). Holism, Chinese medicine and systems ideologies: rewriting the past to imagine the future. In: E. Whitehead & A. Woods (Eds.), *The Edinburgh Companion to the Critical Medical Humanities* (chapter 3). Edinburgh, UK: Edinburgh University Press.

111. Jagtenberg, T., & Evans, S. (2003). Global herbal medicine: a critique. *Journal of Alternative and Complementary Medicine*, 9(2): 321–329.

112. Evans, S. (2009). Challenge, tension and possibility: an exploration into contemporary Western herbal medicine in Australia. Unpublished PhD thesis. Berkeley, CA: Bepress. [http://works.bepress.com/sue_evans/15/]

113. Singer, J., & Fisher, K. (2007). The impact of co-option on herbalism: a bifurcation in epistemology and practice. *Health Sociology Review*, 16(1): 18–26.

114. Fuller, S. (2000). *Thomas Kuhn: A Philosophical History of Our Times*. Chicago, IL: University of Chicago Press.

115. Fuller, S. (2006). *The Philosophy of Science and Technology Studies*. London: Routledge.

116. Mediherb. (2015). *Standard Process*. Palmyra, WI: Standard Process. [http://www.standardprocess.com]

117. Scheid, V. (2006). Chinese medicine and the problem of tradition. *Asian Medicine*, 2(1): 59–71.

118. Law, J. (2004). *After Method—Mess in Social Science Research*. London: Routledge.

119. Law, J., & Mol, A. (2002). *Complexities—Social Studies of Knowledge Practices*. Durham, NC: Duke University Press.

120. Foucault, M. (2001). *The Order of Things: an Archaeology of the Human Sciences*. London: Routledge.

121. Crellin, J., & Philpott, J. (1997). *Trying to Give Ease: Tommie Bass and the Story of Herbal Medicine*. Durham, NC: Duke University Press.

122. Naraindas, H. (2011). Of relics, body parts and laser beams: the German Heilpraktiker and his Ayurvedic spa. *Anthropology & Medicine, 18*(1): 67–86.
123. Langwick, S. (2011). *Bodies, Politics and African Healing: the Matter of Maladies in Tanzania.* Bloomington, IN: Indiana University Press.
124. Carsten, J. (2012). Fieldwork since the 1980s: total immersion and its discontents. In: R. Fardon, O. Harris, T. H. J. Marchand, M. Nuttall, C. Shore, V. Strang, & R. A. Wilson (Eds.), *The SAGE Handbook of Social Anthropology, vol. 2* (pp. 7–20). London: Sage Publications.
125. Rabinow, P., & Marcus, G. E. (2008). *Designs for an Anthropology of the Contemporary.* Durham, NC: Duke University Press.
126. Ingold, T. (2008). Anthropology is *not* ethnography. *British Academy Review, 11*: 21–23.
127. Myers, R. (2011). The familiar strange and the strange familiar in anthropology and beyond. *General Anthropology, 18*(2): 1–9.
128. Inhorn, M., & Wentzell, E. (2012). *Medical Anthropology at the Intersections: Histories, Activisms and Futures.* Durham, NC: Duke University Press.
129. Adams, V., Schrempf, M., & Craig, S. R. (Eds.) (2010). *Medicine between Science and Religion.* Oxford: Berghahn.
130. Heywood, P. (2017). The ontological turn. In: F. Stein, S. Lazar, M. Candea, H. Diemberger, J. Robbins, A. Sanchez, & R. Stasch (Eds.), *The Cambridge Encyclopedia of Anthropology.* Cambridge: University of Cambridge. [https://www.anthroencyclopedia.com]
131. Bloor, D. (1976). *Knowledge and Social Imagery.* Chicago, IL: University of Chicago Press.
132. Denzin, N. (2001). The reflexive interview and performative social science. *Qualitative Research, 1*(1): 23–46.
133. Shukla, N., Wilson, E., & Boddy, J. (2014). Combining thematic and narrative analysis of qualitative interviews to understand children's spatialities in Andhra Pradesh, India. Southampton, UK: National Centre for Research Methods. [http://www.eprints.ncrm.ac.uk]
134. Riessman, C. (2008). *Narrative Methods for the Human Sciences.* London: Sage.
135. Riessman, C. (1990). *Divorce Talk.* New Brunswick, NJ: Rutgers University Press.
136. West, L., Bron, A., & Merrill, B. (2014). Researching student experience. In: F. Finnegan, B. Merrill, & C. Thunborg (Eds.), *Student Voices on Inequalities in European Higher Education.* London: Routledge.
137. Merrill, B., & West, L. (2009). *Using Biographical Methods in Social Research.* London: Sage.

138. Langellier, K. (2001). Personal narrative. In: M. Jolly (Ed.), *Encyclopedia of Life Writing: Autobiographical and Biographical Forms, vol. 2.* (pp. 699–701). London: Fitzroy Dearborn.

139. Bron, A., & West, L. (2000). Time for stories: the emergence of life history methods in the social sciences. *International Journal of Contemporary Sociology, 37*(2): 158–175.

140. Loots, G., Coppens, K., & Sermijn, J. (2013) Practising a rhizomatic perspective in narrative research. In: M. Andrews, C. Squire, & M. Tamboukou (Eds.), *Doing Narrative Research* (pp. 108–125). London: Sage.

141. Deleuze, G., & Guattari, F. (2014 [1987]). *A Thousand Plateaus: Capitalism and Schizophrenia.* London: Continuum Publishing.

142. Sermijn, J., Devlieger, P., & Loots, G. (2008). The narrative construction of the self. Selfhood as a rhizomatic story. *Qualitative Inquiry, 14*(4): 632–650. [http://www.sagepub.com]

143. Bold, C. (2012). *Using Narrative in Research.* London: Sage.

144. Wengraf, T. (2001). *Qualitative Research Interviewing: Biographic Narrative and Semi-structured Methods.* London: Sage.

145. Wengraf, T. (2012). Interviewing for life-histories, lived periods and situations, and ongoing personal experience using the biographic-narrative interpretative method (BNIM). Unpublished personal communication.

146. Jones, K. (2003). The turn to a narrative knowing of persons: one method explored. *Nursing Times Research,* Jan, 8: 60–71.

147. Braun, V., & Clarke, V. (2006). Using thematic analysis in psychology. *Qualitative Research in Psychology, 3*(2): 77–101.

148. Braun, V., & Clarke, V. (2013). *Successful Qualitative Research: A Practical Guide for Beginners.* London: Sage.

149. Barnes, L. (2009). Practitioner decisions to engage in Chinese medicine: cultural messages under the skin. *Medical Anthropology: Cross-cultural Studies in Health and Illness, 28*(2): 141–165.

150. DuBois, T. (2009). *An Introduction to Shamanism.* Cambridge: Cambridge University Press.

151. Saler, M. (2006). Modernity and enchantment: a historiographic review. *American Historical Review,* June, 111(3): 692–716.

152. Hobbes, T. (2014 [1651]). Of the natural condition of mankind as concerning their felicity and misery. In: T. Hobbes, *Leviathan.* London: Bibliophile.

153. Rousseau, J.-J. (1998 [1762]). *The Social Contract.* London: Bibliophile.

154. Marx, K. (2013 [1864 volume 1/1884 volume 2]). *Capital: vols. 1 and 2.* Ware, UK: Wordsworth.

155. Durkheim, E. (2006 [1897]). *On Suicide.* London: Penguin Classics.

156. Whitebook, J. (2002). Slow magic: Psychoanalysis and "the disenchantment of the world." *J Am Psychanal Assoc., 50*(4): 1197–1217.

157. Weber, M. (2004 [1919]). Science as vocation. In: D. Owen & T. Strong (Eds.), *Max Weber. The Vocation Lectures.* Cambridge: Hackett Publishing.

158. Cascardi, A. (1992). *The Subject of Modernity.* Cambridge: Cambridge University Press.

159. Angus, I. (1983). Disenchantment and modernity: the mirror of technique. *Human Studies, 6*: 141–166.

160. Sherry, P. (2009). Disenchantment, re-enchantment and enchantment. *Modern Theology, 25*(3): 369–386.

161. Gane, N. (2005). *Weber and Postmodernism.* London: Palgrave.

162. Ritzer, G. (1975). Professionalization, bureaucratization and rationalization: the views of Max Weber. *Social Forces, 53*(4): 627–634.

163. Braun, S. B. (2011). *Neo Shamanism as a Healing System: Enchanted Healing in a Modern World.* Ann Arbor, MI: ProQuest.

164. Abram, D. (1997). *The Spell of the Sensuous.* London: Vintage.

165. London, J. (2015). The ecology of magic: an interview with David Abram. [http://www.scottlondon.com]

166. Serres, M. (1985). *The Five Senses: A Philosophy of Mingled Bodies.* London: Continuum.

167. Chimisso, C. (2010). *The Five Senses: A Philosophy of Mingled Bodies.* Book review. *International Studies in the Philosophy of Science,* 24(2): 226–228.

168. Connor, S. (1999). *Michel Serres' Five Senses.* [http://www.stevenconnor.com]

169. Josephson-Storm, J. (2017). *The Myth of Disenchantment: Magic, Modernity and the Birth of the Human Sciences.* Chicago, IL: University of Chicago Press.

170. Szerszynski, B. (2004). *Nature, Technology and the Sacred.* London: Wiley-Blackwell.

171. Bennett, J. (2010). *Vibrant Matter: A Political Ecology of Things.* Durham, NC: Duke University Press.

172. Berman, M. (1981). *The Reenchantment of the World.* Ithaca, NY: Cornell University Press.

173. Khan, G. (2012). Vital materiality and non-human agency: an interview with Jane Bennett. In: *Dialogues with Contemporary Political Theorists* (pp. 43–57). London: Palgrave Macmillan.

174. Seigworth, G., & Gregg, M. (2010). An Inventory of Shimmers. In: M. Gregg & G. Seigworth (Eds.), *The Affect Theory Reader* (pp. 1–25). Durham, NC: Duke University Press.

175. Grossberg, L. (2010). Affect's future: rediscovering the virtual in the actual. In: M. Gregg & G. Seigworth (Eds.), *The Affect Theory Reader* (pp. 309–338). Durham, NC: Duke University Press.

176. Shouse, E. (2005). Feeling, affect, emotion. *M/C Journal*, 8(6).
177. Wetherell, M. (2012). *Affect and Emotion: a New Social Science Understanding*. London: Sage.
178. Milton, K. (2002). *Loving Nature*. London: Routledge.
179. Haraway, D. (1991). A manifesto for cyborgs: science, technology, and socialist-feminism in the late twentieth century. In: *Simians, Cyborgs, and Women: the Reinvention of Nature* (pp. 149–182). London: Routledge.
180. Fisher, P. (1998). *Wonder, the Rainbow and the Aesthetics of Rare Experiences*. Cambridge, MA: Harvard University Press.
181. Dawkins, R. (1988). *Unweaving the Rainbow: Science, Delusion and the Appetite for Wonder*. London: Penguin.
182. Watson, P. (2014). *The Age of Nothing*. London: Weidenfeld & Nicolson.
183. Pels, P. (2003). Introduction: magic and modernity. In: B. Meyer & P. Pels (Eds.), *Magic and Modernity: Interfaces of RevelationConcealment* (pp. 1–38). Redwood City, CA: Stanford University Press.
184. Densmore, F. (1974). *How Indians Use Wild Plants for Food, Medicine and Crafts*. New York: Dover.
185. Will, C. (2007). The alchemy of clinical trials. *BioSocieties*, 2(1): 85–99.
186. Brives, C. (2016). What's in the context? Tenses and Tensions in evidence-based medicine. *Medical Anthropology*, 35(5): 369–376.
187. Greyson, L. (forthcoming). *Vital Reenchantments: Biophilia, Gaia, Cosmos, and the Affectively Ecological*. Goleta, CA: Punctum.
188. Daston, L., & Galison, P. (2010). *Objectivity*. London: Zone.
189. McLuhan, T. (1992). *Touch the Earth: A Self Portrait of Indian Existence*. Victoria, BC, Canada: Promontory.
190. Illich, I. (1973). *Tools for Conviviality*. London. Marion Boyars Publishing.
191. Illich, I. (1995 [1971]). *Deschooling Society*. London: Marion Boyars Publishing.
192. Duraffourd, C. (1983–1996). *Cahiers de Phytothérapie Clinique*. Vols. 1–5. Paris: Elsevier Masson.
193. Duraffourd, C., & Lapraz, J.-C. (2002). *Traité de Phytothérapie Clinique*. Paris: Elsevier Masson.
194. Lapraz, J.-C., & Hedayat, K. (2013). Endobiogeny: a global approach to systems biology (Part 1 of 2). *Global Advances in Health and Medicine*, 2(1): 64–78.
195. Lapraz, J.-C. & Hedayat, K. (2013). Endobiogeny: a global approach to systems biology (Part 2 of 2). *Global Advances in Health and Medicine*, 2(2): 32–56.
196. Nicholls, C. (2013). Endobiogenics and the terrain in modern phytotherapy. Presentation. NIMH Conference, Crewe, 2 November.
197. Narby, J., & Huxley, F. (2001). *Shamans through Time: 500 Years on the Path to Knowledge*. London: Thames & Hudson.

198. Backman, L., & Hultkrantz, A. (1978). *Studies in Lapp Shamanism*. Stockholm: Almqvist & Wiksell International.

199. Thomson, S. (1849). *New Guide to Health, or Botanic Family Physician: containing a complete system of practice, upon a plan entirely new: with a description of the vegetables made use of, and directions for preparing and administering them to cure disease. (To which is added): Narrative of the life of Samuel Thomson*. Cornhill: E. G. House.

200. Hall, M. (2011). *Plants as Persons*. Albany, NY: State University of New York.

201. Marder, M. (2013). *Plant-Thinking: a Philosophy of Vegetal Life*. New York: Columbia University Press.

202. Gagliano, M., Ryan, J., & Vieira, P. (2017a). *The Language of Plants: Science, Philosophy, Literature*. Minneapolis, MN: University of Minnesota Press.

203. Karban, R. (2015). *Plant Sensing and Communication*. Chicago, IL: University of Chicago Press.

204. Darwin, C. (1880). *The Power of Movement in Plants*. London: John Murray.

205. Bastin, L. (1908). The intelligence of the plant. *Pall Mall Magazine*, 42(187): 550–558.

206. Trewavas, A. (2015). *Plant Intelligence and Behaviour*. Oxford: Oxford University Press.

207. Myers, N. (2015). Conversations on plant sensing—notes from the field. *NatureCulture*, 3: 35–66.

208. Keller, E. (1983). *A Feeling for the Organism: the Life and Work of Barbara McClintock*. New York: W. H. Freeman.

209. Gagliano, M., & Grimonprez, M. (2015). Breaking the silence—language and the making of meaning in plants. *Ecopsychology*, 7(3): 145–151.

210. Brenner, E. D., Stahlberg, R., Mancuso, S., Vivanco, J., & Van Volkenburgh, E. (2006). Plant neurobiology: an integrated view of plant signaling. *Trends in Plant Science*, 11(8): 413–419.

211. Chamovitz, D. (2013). *What a Plant Knows*. Oxford: One World.

212. Dudley, S., & File, A. (2007). Kin recognition in an annual plant. *Biology Letters*, 3: 435–438.

213. Garzon, P., & Deijzer, F. (2011). Plants: adaptive behavior, root-brains, and minimal cognition. *Adaptive Behavior*, 19(3): 155–171.

214. Mancuso, S., & Viola, A. (2015). *Brilliant Green, the Surprising History and Science of Plant Intelligence*. Washington, DC: Island Press.

215. Pollan, M. (2013). The intelligent plant: scientists debate a new way of understanding flora. *The New Yorker*, 23 & 30 December. [http://www.newyorker.com]

216. Simard, S. W. (2009). The foundational role of mycorrhizal networks in self organization of interior Douglas-fir forests. *Forest Ecology and Management*, 258S: 95–107.

217. Simard, S. W. (2012). Mycorrhizal networks and seedling establishment in Douglas-fir forests. In: D. Southworth (Ed.), *Biocomplexity of Plant–Fungal Interactions, First Edition* (pp. 85–107). London: John Wiley & Sons.

218. Simard, S. W., Beiler, K. J., Bingham, M. A., Deslippe, J. R., Philip, L. J., & Teste, F. (2012). Mycorrhizal networks: mechanisms, ecology and modelling. Invited review. *Fungal Biology Reviews, 26*: 39–60.

219. Trewavas, A. (2005). Plant intelligence. *Naturwissenschaften, 92*, 401–413.

220. Gagliano, M. (2012). Green symphonies: a call for studies on acoustic communication in plants. *Behavioral Ecology, 24*: 789–796.

221. Gagliano, M., Grimonprez, M., Depczynski, M., & Renton, M. (2017). Tuned in: plant roots use sound to locate water. *Oecologia. 184*(1): 151–160.

222. Karban, R. (2017). The language of plant communication (and how it compares to animal communication). In: Gagliano, M., Ryan, J., & Vieira, P. *The Language of Plants: Science, Philosophy, Literature* (pp. 3–26). Minneapolis, MN: University of Minnesota Press.

223. Gagliano, M., Renton, M., Depczynski, M., & Mancuso, S. (2014). Experience teaches plants to learn faster and forget slower in environments where it matters. *Oecologia, 175*(1): 63–72.

224. Gagliano, M., Renton, M., Depczynski, M., & Mancuso, S. (2016). Learning by association in plants. *Scientific Reports, 6*: 38427.

225. Cook, G. (2012). Do plants think? *Scientific American*, 5 June. [http://www.scientificamerican.com]

226. Marder, M. (2013). Of plants, and other secrets. *Societies, 3*: 16–23.

227. Marder, M. (2012). Plant intentionality and the phenomenological framework of plant intelligence. *Plant Signaling and Behavior, 7*(11): 1–8.

228. Marder, M. (2015). The place of plants: speciality, movement, growth. *Performance Philosophy, 1*: 185–194.

229. Marder, M. (2012). Resist like a plant! On the vegetal life of political movements. *Peace Studies Journal, 5*(1): 24–32.

230. Pouteau, S. (2018). Plants as open beings: from aesthetics to plant–human ethics. In: A. Kalhoff, M. Di Paola, & M. Schorgenhumer (Eds.), *Plant Ethics: Concepts and Applications* (pp. 82–97). Oxford: Routledge.

231. Marder, M. (2012). The life of plants and the limits of empathy. *Dialogue, 51*(2): 259–273.

232. Marder, M. (2015). The sense of seeds, or seminal events. *Environmental Philosophy*. doi: 10.5840/envirophil201542920.

233. Marder, M. (2011). Vegetal anti-metaphysics: learning from plants. *Continental Philosophy Review, 44*: 469–489.

234. Houle, K. (2018). Facing only outwards? Plant bodily morphogenesis and ethical conceptual genesis. In: A. Kalhoff, M. Di Paola, & M. Schorgenhumer (Eds.), *Plant Ethics: Concepts and Applications* (pp. 70–81). Oxford: Routledge.

235. Marder, M. (2014). For a phytocentrism to come. *Environmental Philosophy*. doi: 10.5840/envirophil20145110.

236. Marder, M. (2013). What is plant-thinking? *Klesis—revue philosophique*, 25: 124–143.

237. Kalhoff, A. (2018). The flourishing of plants: a neo-Aristotelian approach to plant ethics. In: A. Kalhoff, M. Di Paola, & M. Schorgenhumer (Eds.), *Plant Ethics: Concepts and Applications* (pp. 51–58). Oxford: Routledge.

238. Ryan, J. (2017). *Plants in Contemporary Poetry: Ecocriticism and the Botanical Imagination*. New York: Routledge.

239. Ryan, J. (2017). In the key of green? The silent voices of plants in poetry. In: M. Gagliano, J. Ryan, & P. Vieira (Eds.), *The Language of Plants: Science, Philosophy, Literature* (pp. 273–296). Minnepolis, MN: University of Minnesota Press.

240. Ryan, J., & Giblett, R. (2018). *Forest Family: Australian Culture, Art and Trees*. Leiden, the Netherlands: Brill.

241. Vieira, P., Gagliano, M., & Ryan, J. (2015). *The Green Thread: Dialogues with the Vegetal World*. Lanham, MD: Lexington.

242. Vieira, P. (2016). Phytofables: tales of the Amazon. *Journal of Lusophone Studies*, 1(2): 116–134.

243. Vieira, P. (2017) Phytographia: literature as plant writing. In: M. Gagliano, J. Ryan, & P. Vieira (Eds.), *The Language of Plants: Science, Philosophy, Literature* (pp. 215–234). Minneapolis, MN: University of Minnesota Press.

244. Laist, R. (2013). *Plants and Literature: Essays in Critical Plant Studies*. Amsterdam, the Netherlands: Rodopi.

245. Gibson, P. (2018). *The Plant Contract: Art's Return to Vegetal Life*. Leiden, the Netherlands: Brill.

246. Gibson, P., & Brits, B. (2018). *Covert Plants: Vegetal Consciousness and Agency in an Anthropocentric World*. Goleta, CA: Brainstorm.

247. Head, L., Atchison, J., Phillips, C., & Buckingham, K. (Eds.) (2017). *Vegetal Politics: Belonging, Practices and Places*. New York: Routledge.

248. Myers, N. (2017). Becoming sensor in sentient worlds: a more-than-natural history of a black oak savannah. In: G. Bakke & M. Peterson (Eds.), *Between Matter and Method: Encounters in Anthropology and Art* (pp. 73–96). New York: Bloomsbury.

249. Myers, N. (2017). From the Anthropocene to the Planthroposcene: designing gardens for plant/people involution. *History and Anthropology*. http://dx.doi.org/10.1080/02757206.2017.1289934.

250. Myers, N. (2015). Edenic apocalypse: Singapore's end-of-time botanical tourism. In: H. Davis & E. Turpin (Eds.), *Art in the Anthropocene: Encounters Among Aesthetics, Politics, Environments and Epistemologies*. London: Open Humanities Press.

251. Myers, N. (2016). Photosynthesis. Theorizing the contemporary. *Cultural Anthropology*, 21 January. [https://culanth.org/fieldsights/790-photosynthesis]

252. Pollan, M. (2002). *The Botany of Desire*. London: Bloomsbury.

253. Attala, L. (2014). Conversations over dinner. Botanical Ontologies Conference, Oxford University, 17 May. [http://www.academia.edu]

254. Gagliano, M. (2018). *Thus Spoke the Plant: a Remarkable Journey of Groundbreaking Scientific Discoveries and Personal Encounters with Plants*. Berkeley: North Atlantic Books.

255. Aloi, G. (2018). *Why Look at Plants?* Leiden, the Netherlands: Brill.

256. Nealon, J. (2015). *Plant Theory: Biopower and Vegetal Life*. Redwood City: Stanford University Press.

257. Irigaray, L., & Marder, M. (2016). *Through Vegetal Being: Two Philosophical Perspectives*. New York: Columbia University Press.

258. Irigaray, L. (2017). What the vegetal world says to us. In: M. Gagliano, J. Ryan, & P. Vieira (Eds.), *The Language of Plants: Science, Philosophy, Literature* (pp. 126–135). Minneapolis, MN: University of Minnesota Press.

259. Miller, E. (2002). *The Vegetative Soul: from Philosophy of Nature to Subjectivity in the Feminine*. New York: State University of New York.

260. Marder, M. (2017). To hear plants speak. In: M. Gagliano, J. Ryan, & P. Vieira, P. (Eds.), *The Language of Plants: Science, Philosophy, Literature* (pp. 103–125). Minneapolis, MN: University of Minnesota Press.

261. Hsu, E., & Harris, S. (2010). *Plants, Health and Healing: On the Interface of Ethnobotany and Medical Anthropology*. Oxford: Berghahn.

262. Kirskey, S., & Helmreich, S. (2010). The emergence of multispecies ethnography. *Cultural Anthropology*, 25(4): 545–576.

263. Ogden, L., Hall, B., & Tanita, K. (2013). Animals, plants, people and things: a review of multispecies ethnography. *Environment and Society: Advances in Research*, 4: 5–24.

264. Kohn, E. (2013). *How Forests Think: Toward an Anthropology beyond the Human*. Berkeley, CA: University of California Press.

265. Tsing, A. (2017). *The Mushroom at the End of the World: On the Possibility of Life in Capitalist Ruins*. Princeton, NJ: Princeton University Press.

266. Gibson, D. (2018). Rethinking medicinal plants and plant medicines. *Anthropology Southern Africa*, 41(1): 1–14.

267. Gibson, D. (2018). Towards plant-centred methodologies. *Anthropology Southern Africa*, 41(2): 92–103.

268. Abram, D. (2014). The invisibles: towards a phenomenology of the spirits. In: Harvey, G., *The Handbook of Contemporary Animism* (pp. 124–134). New York: Routledge.

269. Harvey, G. (2005). *Animism: Respecting the Living World*. London: C. Hurst and Co.

270. Harvey, G. (2014). *The Handbook of Contemporary Animism*. New York: Routledge.

271. Grusin, R. (2015). *The Nonhuman Turn*. Minneapolis, MN: University of Minnesota Press.

272. Clifford, J., & Marcus, G. E. (1986). *Writing Culture: the Poetics and Politics of Ethnography*. Berkeley, CA: University of California Press.

273. Palecek, M., & Risjord, M. (2012). Relativism and the ontological turn within anthropology. *Philosophy of the Social Sciences, 43*(1): 3–23.

274. Clough, P., & Halley, J. (2007). *The Affective Turn: Theorizing the Social*. Durham, NC: Duke University Press.

275. Stanson, J. (2016). Ethnography and the choices posed by the "affective turn". In: J. Frykman & M. Povrzanovic Frykman (Eds.), *Sensitive Objects: Affect and Material Culture* (pp. 55–77). Lund, Norway: Nordic Academic Press.

276. Stark, H., & Roffe, J. (2015). *Deleuze and the Non/Human*. Basingstoke, UK: Palgrave Macmillan.

277. Descola, P. (2014). All too human (still). *Journal of Ethnographic Theory, 4*(2): 267–273.

278. Braidotti, R. (2013). *The Posthuman*. Cambridge: Polity Press.

279. Haraway, D. (2008). *When Species Meet*. Minneapolis, MN: University of Minnesota Press.

280. Haraway, D. (1999). *How Like a Leaf*. London: Routledge.

281. Williams, R. (1977). *Marxism and Literature*. Oxford: Oxford University Press.

282. Gramsci, A. (1971). *Selections from the Prison Notebooks of Antonio Gramsci*. New York: International Publishers.

283. Giddens, A. (1979). *Central Problems in Social Theory: Action, Structure and Contradiction in Social Analysis*. Berkeley, CA: University of California Press.

284. Bourdieu, P. (1977). *Outline of a Theory of Practice*. Cambridge: Cambridge University Press.

285. Butler, J. (1997). *Excitable Speech: A Politics of the Performative*. New York: Routledge.

286. Ahearn, L. (2001a). Language and agency. *Annual Review of Anthropology, 30*: 109–137.

287. Gardiner, J. (1995). *Provoking Agents: Gender and Agency in Theory and Practice*. Urbana, IL: University of Illinois Press.

288. Davies, B. (2000). *A Body of Writing, 1990–1999*. Walnut Creek, CA: Altamira Press.

289. Latour, B. (2007). *Reassembling the Social: an Introduction to Actor-Network-Theory*. Oxford: Oxford University Press.

290. Law, J., & Hassard, J. (1999). *Actor Network Theory and After*. Oxford: Blackwell.

291. Callon, M. (1986). Some elements of a sociology of translation: domestication of the scallops and the fishermen of Saint Brieuc Bay. In: J. Law (Ed.), *Power, Action and Belief: a New Sociology of Knowledge?* London: Routledge & Kegan Paul.

292. Ahearn, L. (2001b). *Invitations to Love: Literacy, Love Letters, and Social Change in Nepal*. Ann Arbor, MI: University of Michigan Press.

293. Mahmood, S. (2005). *The Politics of Piety: The Islamic Revival and the Feminist Subject*. Princeton, NJ: Princeton University Press.

294. Latour, B. (1996). *Aramis; or, The Love of Technology*. Cambridge, MA: Harvard University Press.

295. Thoreau, H. D. (1973). *The Writings of Henry David Thoreau: Walden*. Princeton, NJ: Princeton University Press.

296. Spinoza, B. (1667). *Ethics: Treatise on the Emendation of the Intellect, and Selected Letters*. Indianapolis, IN: Hackett, 1992.

297. Bergson, H. (1998). *Creative Evolution*. New York: Dover.

298. Harman, G. (2015). *The Metaphysics of Objects: Latour and His Aftermath*. [http://www.pervegalit.files.wordpress.com]

299. Marder, M. (2016). *Grafts: Writings on Plants*. Minneapolis, MN: Univocal.

300. Wilson, E. O. (1990 [1984]). *Biophilia: the Human Bond with Other Species*. Cambridge, MA: Harvard University Press.

301. Tsunetsugu, Y., Park, B.-J., & Miyazaki, Y. (2010). Trends in research related to "Shinrin-yoku" (taking in the forest atmosphere or forest bathing) in Japan. *Environmental Health & Preventive Medicine, 15*: 27–37.

302. Li, Q. (2010). Effect of forest bathing trips on human immune function. *Environmental Health & Preventive Medicine, 15*: 9–17.

303. Ivens, S. (2018). *Forest Therapy: Seasonal Ways to Embrace Nature for a Happier You*. London: Piatkus.

304. Haller, R., Kennedy, K., & Capra, C. (forthcoming). *The Profession and Practice of Horticulture Therapy*. Boca Raton, FL: CRC Press.

305. Stuart-Smith, S. (forthcoming). *Horticulture Therapy: The Well Gardened Mind*. London: William Collins.

INDEX

321

Printed in the USA
CPSIA information can be obtained
at www.ICGtesting.com
JSHW061419221024
72172JS00018B/135